J. Taylor, R. Simader, P. Nieland (Editors)

Potential and Possibility: Rehabilitation at end of life

T0175632

Jenny Taylor, Rainer Simader, Peter Nieland (Editors)

Potential and Possibility: Rehabilitation at end of life

Physiotherapy in Palliative Care

First Edition

With contributions from:

C. Bausewein, J. van den Broek, S. Cobbe, K. Coe, Y. Dahlin, J. E. Ellershaw, E. Gail, B. Fiechter Lienert, A. F. Goodhead, E. Grünberger, N. Hartley, B. Hewitt, L. Hollander, B. Jaspers, R. Jennings, I.-S. Kim, M.-M. Lippka, L. Malcolm, T. McGlinchey, E. Müllauer, P. Nieland, K. Norman, C. Plath, K. Reckinger, R. Simader, W. Schönleiter, S. Schraut, N. P. Sykes, J. Taylor

Translations provided by: Beverley Taylor, Munich, Germany

Foreword by: Baroness Ilora Finlay of Llandaff, FRCGP, FRCP, Cardiff, UK

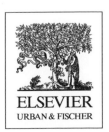

ELSEVIER
URBAN & FISCHER

URBAN & FISCHER München

All business correspondence should be forwarded to:
Elsevier GmbH, Urban & Fischer Verlag, Hackerbrücke 6, 80335 München
physiotherapie@elsevier.de

Important notice for the reader

Practices in physiotherapy and medicine are forever changing due to research and clinical experience. The publishers and authors of this book have taken tremendous care to ensure that the therapeutic advice and information herein (particularly with respect to indications, dosage schedules and adverse effects) confer with the standards accepted at the time of publication. This does not absolve the readers of this book from the obligation to verify, by referring to further written sources of information, that the information is not contradictory, nor does it release them from full responsibility for the therapeutic decisions they make.

The publisher can accept no responsibility for the selection and integrity of the information on the medicinal products listed in this book.

Protected product names (trademarks) are generally highlighted as such (®). The lack of such a reference does not necessarily imply that the names are not protected.

The information on diagnosis and therapy may to some extent differ from standard practices in Great Britain. Caution: The dosage schedules and instructions for use described in such cases may differ from those of the British marketing authorisations.

Bibliographic information published by the Deutsche Nationalbibliothek.

The Deutsche Nationalbibliothek lists this publication in the Deutsche Nationalbibliografie; detailed bibliographic data are available in the Internet at http://dnb.d-nb.de.

All rights reserved:
1. edition 2013
© Elsevier GmbH, Munich, Germany
Urban & Fischer Verlag is an imprint of Elsevier GmbH.

13 14 15 16 17   5 4 3 2 1

All rights, including translation, are reserved. No part of this publication may be reproduced, stored in a retrieval system, or transmitted in any other form or by any means, electronic, mechanical, photocopying, recording, or otherwise without the prior written permission of the publisher.

Acquisition Editor: Rainer Simader, Munich, Germany
Development Editor: Ines Mergenhagen, Munich, Germany
English text revised by: Martin Mellor, Edinburgh, UK
Production Manager: Ute Landwehr-Heldt, Bremen, Germany
Composed by: abavo GmbH, Buchloe, Germany; TnQ, Chennai, India
Printed and bound by: Printer Trento, Trento, Italy
Cover Illustration: © St Christopher's Hospice, London, UK
Cover Design: Spiesz Design, Neu-Ulm, Germany

ISBN Print 978-0-7020-5027-5
ISBN e-Book 978-3-437-16974-8

Current information by **www.elsevier.de** and **www.elsevier.com**

Foreword

Since 1995, when the Calman Hine report on Cancer Services was published, physiotherapy has been recognised as a core component of specialist palliative care. However, it has not been until now that a definitive and accessible textbook on physiotherapy in palliative and end of life care has been written.

The role of the physiotherapist is increasingly recognised as a key element in efforts to improve patients' quality of life and enable the maintenance of independent living in the face of advancing disease. Diagnostic skills mean that physiotherapists are frequently the first to detect conditions such as early spinal cord compression, making the difference between mobility and paraplegia. Investigation and referral allow mobility to be retained through immediate radiotherapy or surgery.

For patients' relatives, being taught how to help a patient move efficiently, stand from sitting or lying, or transfer from bed to chair safely will allow patients to live at home during their final illness. Appropriate breathing techniques can diminish the terror of severe dyspnoea. In these and many other areas, the positive enabling attitude of physiotherapy has brought about real service change and transformed patients' outlook from despair to realistic hope.

The combination of specialist rehabilitation expertise and excellent communication skills make the physiotherapist an indispensable support in the lives of patients who are desperate to maintain or regain independence in the face of progressing disease. Through team working, others are brought in to address issues that may have gone unrecognised or unheeded; so often, as these pages illustrate, the physiotherapist is able to unlock the unique potential of patient and carers as well as detect the unnoticed problems.

The real life case study examples, emphasising the importance of the patients' own views, bring to life the importance of physiotherapy in end of life care, adding quality to those final days, weeks or months of life. Cicely Saunders pointed out that the way that people die lives on in the memory of those left behind – the impact of effective end of life physiotherapy can endure for years after a person has died.

January 2013

Baroness Ilora Finlay of Llandaff, FRCGP, FRCP,
Professor of Palliative Medicine, Cardiff University,
President of the Chartered Society of Physiotherapy, UK.

Editors Comment

This book, published in both German and English versions, is a dream realised. A dream we three co-editors first conceived after an exhilarating physiotherapy pre-meeting at the *European Association of Palliative Care* (EAPC) conference in Vienna in 2009. In recent years physiotherapists from around the world, working in a variety of palliative/end of life care clinical settings, have been seeking to share knowledge and expertise; and it is universally acknowledged that wherever physiotherapists network together, enthusiasm is high! Our dream was consolidated in London when physiotherapists from around the world met at the 'Physio Europe and Beyond' 2 day conference at St. Christopher's Hospice in 2010. By capitalising on our creation of an EAPC Physiotherapy Task Force, strong links had been forged as a specialist professional group. The buzz of physiotherapists at the EAPC conference in Lisbon in 2011 that followed further fuelled our determination to embark on this enterprise.

This publication has come to print at a time when the barriers between countries, cultures and approaches are breaking down. More physiotherapists are being drawn to palliative care as a specialty, and the conviction grew that if we are to enhance our important role as specialist physiotherapists improving the quality of life for patients at the end of life, we can do much more together than we can in isolation.

Moreover, in a context of improved survivorship, growing numbers of physiotherapists in all specialties will encounter precisely the challenges demanding and benefiting from the knowledge, and most of all, skills we can share. Palliative care clinical skills of the specialist physiotherapist are ever more widely applicable; from paediatric to elderly care, from acute hospital settings to hospices, and from the bedside to the gymnasium. But aside from that, there is also a particular attitude needed from the health professional towards patients at the end of life. The palliative care physiotherapist exemplifies the empathetic and holistic approach needed to reach complex, changing, and realistic goals. Patient empowerment and self-help is key, and in the more pressured and constrained climate in health care generally today, this is a model that can be usefully taught. Future research and education in this field will always be paramount, and hopefully this publication will contribute to engender ideas and discussion. While the development of physiotherapy techniques and best practice at end of life is the primary aim, disseminating our skills, many of them transferable, to other multi-professional clinicians is a worthy goal.

We have endeavoured to include a comprehensive range of topics, presented in a case-specific, accessible, and user-friendly format, which aims to be a useful resource in a variety of settings. In view of the many nationalities and contexts of our contributors, the editors have utilised red 'Caution' and green 'Guidance' boxes as a continuous theme running through many of the chapters to highlight key precautions and helpful strategies. We hope that this format really helps to direct and assist the reader. Our intention is that this volume is not only a source of clinical knowledge, but also opens up debate and thinking around physiotherapy education and training, both given and received.

Educational requirements for entry to the physiotherapy profession vary from country to country. Professional autonomy differs. In some countries rehabilitation, if not contra-indicated, is seen as revolutionary to patients at end of life. Differences in approach are a 'given' and rather than feeling defensive as a profession we must embrace these differences and use them as a catalyst for ongoing analysis and re-evaluation. But beyond these considerations, we know that wherever physiotherapists are privileged to work alongside these universally vulnerable patients, our clinical practice constantly evolves. So, to encourage the development of practice in the workplace, reflective questions have been included in the case studies with the intention of provoking discussion and analysis. As co-editors we have aimed to stimulate debate and inspire innovation. Practice for all of us evolves in a changing landscape; so by challenging our own thinking maybe we will contribute to creating a powerful vision towards growth and change for future models of physiotherapy practice?

Importantly, we also hope to attract interest from other professionals in the field to enhance their understanding of our role. It is without doubt that we must raise our profile to encourage health care commissioners in every country to recognise the major contribution we can make as a professional group to end of life care; not only in delivering symptom control and rehabilitation excellence but, significantly in these challenging times, in overall patient cost-effectiveness.

London, Wallern, Bonn in January 2013
Jenny Taylor, Rainer Simader, Peter Nieland

Acknowledgements

Working on this book has been both a joy and a challenge. Our remit has been broad and the range of contributors wide. There have been intricacies of language to grapple with, and initial misunderstandings or misinterpretations have invariably been patiently resolved. It has all been hugely rewarding and we are so grateful to the 29 authors from around 9 different countries who have brought their experience, passion, and commitment to this exciting publication. We would like to thank Ines Mergenhagen, Elsevier, Munich, Germany, who managed to steer us on a safe path throughout with her optimism, patience and good humour. Thanks are also due to our dedicated editorial team, in particular to Beverley Taylor for translations and to Martin Mellor for extensive copyediting.

In the UK the editors have been most grateful for constant encouragement from colleagues at St. Christopher's Hospice, who by unstintingly sharing their wealth of experience in both writing and editing have given us invaluable support. Grateful thanks are due particularly to Dr. Emma Hall, consultant in palliative medicine, for her advice and expertise for the English language edition in ensuring the 'Pharmacological Management of Pain' section conforms with standard UK practice.

Last, but by no means least, we are hugely indebted to all our many patients, both past and present, who have so generously given their commitment, impressions and feedback not only directly for this book, but indirectly in shaping our views, informing our practice and being our inspiration. We thank them all for their courage and resilience in the face of suffering, and especially for their belief and trust in us.

London, Wallern, Bonn in January 2013
Jenny Taylor, Rainer Simader, Peter Nieland

Editors and contributing authors

Editors

Jenny Taylor, Honorary consultant Physiotherapist; former Head of Allied Health Professional (AHP) team, St Christopher's Hospice, London; Founder Chair of the Physiotherapy Task Force of the European Association of Palliative Care (EAPC); London, UK

Rainer Simader, Physiotherapist; Lecturer for physiotherapy; Chair of the task force physiotherapy in palliative care (Austrian Physiotherapy Association); member of the Physiotherapy Task Force of the European Association of Palliative Care (EAPC); Dance and movement psychotherapist; Wallern, Austria

Peter Nieland, Physiotherapist; Head of physiotherapy department Malteser Hospital Bonn/Rhein-Sieg; Chair of the task force physiotherapy in palliative care (German Palliative Care Association); member of the Physiotherapy Task Force of the European Association of Palliative Care (EAPC); Bonn, Germany

Contributing authors

Bausewein, Claudia, Professor of palliative medicine and Director of the multiprofessional centre for palliative care, University Hospital Munich, Germany; visiting Professor King's College, London, UK

van den Broek, Jacob, Physiotherapist in Palliative Care, Hospice kuria; Chair of the Physiotherapy Task Force in European Association of Palliative Care (EAPC); Amsterdam, The Netherlands

Cobbe, Sinead, Senior Physiotherapist, Milford Care Centre, Limerick, Ireland

Coe, Kristina, Neuro-Oncology Physiotherapist, The Christie NHS Foundation Trust, Manchester, UK

Dahlin, Ylva, Head surgical/oncology Physiotherapist, Karolinska University Hospital, Stockholm, Sweden

Ellershaw, John E, Professor of Palliative Medicine, Director Marie Curie Palliative Care Institute, Liverpool, UK

Eva, Gail, Research Fellow, Department of Brain Repair and Rehabilitation, UCL Institute of Neurology, London, UK

Fiechter Lienert, Brigitte, Physiotherapist; Lecturer for Physiotherapy at the University of Applied Science Winterthur/Zurich, Switzerland

Goodhead, Andrew F, Chaplain and Spiritual Care lead, St Christopher's Hospice, London, UK

Grünberger, Elisabeth, Psychotherapist; Gerontologist; Physiotherapist; Supervisor; Vienna, Austria

Hartley, Nigel, Director of Supportive Care, St Christopher's Hospice, London, UK

Hewitt, Bronwen, Senior Physiotherapist, Sacred Heart Palliative Care Service, St Vincent's Hospital, Sydney, Australia

Hollander, Louis, Physiotherapist, specialist in elderly care, Livio nursing home „De Cromhoff"; Senior lecturer for physiotherapy, University of Applied Science, Enschede, The Netherlands

Jaspers, Birgit, Philosopher, medical scientist, linguist; Research Fellow for ethical issues, Department for Palliative Care University Bonn and University Göttingen, Germany

Jennings, Rebecca, Specialist Physiotherapist and Therapy Services Manager, St Joseph's Hospice, London, UK

Kim, In-Sun, Nurse and theologian; founder member of „Dong Heng" intercultural hospice, Berlin; Director of „Dong Ban Ja" intercultural hospice service, Berlin-Brandenburg; Chair of "Dong Heng" hospice foundation; Berlin, Germany

Lippka, Michael-M., Social worker; Lecturer for communication; Linz, Austria

Malcolm, Lorna, Senior Physiotherapist, St Christopher's Hospice, London, UK

McGlinchey, Tamsin, Research Assistant, Marie Curie Palliative Care Institute, Liverpool, UK

Müllauer, Eva, Physiothererapist, specialised in pulmonary rehabilitation, Pulmonary Hospital Hitzing/Neurological Hospital Rosenhügel, Vienna; Lecturer for Physiotherapy at the University of Applied Science, Salzburg and Vienna, Austria

Norman, Kate, Senior Physiotherapist, St Christopher's Hospice, London, UK

Plath, Christina, Freelance Physiotherapist in home care setting, Göttingen, Germany

Reckinger, Klaus, Consultant for internal medicine, pain therapy and palliative care; Director of 'Gildas Akademie' (Centre for further education and training in palliative care); Herten, Germany

Schönleiter, Wolf, Sociologist; Lecturer at the University of Applied Science Hamburg; Supervisor and Counsellor, St. Augustin/Bonn, Germany

Schraut, Sabine, Consultant for paediatric medicine, neuropaediatrics and palliative care, Childrens' Hospice „Bärenherz" Wiesbaden; private practice, Niederhausen, Germany

Sykes, Nigel P, Medical Director and Consultant in Palliative Medicine, St Christopher's Hospice, London, UK

Picture Credits

The credits for each figure are enclosed in square brackets at the end of the caption. Any graphics and figures not specifically identified © Elsevier GmbH, Munich.

F148	Reprinted with kind permission of the International Association for the Study of Pain® (IASP®)
F323	Smith, C., Hale, L., Olson, K., Schneiders, A. (2009) 'How does exercise influence fatigue in people with multiple sclerosis?', Disability and Rehabilitation, 21(9), 685–692
F324/L157	Noble, B., Borg, G., Jacobs, I, Ceci, R., Kaiser, P (1983) 'A category-ratio perceived exertion scale: relationship to blood and muscle lactates and heart rate', Medicine and Science in Sports and Exercise, 15(6), 523–528
L157	Susanne Adler, Lübeck, Germany
M540/L157	Jenny Taylor, London, UK/Susanne Adler, Lübeck, Germany
M541/L157	Ylva Dahlin, Johanneshov, Sweden/Susanne Adler, Lübeck, Germany
M542/L157	Bronwen Hewitt, Ashfield, Australia/Susanne Adler, Lübeck, Germany
M543/L157	Kristina Coe, Manchester, UK/Susanne Adler, Lübeck, Germany
M544	Eva Müllauer, Vienna, Austria
M545/L157	Sinead Cobbe, Castleroy Limerick, Ireland/Susanne Adler, Lübeck, Germany
M546/L157	P. Nieland, Bonn, Germany/Susanne Adler, Lübeck, Germany
M547/L157	Rainer Simader, Wallern, Austria/Susanne Adler, Lübeck, Germany
M548	Christina Plath, Göttingen, Germany
M548/L157	Christina Plath, Göttingen, Germany/Susanne Adler, Lübeck, Germany
M549/L157	Michael Lippka, Linz, Austria/Susanne Adler, Lübeck, Germany
O596	Antonie Colijn, Enschede, The Netherlands
O597	M. Scharrenbroich, Bonn, Germany
O598	Fam. Maywald, Alzey, Germany
T440	St Christopher's Hospice, London, UK
W798/L157	WHO, Genf, Switzerland/Susanne Adler, Lübeck, Germany
W825/F322	Greater Manchester and Cheshire Cancer Network/Greenhalgh, S. Turnpenney, J. Richards, L & Self, J (2010): Metastatic spinal cord compression (MSCC) key red flags

Table of Contents

Approaching the topic of physiotherapy in palliative care

1.1 Definition of palliative care and end of life care
Nigel Sykes

The World Health Organization (WHO) defines palliative care as *'an approach that improves the quality of life of patients and families facing the problems associated with life-threatening illness through the prevention and relief of suffering by means of early identification and impeccable assessment and treatment of pain and other problems, which are physical, psychosocial and spiritual.'* To claim impeccability seems a tall order for any service, but the attention to detail on every level of assessment and treatment, including relationship with both patients and those close to them, is an accepted hallmark of specialist palliative care practice.

'Palliative care' as a term was coined by Professor Balfour Mount when he sought to replicate in Quebec the style of care pioneered by Dr (later Dame) Cicely Saunders at St Christopher's Hospice, which she had set up in London UK in 1967. 'Hospice' did not translate well into French, but a type of care that attempted to cloak the symptoms of incurable, progressive diseases ('palliative' derives from the Latin *pallium* meaning 'a cloak') was certainly what the hospice did. 'Hospice' is therefore now an organization – with or without a building – that exists to practise palliative care.

However, although palliative care (and especially hospice organizations) have been associated with caring for patients who are dying from cancer, elements of the definition of palliative care are relevant much earlier in the disease trajectory and to diseases other than malignancy. On the one hand, specialist palliative care has been gradually opening up to a range of other end stage conditions, such as heart failure, chronic obstructive pulmonary disease and degenerative neurological states and, on the other hand, it is increasingly recognized that the essentials of palliative care should be part of the skill set of any clinician and have applicability both to the earlier stages of cancer, for instance, and to people dying from the frailty of old age. Sometimes this is called 'supportive care' or 'generic palliative care'. Palliative care also makes up the content of 'end of life care', and it is a tribute to the work of the specialty in the UK that since 2008 this has been the subject of a government strategy (Department of Health 2008). As to what 'end of life' means, the *Gold Standards Framework* (Thomas/Sawkins 2008) – one of the tools promoted by the British strategy – features an end of life care register to which access is triggered by a 'no' answer to the so-called surprise question, viz. 'Would you be surprised if this patient died within the next year?'

Where palliative care is better established, the question of whether it should have specialty status remains contentious, but experience from countries where it has a recognizable presence suggests that it raises the consciousness of the wider clinical community about the fact that ultimately all their patients die and that a multifaceted, holistic mode of care is widely appreciated. Such a mode of care is not just appreciated by dying people and their families but also by a far wider range of those who are ill. So while palliative care deals with dying like no other clinical group does, it is not solely about the very end of life but, as its founder said, it is about *'living until you die'* (Saunders 1973). The author has encountered doctors who were nonplussed that a hospice should employ a physiotherapist but, of course, while a patient may be dying they are not dead yet, and help in remaining as safely active as possible improves morale, alleviates musculoskeletal discomfort and assists achievement of whatever life goals remain unfulfilled. Access to physiotherapy is therefore a key requirement for a properly comprehensive palliative care service.

1.1.1 Development of palliative care

Palliative care has progressed a long way from its origins in the 1960s. Clinical services exist in over 115 countries; it is a recognized medical specialty or sub-specialty in Australia, Ireland, New Zealand, the UK, and the USA. Thirteen professorial chairs related to palliative care exist in the UK and over 30 internationally; there are at least 12 peer-reviewed English-language journals primarily devoted to palliative care research and development. Yet this progress masks huge deficiencies: more than half of the world has no access to palliative care; where it does exist, integration with the national health system is rare and funding is correspondingly erratic; standards of service are highly variable; availability of opioid analgesia is often restricted.

In many places there is therefore an immediate challenge to expand the availability of palliative care, in terms both of service provision and of medicines access. In 1987, WHO published its Analgesic Ladder, which identified morphine as the single most effective analgesic for cancer pain (WHO 1987) and effectively made a nation's per capita consumption of morphine a proxy for the extent to which its citizens have access to pain relief and palliative care. Advocacy since that time by the WHO and its *Pain and Policy Studies Collaborating Group* at the University of Wisconsin can take much credit for the increase in willingness to prescribe opioids more often and more generously (Kuehn 2007). Global morphine consumption has risen from about two tons in 1985, before WHO intervention, to around 25 tons in 2012.

Nonetheless obstructions to patients actually obtaining the pain relief they need remain, particularly in developing countries where access to morphine is minimal or absent but where most people dying from cancer or AIDS live. Governmental fears of illicit trafficking of morphine are part of the problem, but so are medical anxieties about adverse effects. The opiophobia that disallows all opioid drugs can modify into specific morphine phobia, with the result either that only very expensive alternative opioids – with the same potential side effects – are allowed. Either way the poor get nothing. Yet morphine, properly used, is safe and 10 mg of it should not cost more than one US cent.

Two examples of palliative care groups taking the initiative to improve access to opioid analgesia are Romania and Uganda. In Romania successful lobbying persuaded the government to reform the previously highly restrictive laws on opioid prescribing (Mosoiu et al. 2006). In Uganda, similar lobbying achieved permission for appropriately trained nurses to supply morphine, transforming the situation for patients in country areas who had previously been able to obtain pain relief only by dint of themselves or a relative making a long trek to the nearest town with a hospital (Jagwe 2006). In both countries there have also been systematic efforts to provide education in palliative care for the healthcare workforce (Landon/Mosoiu 2010).

The challenges in developed countries have increasingly moved beyond the essentials of getting palliative care established. Even where dedicated palliative care services exist they cannot serve all those who are dying, still less all who have some need for palliation. This situation will worsen in future because of the ageing of western society. Typically, the number of people over 65 will double by 2040, and the number of deaths will increase by a third by 2025. It has been estimated that 80 % of those over 65 have some form of chronic illness and around 60 % have two or more chronic illnesses (CHPCA 2011). At the same time even cancers are assuming more of the character of chronic diseases, with those affected living for an increasing number of years but often with some degree of disability caused by residual disease or their original treatment. Palliative care in countries such as these faces a threefold challenge to:

- maximize the number of patients who can be seen with the resources available;
- have a strong focus on education in order to spread the essential skills of palliation around the health and social care professional community;
- be a catalyst for public education so that society gains greater ease not only in discussing and planning for

the end of life but also in caring for relatives and friends who are terminally ill, in an era when shifting age structures means that the pool of professional carers is set to shrink compared to the number who will need to be cared for.

This agenda demands not only attention to the palliative care organization's service but also to its relationship with other organizations and services. The vision must be that it should be possible to die well wherever that death occurs: home is the preferred choice of most, but more and more will die in care homes, and many are likely to continue to die in hospitals. At the same time, those who are dying should be enabled to live well until they die, and here lies the key contribution of physiotherapy. **Rehabilitation and maintenance of function are needed to underpin 'living well', which may mean a shift of approach on the part of physiotherapists accustomed to full restoration of function as the goal of their interventions.** The practitioners of palliative care and rehabilitation often do not know each other well, and yet they have complementary skills that if brought together could benefit many patients, particularly those with progressive neurological disorders (Turner-Stokes et al. 2007), and probably others as well.

To have a rehabilitative approach to care, modulated to the individual's changing capability, is counter-cultural for the many members of the public who continue to see referral to palliative care as in itself a death sentence. All those who work in hospices have stories of those who could have benefited from the service much earlier had they and, often their families, not been too afraid to attend. Palliative care services must find ways to reach out to these groups, and the development of groups resembling conventional gym sessions can be one method. Such clinical initiatives can be complemented by national campaigns of public awareness-raising such as the UK *Dying Matters* project that has adopted a wide variety of methods – from print to video, from personal testimony to professional comedians – to encourage people to talk about their death, plan for it and become more comfortable with considering all aspects of death and dying (http://www.dyingmatters.org/).

1.1.2 Conclusion

Palliative care is about living as well as dying, about diseases well beyond cancer, and about far more people than just those directly affected through disease. Indeed, through its care of families it has the potential to affect attitudes towards healthcare and incurable illness across generations. But there is far to go before these ideals of care will be available to all who need them.

REFERENCES

Canadian Hospice Palliative Care Association (CHPCA). Hospice palliative care in Canada. Fact sheet. Ottawa: CHPCA, 2011.

Jagwe J. The introduction of palliative care in Uganda. J Palliat Med 2006;5:159–163.

Kuehn BM. Opioid prescriptions soar: Increase in legitimate use as well as abuse. JAMA 2007;297:249–251.

Landon A, Mosoiu D. Hospice 'Casa Sperantei': Pioneering palliative home care services in Romania. Prog Palliat Care 2010;18:23–26.

Mosoiu D, Ryan KM, Joranson DE, Garthwaite JP. Reform of drug control policy for palliative care in Romania. Lancet 2006;367:2,110–2,117.

NICE. Improving Supportive and Palliative Care for Adults with Cancer. London: National Institute for Clinical Excellence, 2004.

Saunders C. A death in the family: A professional view. Br Med J 1973;1(5844):30–31.

Thomas K, Sawkins N. The gold standards framework in care homes training programme: Good practice guide. Walsall: Gold Standards Framework Programme, 2008.

Turner-Stokes L, Sykes N, Silber E, Khatri A, Sutton L, Young E. From diagnosis to death: exploring the interface between neurology, rehabilitation and palliative care in the management of people with long-term neurological conditions. Clin Med 2007;7:129–136.

UK Department of Health. End of life care strategy: Promoting high quality care for all adults at the end of life. London: UK Department of Health, 2008. Available at http://www.dyingmatters.org (last accessed November 2011).

WHO. Cancer Pain Relief. Geneva: WHO, 1987.

1.2 Who is the palliative care physiotherapist?

Rebecca Jennings

To some, the place of the physiotherapist in palliative care may appear a contradiction: a profession dedicated to the rehabilitation, enablement and empowerment of patients juxtaposed with the domain of terminal illness, death and dying. However, it is essential to distinguish that just because a person has a terminal diagnosis does not mean that they have lost potential for some functional improvement, which is indeed possible in most patients with advanced disease (Cheville 2001). The professional profile of the physiotherapist working in palliative care is characterized by the potential to **offer patients realistic hope, integrated with a pragmatic approach to support them and their carers.** Regaining a sense of control supports patients to make choices that lead to adaptation and empowerment in the changing situations encountered on their illness journey (Platt-Johnson 2007).

Palliative care physiotherapists work with patients at the interface between life and approaching death, so must navigate a balance of wellness and health promotion with the realities of advancing illness. Additionally, physiotherapists encounter a diversity of diagnoses and functional impairments, contextualized within the complex layers of each individual patient's personal, psychosocial and existential experience as they approach the end of life. These factors combine to demand a truly holistic approach that makes palliative care a challenging and rewarding specialty.

This chapter presents the professional profile of the palliative care physiotherapist, their skills, knowledge and personal characteristics. It illuminates the growing recognition of this profession as an integral component of high quality palliative care provision.

1.2.1 Professional profile: The value of the physiotherapist in palliative care

In today's society where personal autonomy is paramount, patients are increasingly expressing the importance of maintaining functional independence as a major component of dignity in the face of advancing illness. As a result the concept of rehabilitation in hospice and palliative care is gaining more attention (Javier/Montagnini 2011). There is growing recognition of the indispensable role that physiotherapists play in leading the evolution of palliative care towards a more empowering, rehabilitative approach to care provision.

The professional profile of physiotherapy in palliative care is gaining importance and cognisance as we look to respond to the escalating needs of an ageing population as growing numbers of individuals approach the end of life. Future projections indicate that mortality rates are likely to increase significantly over the next twenty years, with an expected rise of 17% in the UK between 2012 and 2030 (Gomes/Higginson 2008). Additionally, people are dying at older ages with 44% of the total UK deaths in 2030 expected to be aged over 85 (Gomes/Higginson 2008). Such trends are representative of developed countries internationally where greater numbers of people are living with, and dying from, chronic diseases such as heart failure, chronic obstructive pulmonary disease (COPD) and dementia. However, this rise in life expectancy comes at a potential cost as longevity is frequently compromised by increasing levels of disability, especially in the last year of life (WHO Europe 2011).

The physiotherapy profession is uniquely placed to respond to the challenges posed by an ageing population. Through positive blurring of the boundaries between chronic condition management and palliative care support, physiotherapists are increasingly being recognized as leaders of a rehabilitative approach to palliative care within the interdisciplinary team as it embraces health promotion and self-management across the spectrum of advanced conditions (Cane et al. 2011).

The physiotherapist has potential to impact widely not only clinically but also strategically: the physiotherapist can help to optimize quality of life for patients with advanced illness, whilst reducing dependence on carers and support services, representing important cost savings. In this context they must represent an integral dimension of the interdisciplinary palliative care team (Kumar et al. 2011) and have a pivotal role to play in the development of palliative care services of the future.

'Specialist generalist': Defining attributes of the palliative care physiotherapist

From many perspectives the profile of the palliative care physiotherapist may be viewed as 'specialist generalist': distinguished by a combination of expert knowledge, diverse therapeutic skills, and varied clinical experience, which come together to support the holistic, often complex, needs of patients with advanced illness. We will see that while the philosophy of physiotherapy in palliative care is clearly underpinned by robust clinical assessment and reasoning with attention to detail of anatomy and physiology (➤ Chapter 2.1), what differentiates it from other professions is the ability to contextualize this knowledge in the domains of functionality to accurately reflect the patient's lived experience.

For example, consider a patient's pain. The sensation of pain itself is a problem, and the strategies we can use for managing this complex symptom are explored in depth in ➤ Chapter 2.2. However physiotherapists also acknowledge that the true magnitude of pain can only be fully understood by going beyond the symptom to explore the wider context of what it means to each patient, to understand how the "total pain" experience (➤ Chapter 1.3) impacts on that person's function and ability to interact with their environment

and others (Jennings unpublished 2012). This is the interface where disease renders the body conscious, where the symptoms and impairments of advancing illness mean that the ability to function, once taken for granted, is compromised (Williams/Bendelow 1998). This is the domain of the palliative care physiotherapist. Through a whole person approach, bridging both medical and psychosocial disciplines, physiotherapists work alongside patients and their carers to help:

- maintain independence;
- adapt to functional losses engendered by advancing disease;
- redefine interaction with the world;
- preserve a sense of self until the moment of death.

1.2.2 Clinical skills and knowledge

Knowledge of anatomy and pathophysiology of advanced, life-limiting conditions

Whilst the speciality of palliative care has traditionally grown out of oncology (Addington-Hall/Higginson 2001), over recent decades palliative care services have widened to embrace the spectrum of life-limiting conditions. Access to palliative care is determined by patient need rather than diagnosis or stage of disease. As a result in any given day the palliative care physiotherapist may encounter patients with a range of diagnoses, including cancer, chronic obstructive pulmonary disease (COPD), dementia, heart failure, HIV, motor neuron disease, multiple sclerosis, or renal failure, in addition to other less prevalent conditions that limit life expectancy. Despite the high prevalence of symptoms in advanced disease (➤ Figure 1.1), many can be improved through timely and effective physiotherapy intervention. Increasingly non-pharmacological approaches to pain, breathlessness, fatigue, oedema and anxiety are recognized by all the medical teams as an es-

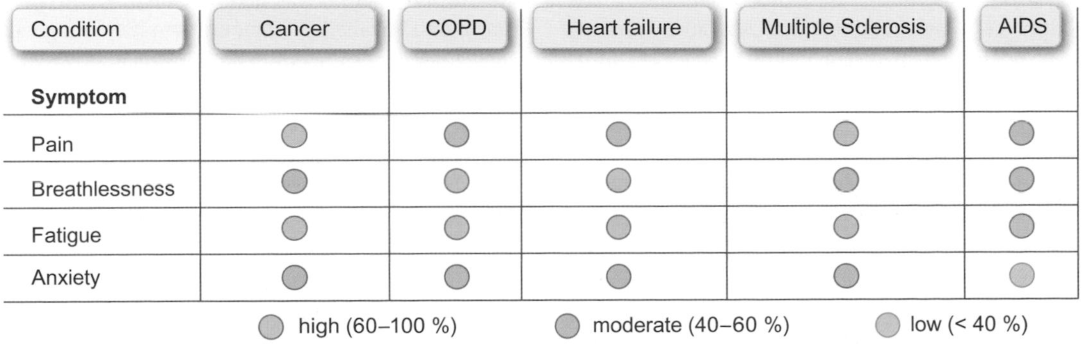

Condition	Cancer	COPD	Heart failure	Multiple Sclerosis	AIDS
Symptom					
Pain	●	●	●	●	●
Breathlessness	●	●	●	●	●
Fatigue	●	●	●	●	●
Anxiety	●	●	●	●	●

● high (60–100 %) ● moderate (40–60 %) ● low (< 40 %)

Figure 1.1 The profile of physiotherapy-responsive symptoms in common conditions in palliative care (based on data from Saleem/Leigh/Higginson 2007 and Solano/Gomes/Higginson 2007) [M541/L157]

sential component of symptom management. In many situations, such as the control of refractory breathlessness (➤ Chapter 2.3, ➤ Chapter 2.4), they are considered equally as important as pharmacological treatments (Booth et al. 2008). Specific chapters in Part 2 of this book address many of these symptoms directly and, using case studies, illustrate the valuable role of the physiotherapist in symptom control at the end of life.

Physiotherapists possess sound clinical knowledge of the anatomy and pathophysiology of cancer, neurological conditions and organ failure to provide a platform for robust clinical reasoning, which underpins every dimension of clinical practice. The communication of this knowledge to educate patients represents a major component of the rehabilitation process (Platt-Johnson 2007) through which the physiotherapist empowers patients and their carers. **A key attribute of the physiotherapist profile is the ability to explain how the disease processes affect physical functioning in a clear, non-threatening way.** This helps them to understand their condition, and by facilitating the exploration and alleviation of patients' fears, promotes informed self-management.

Attention to the interface between symptoms and function: Emphasis on early detection and proactive response

As the profession working most closely with patients to optimize functional ability, physiotherapists effectively establish how their physical symptoms impact on activities of daily living and normal day-to-day existence. Early presentation of symptoms is often evident on exertion, and physiotherapists are well placed to detect and diagnose subtle changes in a patient's condition. Frequent opportunities for detection may arise throughout the disease trajectory depending on the timing of physiotherapy interventions (➤ Chapter 1.4). This enables proactive identification of certain reversible or treatable conditions, such as chest infections, steroid induced myopathy or dependent oedema, which when accurately differentiated from disease progression can be successfully treated to make a significant impact to patients' health and quality of life.

This close association with patients also puts physiotherapists in an advantageous position to screen for palliative care emergencies, such as malignant spinal cord compression, pathological fractures, superior vena cava obstruction and pulmonary emboli (Smith 1994; Watson et al. 2005). Physiotherapists – through a good working knowledge of signs and symptoms and comprehensive physical assessment skills – can accurately sus-

pect the onset of these conditions, elicit formal diagnosis and, in so doing, activate appropriate treatment pathways to avert the risk of irreparable decline for patients including irreversible paralysis and premature death (Watson et al. 2005).

The above examples reflect the emphasis on proactive rather than reactive care: a hallmark of the physiotherapy profession. Some of the most challenging palliative care emergencies are discussed further in ➤ Chapter 2.1. **By educating patients to understand their disease process and encouraging them to proactively detect changes in their condition, patients are empowered to become experts in their own well-being.** In this way physiotherapists play an important role in facilitating health promotion and foster a growing sense of control.

The impeccable holistic assessment of function

Despite the myriad losses encountered in advanced disease, physiotherapists have potential to make a significant difference to many of these dimensions of quality of life (Javier/Montagnini 2011; Oldervoll et al. 2011; Yoshioka 1994).

These include biographical disruption in which independence and autonomy, social participation, social roles, vocation, self-esteem and self-worth may be compromised (Bury 1982; Reeve et al. 2010). The key lies in impeccable holistic clinical assessment. How this is implemented is detailed in ➤ Chapter 2.1. The aims are to identify the combination of factors impacting on a patient's ability to function and to explore the significance of such factors for that person within their own life context. This process is unique to each individual. It provides an insight to who that person is, what motivates them, what worries them, and what their priorities are at that moment and for their future. Through this growing understanding the physiotherapist is perfectly placed to develop a relationship with their patient as a whole person, and to formulate a collaborative plan through which physiotherapy can make a real difference.

Physiotherapists also play a key role in advocating for patients' independence and empowerment. By feeding back their assessment findings to the wider team, physiotherapists voice the real concerns of patients, helping to ensure that their personal goals and fears remain firmly at the centre of holistic care. Patient views inform physiotherapists' practice, and more can be learnt on this subject in ➤ Chapter 1.5.

Clinical approach

A defining characteristic of the professional profile of the physiotherapist working in end of life care is their role in supporting patients to 'habilitate'; that is to adapt to and come to terms with changes encountered on their illness journey, stepping beyond unrealistic expectations of returning to premorbid levels of function which the 're' of rehabilitation implies. Physiotherapists champion a rehabilitative approach to palliative care provision across the interdisciplinary team. This supports patients to make functional improvements in the face of multiple losses encountered in advancing disease (Cheville 2001), and regardless of how small, these can offer patients realistic hope and a positive focus through which patients can exert some control over their illness.

Pragmatic outlook

A pragmatic 'can do' approach is often characteristic of physiotherapists working in palliative care who think 'outside of the box' to find creative rehabilitative approaches. When time is of the essence, perspective on risk must whenever possible be adjusted to support patients' wishes, which may be their last. There is often a small window of opportunity, and without pragmatic action that window may close with deterioration and no opportunity for a second chance. **Physiotherapists contributing innovative solutions and a willingness to take considered risks can make all the difference to patients' quality of life.** Scenarios include mobilizing a patient with metastatic bone disease at high risk of pathological fracture or spinal cord compression who wishes to remain independent, or negotiating the balance between safety and independence to support a patient's wish to go home, even if the discharge is only likely to last a few days. These are examples of the complex scenarios to which the palliative care physiotherapist routinely applies sound clinical reasoning skills (➤ Chapter 2.1).

Interdisciplinary working and shared leadership

Teamwork is an integral part of the philosophy of palliative care (Saunders 1976) with the model of interdisciplinary working firmly embedded in clinical practice (NICE 2004). Increasingly the physiotherapist is recognized as a core member of the specialist palliative care team (Kumar et al. 2011) together with doctors, nurses, social workers, spiritual care workers and a range of other professionals, where each professional group contributes expertise such that the collective expertise of the team is greater than its individual parts (Crawford/Price 2003).

The interdisciplinary model of palliative care promotes collaborative working between professions in a non-hierarchical working style (Connor 2009). Leadership is task dependent, determined by the individual patient's situation (Crawford/Price 2003). By providing realistic guidance regarding patients' functional abilities, goals and aspirations to inform discharge planning and support the team in a unified rehabilitative approach to care, the physiotherapist enables patients to live actively until they die (Saunders 1976). These evolving approaches to end of life care are discussed further in ➤ Chapter 1.3.

Physiotherapists have a key educational role (Platt-Johnson 2007) in promoting non-pharmacological strategies and rehabilitative approaches to care both to palliative care colleagues and professionals working in generalist roles such as district nurses, general practitioners and community teams. **Skilful in problem-solving, their experience is frequently sought to contribute pragmatic solutions and practical perspectives to team debriefs and patient case reviews.**

Furthermore physiotherapists increasingly embrace opportunities for leadership and management that provide a platform for physiotherapists to influence patient care at a more strategic level, to look beyond the individual patient, and to consider the big picture of palliative care delivery. The undertaking of postgraduate courses can be supportive to this progression. Such enhanced roles offer unique challenges in creative service development and require a combination of vision, ability to inspire and motivate others, and a commitment to transform patient care.

Personal attributes

This specialist field attracts physiotherapists with a desire to address the whole person. They build close rapport with their patients through a focus on 'real' lived functional problems that bring the impact of advancing illness on day to day life out into the open. This facilitates a relationship of trust and respect in which patients feel safe to let down their barriers and share their inner thoughts and fears. Physiotherapists are well advised to pay close attention to patients' views; an exposition of these can be found in ➤ Chapter 1.5. By grasping the opportunities presented during physiotherapy sessions to support patients and their families to have open, honest conversations, their wishes and concerns regarding the end of life can be fully explored. This is essential to ensuring such wishes can be planned for and met (Barclay/Maher 2010).

Physiotherapists working in this field possess advanced communication skills, which enable them to 'go there' with patients to explore their psycho-emotional and spiritual needs (➤ Chapter 3.1, ➤ Chapter 3.2, ➤ Chapter 4.2). This must be balanced with accurate empathy, i. e. the ability to sensitively understand patients' feelings in the immediacy of the moment, without being lost in their own feelings (Rogers 1957, Rogers 1967; Watson et al. 2005). It is crucial to develop the art of maintaining sufficient emotional distance to provide appropriate support, while building professional resilience (➤ Chapter 5.1) to work effectively in a challenging field. This emotional intelligence enhances our profile both with patients and colleagues.

1.2.3 Education opportunities for physiotherapists in palliative care

Although physiotherapy education varies in different countries, it ranges mostly from the undergraduate degree – the necessary qualification to practise as a physiotherapist – through to postgraduate masters and doctorate courses, which facilitate the academic expertise of physiotherapists specializing in palliative care.

Undergraduate physiotherapy degrees

Undergraduate physiotherapy degrees internationally range in duration from 3–4 years. Although little attention has been dedicated historically to palliative care in the undergraduate curriculum, palliative care physiotherapists are increasingly being invited to deliver lectures on these degree courses, and students are offered the opportunity to undertake palliative care placements for their elective clinical options. Developing close relationships between experienced palliative care physiotherapists and training colleges provides scope to raise the professional profile and promote physiotherapy career opportunities in palliative care.

Continuous professional development

Physiotherapists are committed to the pursuit of evidence-based practice and evolving professional knowledge to ensure that they provide current best practice to patients. For palliative care physiotherapists this may include:
- keeping up to date with current evidence relating to physiotherapy and palliative care;
- attending and contributing to in-service presentations or educational lectures within their physiotherapy team or organization;
- pursuing specialist knowledge by undertaking training courses specific to physiotherapy or palliative care;
- attending or presenting at palliative care conferences (nationally and internationally);
- reflecting on current personal physiotherapy practice in palliative care;
- participating in palliative care research;
- contributing to local, national and international committees that influence physiotherapy or palliative care development at a strategic and policy level.

Postgraduate study

Increasingly physiotherapists pursue postgraduate study to attain masters or doctorate qualifications in palliative care. In the UK these courses are multiprofessional, offering a unique learning environment that replicates the interdisciplinary nature of palliative care in practice. Such courses allow physiotherapists to develop expert knowledge in their chosen field of palliative care, to undertake research to support the effectiveness of physiotherapy interventions, to develop leadership and management skills, and to raise the profile of physiotherapy in this field.

In this chapter an example is given from Austria and Germany showing the development of having physiotherapy in palliative care integrated into the undergraduate education course and how the profile of palliative care as a specialty has been raised amongst physiotherapists (➤ Box 'Germany and Austria').

Germany and Austria – a model for training, further education and professional teaching
Rainer Simader

History

In 1996, the first foray into the world of teaching palliative physiotherapy was made by Peter Nieland at the Dr Mildred Scheel Academy in Cologne. The experience thereby gained was gradually expanded, from 1999 onwards, in order to create and develop a curriculum for palliative physiotherapy under the auspices of the *Physiotherapy Working Group* of the *German Society for Palliative Care* (DGP). Initial data confirmed that in many practical clinical placements – primarily in the areas of intensive care, oncology and geriatrics – students of physiotherapy are confronted by the subject of "death and dying" (Katamay 2003). In 2005, an analysis commissioned by the DGP questioned the extent to which the subjects such as 'dealing with patients who are seriously and terminally ill', 'handling loss and grief', 'palliative medicine' or 'ethics', for instance, are integrated into physiotherapy training (Simader 2005). To this end, questionnaires were sent to all educational establishments in Germany, Austria and Switzerland. Half of those surveyed initially claimed that the said topics were covered in various lessons. On closer inspection, however, it became clear that palliative care skills were hardly being touched upon; legal or pathophysiological aspects, for example, were more likely to be addressed. Only at two educational institutes was the subject of palliative care mentioned in the curricula. Overall, the assumption was confirmed that despite a considerable need, knowledge of palliative care was minimal and regulated teaching of the subject was lacking (Simader 2005, Nieland 2008).

Consequences

As a consequence, a 40-hour basic curriculum for physiotherapists was developed (Mehne/Nieland/Simader 2007), serving as the foundation for training and further education of physiotherapists. It encompasses both palliative care, nursing and psychosocial, as well as ethical, spiritual and physiotherapeutic approaches to the reasoning and practical concepts specific to palliative physiotherapy.
In order to integrate such content into programmes for basic training as well as continuing professional development (CPD), resources were used from the taskforces of *Physiotherapy in Palliative Care* and

Hospices of the *German Society for Palliative Care* (DGP), and of the *Association of Austrian Physiotherapists* (PhysioAustria) as well as the *Central Association of German Physiotherapists* (ZVK e. V.).

Advanced and further education/CPD

Since 2007, diverse private and state educational establishments in Germany and Austria have been offering 40-hour basic courses as well as a number of shorter introductory and advanced courses aimed at physiotherapists and palliative care teams. During these often one-week courses, physiotherapists are taught by members of the various palliative care professions (medicine, nursing, psychosocial professions, pastoral care, etc.), whilst course administration is the responsibility of a physiotherapist experienced in palliative care. 'Physiotherapy in Palliative Care' has been integrated as a model into physiotherapy master programmes (e. g. at the University of Applied Sciences of Hildesheim and University of Applied Sciences of Vienna).

Basic training

By linking a large number of physiotherapy teachers and study directors with the Taskforce[1], the subject 'Physiotherapy in Palliative Care' was incorporated in 80 % of all bachelor programmes in Austria by 2012, at 15 to 40 teaching units – in most cases as a compulsory subject, and in a few institutions as an option. The curricula were modified, accordingly, as part of educational reforms. In Germany, the state subsidised changes were made in 2010 in the federal state of Bavaria.
The response of the students has mostly been very positive and beyond the technical level the subject is judged to be very useful (➤ Chapter 1.6). The palliative approach (in addition to rehabilitation and prevention) has now become part of the professional profile of a physiotherapist.

Continuous interprofessional education

Owing to the increasing involvement of physiotherapy in palliative care, more and more therapists are being invited to provide advanced and continuous education courses to interdisciplinary teams. In turn, this broadens the awareness of potential referring doctors as regards physiotherapeutic skills and promotes the necessary exchange.

---

[1] TN: Taskforce Palliative Care of the Austrian federal association of physiotherapists (PhysioAustria)

The following aspects were, and are helpful in successfully integrating physiotherapeutic components into further and continuous education programmes:

- Creation of specialised physiotherapy groups (with therapists working in clinical, teaching and research environments)
- Networking and close cooperation with professional associations of physiotherapists as well as palliative care and hospice organisations
- Working with and advising training establishments
- Working with and advising associations and expert panels

- Attendance at events
- Publications
- Certification and quality assurance

INTERNET LINKS

German Society for Palliative Care [Deutsche Gesellschaft für Palliativmedizin]: www.dgpalliativmedizin.de

German Physiotherapy Association [Deutscher Verband für Physiotherapie] – Central Association of German Physiotherapists [Zentralverband der Physiotherapeuten/Krankengymnasten]: www.zvk.org

Physio Austria, Association of Austrian Physiotherapists [Bundesverband der PhysiotherapeutInnen Österreichs]: www.physioaustria.at

1.2.4 Conclusion

The profile of physiotherapists in palliative care is evolving internationally. The reader will encounter perspectives from different countries where the physiotherapists' clinical status differs from their own. Some are fortunate to work in well-integrated multiprofessional teams; others in isolation. A common factor that unites physiotherapists is, however, that they are recognized as experts in non-pharmacological and rehabilitative support for their patients and, consequently, respect for the profession is increasing. Physiotherapists working in this field are 'specialist generalists' and have much to offer patients through their pragmatic approach, with an emphasis on empowerment, enablement and self-management. This ethos puts health promotion and positive adaptation to disability at its heart.

Physiotherapists are in a unique position to work at the interface of chronic disease and palliative care. The profession is likely to grow in prowess as physiotherapists see greater numbers of patients with chronic conditions benefiting from palliative care in the future.

Increasingly physiotherapists are stepping forward for leadership positions to creatively raise the profile of physiotherapy as an integral component of high quality end of life care provision. Promoting a rehabilitative approach to palliative care, with continuing close attention to education and psychosocial well-being, the physiotherapy profession can shape both the dignity and quality of life of patients as they navigate the challenges of disease progression, supporting the patients to live fully until they die.

REFERENCES

Addington-Hall JM, Higginson IJ. Palliative care for non-cancer patients. Oxford: Oxford University Press, 2001.

Barclay S, Maher J. Having the difficult conversations about the end of life. Br Med J 2010;341:c4862.

Booth S, Moosavi SH, Higginson IJ. The etiology and management of intractable breathlessness in patients with advanced cancer: a systematic review of pharmacological therapy. Nat Clin Pract Oncol 2008;5:90–100.

Bury M. Chronic illness as biographical disruption. Sociol Health Illn 1982;4:167–182.

Cane F, Jennings R, Taylor J. A rehabilitation training programme at the end of life. End of Life Care Journal 2011;1(1). Available at http://endoflifejournal.stchristophers.org.uk/clinical-practice-development/a-rehabilitation-training-programme-at-the-end-of-life.

Cheville A. Rehabilitation of patients with advanced cancer. Cancer 2001;92(Suppl 4):1,039–1,048.

Connor SR. Hospice and Palliative Care: The Essential Guide. New York: Taylor and Francis, 2009.

Crawford GB, Price SD. Team working: Palliative care as a model of interdisciplinary practice. Med J Australia 2003;179: S32–S34.

Gomes B, Higginson IJ. Where people die (1974–2030): Past trends, future projections and implications for care. Palliat Med 2008;22:33–41.

Hall S, Petkova H, Tsouros AD, Constanti M, Higginson IJ (eds). Better palliative care for older people: Better practices. Copenhagen: World Health Organization Europe, 2011.

Javier NSC, Montagnini ML. Rehabilitation of the hospice and palliative care patient. J Palliat Med 2011;14:638–648.

Jennings R. Palliative care and rehabilitation: The meaning of pain for patients with advanced cancer and how it influences behaviour. London: Kings College, 2012 (unveröffentlicht).

Katamay A. Die Rolle von Tod und Sterben in der Ausbildung zum Physiotherapeuten. Wie gehen Studenten damit um? Diplomarbeit, Akademie für Physiotherapie, Wels, 2003.

Kumar SP, Jim A, Sisodia V. Effects of palliative care training program on knowledge, attitudes, beliefs and experiences among student physiotherapists: A preliminary quasi-experimental study. Indian J Palliat Care 2011;17:47–53.

Mehne S, Nieland P, Simader R. Basiscurriculum Physiotherapie in Palliative Care. Bonn: Pallia Med Verlag (Akademie für Palliativmedizin, Malteser Krankenhaus Bonn), 2007.

NICE. Improving supportive and palliative care for adults with cancer. London: National Institute for Clinical Excellence, 2004.

Nieland P. Da-Sein. pt_Zeitschrift für Physiotherapeuten 2008;60:7.

Oldervoll LM, Loge JH, Lydersen S, et al. Physical exercise for palliative care cancer patients: A randomized clinical phase II trial. Trondheim: Norwegian University of Science and Technology, 2011.

Platt-Johnson K. Rehabilitation: Imperatives in cancer and palliative care education. In: Foyle L, Holstad J (eds). Innovations in Cancer and Palliative Care Innovations. Milton Keynes: Radcliff Publishing, 2007.

Reeve J, Lloyd Williams M, Payne S, Dowrick C. Revisiting biographical disruption: Exploring individual embodied illness experience in people with terminal cancer. Health (London) 2010;14:178–195.

Rogers CR. The necessary and sufficient conditions of therapeutic personality change. J Consult Psychol 1957;21:95–103.

Rogers CR. Accurate empathic understanding. Presentation, 1967. Available at http://www.centerfortheperson.org/pdf/1967__Accurate_Empathic_Understanding.pdf (last accessed June 2012).

Saleem T, Leigh PN, Higginson IJ. Symptom prevalence in people affected by advanced and progressive neurological conditions: A systematic review. J Palliat Care 2007;23:291 299.

Saunders CM. The challenge of terminal care. In: Symington T, Carter RL (eds). Scientific foundations of oncology. London: Heinemann, 1976: pp. 673–679.

Simader R. Die Rolle von Tod und Sterben in der Ausbildung zur Physiotherapeutin. pt_Zeitschrift für Physiotherapeuten 2005;57(11):77–82.

Smith AM. Emergencies in palliative care. Ann Acad Med Singapore 1994;23:186–190.

Solano JP, Gomes B, Higginson IJ. A comparison of symptom prevalence in far advanced cancer, AIDS, heart disease, chronic obstructive pulmonary disease and renal disease. Journal of Pain and Symptom Management, 2006;31:58–69.

Watson MS, Lucas C, Hoy A. Oxford Handbook of Palliative Medicine. Oxford: Oxford University Press, 2005.

Williams SJ, Bendelow G. The Lived Body: Sociological Themes, Embodied Issues. London: Routledge, 1998.

Yoshioka H. Rehabilitation for the terminal cancer patient. Am J Phys Med Rehab 1994;73:199–206.

1.3 From symptom control to rehabilitation: Physiotherapy approaches to end of life care

Jenny Taylor

The role of the physiotherapist in palliative/end of life care embraces a wide range of both core and specialist skills, and a well-developed ability to engender trust, confidence and coping strategies in very vulnerable patients. This chapter presents an overview of the current palliative care approach to both patients and their carers. Many of the topics raised are addressed in detail by other authors in subsequent chapters. The complexity of multi-factorial symptoms, the challenge of establishing appropriate and collaborative goals, patient expectations, and how all these affect the role of the physiotherapist in this specialty are discussed. Models of treatment evolve, and previous conventional specific symptom-control measures are developing into a 'whole person' approach. Reference is made to the importance of inter-professional collaboration and advanced communication skills. Expert teamwork, case reviews and support for all team members are all noted. Excellent psychosocial skills play a key role in advising patients and families both practically and emotionally. Of growing importance is the educational role of the physiotherapist; above all, the importance to equip the patient, family and professional colleagues with the skills to transfer control into the hands of the patient (Wells 1990). Finally, in recognition of the fact that we are subject to a changing landscape with limited resources in a continually developing field, we explore potential innovation for the physiotherapist in this growing specialty.

1.3.1 Physiotherapy then and now

During the 1960s, in many countries rehabilitative physiotherapy for cancer patients was largely considered to be contra-indicated. Primarily it was deemed appropriate only for a few patients whose disease was considered stable and prognosis relatively positive. Dietz (1969) stated that the principle goal of rehabilitation for people with cancer was improvement in life quality irrespective of time remaining, and with emphasis on maximum productivity with minimum dependence. While this philosophy remains true, the scope of physiotherapy in end of life care has broadened considerably. Palliative care now embraces a wider range of diseases besides cancer, and boundaries with long-term conditions are blurring. With the development of more advanced symptom control, patients are active and 'well' for longer. More freedom to interpret rehabilitation and service delivery provision has emerged as the physiotherapist's professional identity has continued to evolve. In the UK physiotherapists have been autonomous practitioners since 1977, enabling them to use their own clinical judgement and choose treatments without prescription from a medical practitioner. However in many countries medical referral for physiotherapy remains obligatory. The ICF (*International Classification of Func-*

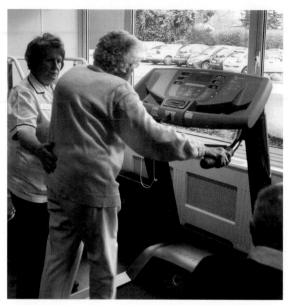

Figure 1.2 A gentle workout on the treadmill (© St Christopher's Hospice, London, UK) [T440]

Table 1.1 Comparison of physiotherapy approaches at end of life

Previous service delivery model	Current service delivery model
Symptom-specific intervention	Whole body approach addressing deconditioning
Prescriptive and didactic	Problem and solution focused
Almost exclusively one to one	Reflecting open and interactive approach
Highly experienced specialist therapists predominant	New therapists nurtured and developed
Privacy focused	Mutually supportive, attractive and fun
Conclusion	
Patient who may be too dependent on physiotherapist	Patient who is confident, independent and empowered

tioning, *Disability and Health*) includes social disability, which is particularly pertinent to palliative care. This WHO (World Health Organization) standard framework model mirrors a physiotherapy service delivery that has shifted from a specific symptom control model to today's active functional and participative model. Moreover, in more recent years it has extended to include aspirational general fitness (➤ Figure 1.2). Many patients have been involved in sport or active gymnasium membership as part of a previous lifestyle. Now that rehabilitation expertise is accessed for longer periods and often sporadically throughout patients' longer disease trajectory, exciting opportunities exist to raise the professional profile of physiotherapists. The physiotherapist is perfectly placed, therefore, to sit right at the heart of good rehabilitative palliative care.

1.3.2 Current context and aim of intervention

The founder of the modern hospice movement, Dame Cicely Saunders (1918–2005) succinctly described the aims of the palliative care professional: *'to enable the dying person to live until he [or she] dies, at his own maximal potential performing to the limit of his physical and mental capacity with control and independence whenever possible'* (Saunders 1998). There could be no better quotation to serve as a model for the physiotherapist. The *National Institute for Clinical Excellence* (NICE), which provides guidance in health issues in the UK, states that

'palliative rehabilitation attempts to maximize patients' ability to function, to promote their independence and to help them to adapt to their condition' (NICE 2004). Both statements embody the key challenges placing end of life care approaches apart from the conventional, more traditional, symptom specific and time-focused approaches (➤ Table 1.1). In the palliative care setting the physiotherapist is presented with a more complex scenario than in the acute setting, where the intended outcome is to return the patient to full pre-morbid power, range and function. Patients display a wider range of symptoms, drawing on the entire range of physiotherapeutic skills, reflective and analytical abilities and personal resources.

After scrupulous attention to a full assessment and details of medical history, the physiotherapist must be ready to apply not only a thorough knowledge of palliative care but also a range of specialties including elderly care, musculoskeletal, neurology, oncology, orthopaedics and respiratory care. In end of life care a more problem-orientated, confidence-building and enabling approach is applicable. 'Problem' in this context is used as a subjective concept. Disability and impairment carry major intractable implications for the patient requiring analysis and interpretation far beyond purely symptom control. By enhancing function, adaptive coping and independence within progressive disease constraints, the focus shifts towards a more patient-centred, holistic approach and includes addressing progressive general fatigue and weakness. Primary emphasis is on discovering how the patients perceive their problems, not only how the therapist perceives them. Furthermore the approach is often heuristic (that is, explored and managed by trial and error) and developing strong clinical relationships with these very vulnerable patients engenders considerable trust. A compassionate and sensitive attitude is the firm foundation for meeting patient needs to reduce dependency. Gradual patient empowerment builds towards a goal of self-reliance and self-efficacy.

While committed to protecting patients from a sense of failure or self-delusion, the physiotherapist must always be mindful that *'people in authority tend to forget that many patients are able, and want to talk about their own fear'* (Mr R. F., a patient reflecting on successful physiotherapy intervention) (➤ Chapter 2.7). Recently, a new reality has emerged for consideration: survivorship. This has a huge impact on service provision commissioners in the UK (Department of Health et al. 2010). According to Webster et al. (1995) emphasis rests on being as fit and well as possible while surviving, and rehabilitation is key. **Patients now living with dying for longer periods present with higher expectations of life quality.** They proactively seek access to rehabilitation services and often have episodic treatments throughout an extended illness trajectory (Platt-Johnson 2007). Physiotherapy in this specialty extends beyond the traditional care of the patient to include consideration of family concerns and environmental needs. Objective aims for the physiotherapist may appear clear, but the emphasis on listening to the patient's unique needs is supremely important.

⚠ **CAUTION**
- Look for symptoms presented in complex and unexpected combinations.
- Is the physiotherapist's problem the patient's problem?
- Is the disease managing the patient, rather than the reverse?

✓ **GUIDANCE**
- Ensure listening is 'active' (➤ Chapter 3.1).
- Ensure that treatment sessions are patient-directed.
- Think holistically with the patient at the centre.

1.3.3 Patient goals and outcomes

Patients at end of life are faced with complex and challenging symptoms associated with their physical decline and loss of function (Eva/Wee 2010). An uncertain disease trajectory and consequent adjustment process compound their increasing dependence and sense of loss of control. The evidence shows, above all, a worry of becoming a burden to others (Cheville 2001; Chochinov et al. 2002; Seale/Addington-Hall 1994). The physiotherapist improves life quality by employing strategies to maximize ability and function within restrictions imposed by disease. Encouraging the use of adaptive techniques, patients are helped to move – in as far as potential allows – from debility to ability.

'I think physiotherapy is wonderful. I feel pleased with myself when I've been in the gym. I didn't think I would manage to walk up stairs again. But it's so nice to be with other people who have similar problems that it makes it easier to try with support from the staff. It's good not to feel alone, as I often can feel quite isolated at home' (Mrs J. M., a patient with primary brain tumour).

Developing high levels of mutual trust and understanding is the firm foundation of physiotherapists' professional relationship. Self-esteem is often very low. Impaired ability to perform even simple everyday tasks strikes at the heart of patients' dignity and provokes feelings of isolation, not just from close family but wider society in general (Hilario 2010). Widely varying symptoms both challenge and compromise expected outcomes. Devising programmes of therapy to maximize limited functional potential demands a high level of professional skill. Strategies are modified to work within a realistic time framework, and withdrawal of therapy as the patient's disease status changes needs to be sensitively managed.

Underlying these considerations is the importance of excellent psychosocial skills to negotiate changing goals and uncertain outcomes. Outcome measures are fraught with difficulty. Many are unwieldy, and there is unease when applying outcome measures to terminally ill patients. An additional problem is response shift: perceived patient outcomes will be influenced by a multitude of factors both over time and in the context of disease progression. This makes perceived patient outcomes very difficult to interpret accurately.

⚠ **CAUTION**
- Set realistic and achievable goals in collaboration with the patient.
- Too high goals result in compromised commitment to physiotherapy.

✓ **GUIDANCE**
- Observe patient's demeanour and body language.
- Building trust is the key to managing changing goals.

1.3.4 Understanding the patient in depth

The first encounter between patient and therapist is pivotal. Patients are subject to a complex mix of emotions

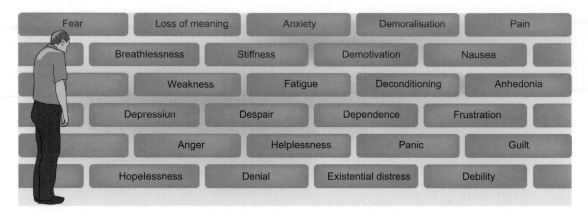

Fear	Loss of meaning	Anxiety	Demoralisation	Pain
Breathlessness	Stiffness	Demotivation	Nausea
Weakness	Fatigue	Deconditioning	Anhedonia
Depression	Despair	Dependence	Frustration
Anger	Helplessness	Panic	Guilt
Hopelessness	Denial	Existential distress	Debility

Figure 1.3 It's a huge wall to climb … [M541/L157]

influenced by losses, hopes and fears (➤ Figure 1.3). A distraction-free environment, where possible, is best. In the author's experience, this need not be in complete privacy; the presence of other patients and physiotherapists can often reduce anxiety or apprehension by 'normalizing' the experience. The physiotherapist attends closely to the patient's insight, to acceptance of the diagnosis, and to the apparent adjustment to its physical implications. As Saunders notes, *'We have to listen to the details of symptoms, giving constant attention to changing needs. We are concerned both to relieve suffering and that our patients should maintain their own character and style to the end'* (Saunders 1988, p. 11).

Patients often have a relative or carer in attendance. Supplemental information provided helps understanding of the patient's temperament and their place in the wider family group, and can ensure a more effective and individualized treatment strategy. But caution is advised, as emotional stress or a well-meant desire for a positive outcome for the patient can influence a relative's perspective. This can distract the therapist from the gold standard 'impeccable' assessment (WHO). When physically assessing the patient, addressing pain is of primary importance. The therapist needs to have a sound working knowledge of the 'total pain' concept (➤ Figure 1.4) as this will impact on patient management.

In a study of 100 patients in a palliative care unit, 90 % of patients with a functional disability reported deconditioning. This is broadly an umbrella term for a combination of muscle weakness, fatigue and breathlessness and is very prevalent in this patient group; 56 % of these patients gained functional improvement after 2 weeks of intervention, and 33 % continuing improvement towards physiotherapy goals (Montagnini et al. 2003). Reassurance is vital to ensure the patient is not

over-exhausted by a first assessment. If confidence is undermined, commitment to ongoing sessions will be compromised.

Total pain

Dame Cicely Saunders developed the 'total pain' model from her own experience working with patients at the end of life. Her unique multiprofessional perspective as a nurse, social-worker and finally physician, brought a new understanding to the complex suffering she observed in her patients. This pain was perhaps most succinctly described in 1963 by one of her patients: *'It began in my back, but now it seems all of me is wrong'* (du Boulay 2007, p. 137). It became clear to Dr. Saunders that as well as addressing the more obvious physical symptoms,

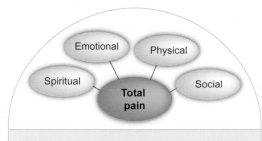

"Total pain was presented as a complex of physical, emotional, social and spiritual elements. The whole experience for a patient includes anxiety, depression and fear; concern for the family who will become bereaved; and often a need to find some meaning in the situation, some deeper reality in which to trust." (Cicely Saunders 1963, Clark 1999)

Figure 1.4 Total pain concept [M541/L157]

many underlying issues of social, emotional, and spiritual pain all conspired to exacerbate the patient's pain experience. These components were therefore of equal importance to consider in ensuring a 'whole person' approach. The categories of 'total pain' could in practice be further broken down to include such factors as isolation, financial worries, societal and cultural concerns, family tensions, anxiety, depression, anger, and fear. Implicit to this new understanding was that a collaborative approach would be needed if symptoms were to be effectively managed. Consequently physiotherapists, when assessing patients, must pay careful attention to the broader implications of symptoms presented.

This 'total pain' concept is now widely recognised throughout the palliative care world and is the foundation of all end of life care.

Fundamental to implementing this approach, Cicely Saunders passionately believed, too, that on-going education and research must always be central as this would guarantee that palliative care would hold its place firmly in the mainstream of medicine.

⚠ **C A U T I O N**
- Pace assessment while monitoring patient closely.
- Balance individual components of treatment sessions.
- Consider and analyse carer's perspectives, but keep the patient central at all times.
- Allow for 'deconditioning': it lowers energy levels.

✓ **G U I D A N C E**
- Plan environment carefully for first assessment.
- Outline strategic treatment plan in discussion with patient.
- Define lower goals to ensure over-achievement for patient morale.
- Keep 'total pain' concept central to all interventions.
- Be optimistic and positive, but realistic and honest.

1.3.5 Team-working

'Blurring of boundaries is to be expected' (Platt-Johnson 2007, p. 243)

A holistic approach to the patients' needs is crucial. This is best delivered by a multiprofessional team collaborating effectively and seamlessly to provide an integrated and coordinated package of care. Hopkins and Tookman (2000) formulated that patients are faced with reconstruction of a new 'self', and this needs support from all members of the multiprofessional team. The patient's past life has to be reconfigured through appropriate aims and goals in order to

shape a future that can be made sense of. This approach challenges the physiotherapist to tailor services appropriately in discussion with other professionals. **Where teams are fortunate to work with a non-hierarchical ethos, the physiotherapist's attitude is non-isolationist, honouring other colleagues' skills. Mutual support can be given with a readiness to cross-refer to other clinicians.**

The mode and source of referral vary around the world, and depend upon various factors, e.g. the palliative care team, specialist doctors, general doctors, community services, and the setting (an acute setting, or self-referral). Team discussions and regular case reviews can ensure that a holistic approach is maintained. Opportunities exist to share problems, reappraise symptom management and ensure a right balance of each professional's input. In contexts where professional autonomy is more restricted, proactive team-working presents a golden opportunity to show-case the considerable skills of the palliative care physiotherapist. Developing supportive and trusting relationships amongst colleagues is crucial. Physiotherapists working outside more formal structures can usefully network with SIGs (specialist interest groups), accessed via national professional organizations; physiotherapists can also consider setting up informal meetings with colleagues involved in patient end of life care. Complex cases can take their toll on emotions, and working in this specialty is both challenging and stressful; clinical supervision for the therapist is therefore paramount.

1.3.6 The collaborative physiotherapy model

Patients are treated as outpatients, in an inpatient unit, either on a one-to-one basis or, increasingly in hospice and palliative-care day units, patients attend group sessions. Interviews conducted with palliative care patients (Enes 2003) established that a major feature in a patient's sense of dignity was to feel able to exert a sense of control over his or her own body. **Throughout physiotherapy sessions the therapist approach is collaborative, not paternalistic.** By focusing more on self-direction, and by encouraging 'ownership' of their rehabilitation, patients are inspired to aim for, and often achieve, their goals, however small. Many patients receiving palliative care experience low self-esteem and diminishing self-worth, described as *'dignity of self'* (Jacobson 2007), which has implications for socialization with others and a feeling of dissociation or exclusion from interactive relationships. In the author's experience, more able patients relish the opportunity to gently 'work out' in a small group, supervised in a contemporary fitness gym

(➤ Figure 1.5). The camaraderie that develops is mutually supportive, motivation is often high, and patients support and encourage each other in an inspirational way. This approach has the added advantage that a greater number of patients can gain access to physiotherapeutic services. See also "Group therapy" in ➤ Chapter 2.6.

1.3.7 Physiotherapy at end of life

A significant proportion of physiotherapists' work continues to be with the dying patient, who is mainly confined to bed and with very limited potential for active rehabilitation. Physiotherapeutic strategies remain central to implement aspects of terminal care. These include pain relief, respiratory care, optimum positioning, increasing joint range, gentle muscle strengthening and contracture reduction techniques. **Although rehabilitation strategies will be modified, mobility should be understood as a spectrum.** Goal defining is always patient-specific. When represented diagrammatically, it can be seen that mobility includes all movement, however limited that may be (➤ Figure 1.6); when broken down into components, every level of ability has equivalent value for the individual patient.

While empathizing with the patient's deterioration, the optimum treatment model continues to address key symptoms, allowing space for the patient's autonomy in discovering remaining potential and drawing on the patient's inner resources. The physiotherapist can advise nursing teams and carers on moving and handling issues and transferring techniques where applicable. This blurs the boundaries of the multiprofessional team in a positive way.

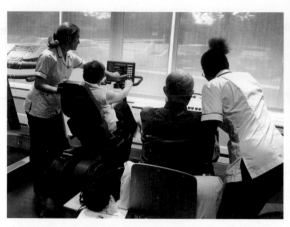

Figure 1.5 Exercising together with professional support (© St Christopher's Hospice, London, UK) [T440]

1.3.8 Alternative contexts for physiotherapy intervention

Through the establishment of home-care teams, many patients receive physiotherapy in the community, in their own homes or – in some countries – in nursing homes. Functional needs can be judged in the patient's own environment, and family concerns can be more thoroughly explored. However, many therapeutic modalities are difficult to implement in a non-clinical environment and home visits present staffing and time challenges. Good networking with community services plays a vital role, and valuable opportunities exist for liaison with a wide range of different professional colleagues. A home visit presents an ideal opportunity for the physiotherapist to give advice and education in activities of daily living, not only to the patient but also to the family and carers.

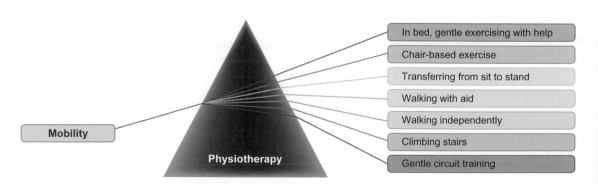

Figure 1.6 The spectrum of mobility [M541/L157]

⚠ **C A U T I O N**

Work *with* the patient, and do not 'do *to*' the patient!
• Mobility is a spectrum: place equal value on all goals.
• Regular clinical supervision must be prioritized.
• Potential therapist 'burn-out' is a risk in this field, due to continuous attrition.

✓ **G U I D A N C E**

• Group work lifts morale and encourages mutual support.
• How to empower a more functional patient who feels helpless? Help less!
• Regular team de-briefs can review what worked (and what did not).
• Set up informal and confidential case review meetings with colleagues.

1.3.9 The educational role of the physiotherapist

Delivering education is a growing priority for the physiotherapist working in palliative care. Staffing and rehabilitation service access constraints exist in most community services and palliative-care units. Rehabilitation programmes designed to teach nurses the basics of assisting inpatient-directed mobility and functional activity can help to maximize the patients' capacities, however limited they may be (Cane et al. 2011). Based on the understanding that rehabilitation starts at the bedside, the workload of nursing teams in facilitating patient care is reduced, and the physiotherapy role gains a higher profile within the multiprofessional team through better mutual understanding. Nurses develop their own formal competencies and physiotherapists are thus enabled to implement and focus on more specialist input. *'To deal with complexity you need a well-functioning team. Rehabilitation is not uniquely the domain of the Allied Health Professional'* (Tookman, unpublished observation, 2007). Student placements in palliative care are mutually rewarding, challenging misconceptions about rehabilitation for the dying, demonstrating holistic, problem-focused assessments, and updating current clinical development. Opportunities to present seminars and case studies to physiotherapy undergraduates, if enthusiastically grasped, sow the seeds of palliative care as a possible future career choice. Ongoing commitment to continuous professional development (CPD) is key to ensuring a firm foundation of palliative care knowledge and maintains current best practice. The educational role of the physiotherapist is extended effectively by delivering teaching presentations to both carers' and professional groups. Possible practical topics to include are fatigue management, falls prevention, moving and handling, pacing and coping, transfer assistance, and advice on general activities of daily living. When a carer is directly involved in the techniques and strategies that have been taught to the patient through their physiotherapy sessions there is an opportunity for solidarity in coping and in managing disease progression creatively.

1.3.10 Innovation

In this continually growing specialty it is important for physiotherapists to embrace new models of clinical intervention, and to be prepared to take risks by not being possessive of their own skills. The effective physiotherapist can grasp new and imaginative initiatives, and always be ready to broaden approaches through working with other professional colleagues in alternative settings, where appropriate (Wu/Quill 2011). To maintain currency as a profession, there is an imperative for the physiotherapist to strive to reflect up-to-date models of fitness. This includes using the latest modern sports equipment and interactive technology, selecting those that are attractive but non-intimidating for the palliative care patient. New models of practice emerge from an open attitude to contemporary and creative approaches. There is potential for input to a range of multiprofessionally-led group sessions, designed for patients both with and without carers. The innovative physiotherapist is wise if receptive to new concepts and fresh ideas suggested by physiotherapists new to the specialty. Integrating motivational and anxiety management techniques can help meet the complex physical needs of these patients. In the author's experience strategies in cognitive behavioural therapy (CBT), for example, are invariably useful. The patient is enabled to gently challenge any faulty beliefs or perceptions around mobility and function. By reducing fear and improving both confidence and outlook, very positive outcomes result.

A key priority is conducting audit and evidence-based research. Ongoing reviews of appropriate outcome measures ensure effective evaluation of physiotherapeutic interventions. These will play a major role in helping commissioners of palliative care service delivery in all countries to perceive physiotherapy as a key profession in this field.

Possibilities and opportunities in palliative/end of life care with physiotherapy as a key role: Future models

Nigel Hartley

I write this as someone who has worked in end of life care for over 20 years. In more recent years, I have worked in a Senior Management position at St Christopher's Hospice, London, UK, where, amongst other things, I am responsible for the management and future direction of the Allied Health Professions Team, which includes physiotherapists.

In the 2010s there is unprecedented change and challenge in the health service. As well as the turmoil caused by global financial uncertainty, there are also many societal issues that force us to think differently about how we deliver good, cost-effective health and social care.

For many people, both living longer with multiple chronic illnesses and becoming increasingly isolated within the places that they live will only add to the complexity of their lived experiences. These challenges are not only facing physiotherapists in specialist palliative care, but every part of every service delivery setting in end of life care. The challenge for end of life care is how to think creatively about filling the gaps and stepping across the divides that exist between end of life care rehabilitation, chronicity and survivorship; this needs to be carried out cost effectively and without a decline in quality.

There is no doubt that physiotherapy is central to developing our understanding in all of these areas and to initiating the kind of service innovation that will be able to move things forward. For any healthcare profession to be seen as an essential part of the health and social care services of the future, they will certainly need to be broad in outlook and creative in practice. **A useful question for physiotherapy practitioners is this: 'What kind of physiotherapist will the future need me to be?'** What is meant by this is that as professionals we need to be not only flexible and committed, but also to be able and willing to go beyond the regular call of duty, developing creative responses to challenging questions whilst working to fuller capacity. At St Christopher's Hospice our physiotherapy team is an integral part of an ongoing development programme in order to deliver high quality services to more people. It is not possible to simply employ additional physiotherapists to meet increasing demand. There is no new money, and more and more people need access to good quality care. Therefore, the development of gym group programmes has been an inventive response to meet demand in an innovative and resourceful way. We live in a 'gym culture'. Because of this, there is an ever stronger likelihood that people coming to the end of life will understand the benefit of well-planned exercise under the observation and guidance of competent and confident physiotherapists. Most people also recognize the importance of exercising together with others. The social experience for those people coming to the end of their life, being 'in the same boat' together, takes on extra significance when those people strive together towards a common goal. The possibility for camaraderie and peer support offers vital encounters for many who, because of their illness, can experience social isolation and social death. Being supported to retain the physiological abilities needed in order to continue to get out and about for as long as possible – whether to hospital appointments, the shop or the pub, for a walk, or to a group in a hospice gym – can be a fundamental part of preserving meaning, hope and belonging.

I have observed the goal to remain motivated both emotionally and physiologically being lived out on a daily basis through gym group programmes at St Christopher's Hospice supported by our team of physiotherapists. The role of the physiotherapist is not only that of a 'high street' gym fitness instructor: the experienced and knowledgeable physiotherapist brings an expertise drawn from rigorous clinical training, which is essential when applied to working with vulnerable people with incurable disease. These patients need to be supported, guided and motivated in order to recognize limitations as well as to strive to bring out the best in themselves and others.

In the 2010s, all health and social care professionals are challenged to change and remould their craft in order to remain relevant and useful in what will definitely be an altered future. **Physiotherapists have a unique opportunity here. This is because the craft of physiotherapy, when practised effectively, has the prospect to overarch the medical and the social, the psychological and the spiritual.** The challenge is simply to be 'the complete professional'. However, this is not a simple task, as too many professionals in this field will hold on to a set of specific defences and cultures. Many will fear losing an autonomy, a confidence, and a set of competences that have been hard won. However, part of the maturing process of the profession is the need to embrace what has been achieved without losing a sense of what else is possible. In short, it is important not to ignore and lose more general skills within a specialist area of practice.

A physiotherapist may ask what kind of physiotherapist the future will need him or her to be. I believe that there are four important areas for consideration:

- Quick assessment: In-depth assessment on a one-to-one basis is costly and time consuming. Although important, it will be essential for the physiotherapist of the future to develop strategies and systems for quick, safe and effective assessments.
- Sharing knowledge: Physiotherapists will need to learn how to – and be willing to – give away information that they know. For example, patients who are not able to attend group programmes in gyms need exercise and physiotherapy packages of support, which will be required to be delivered by other health and social care professionals. Teaching and passing on the skills to do this effectively must become a crucial part of the future physiotherapist's craft. Nurses and other care workers should be supported in order to develop the competence needed to work with these people within the home, the care home, the inpatient setting or other environment.
- Working with groups: Incorporating group therapy models must now be an essential component in palliative/end of life care for the physiotherapists of the future. Understanding the complexities and benefits of working with groups, and the possibility of working safely with as many people as possible in different environments will need to be crucial tools within the future physiotherapist's toolbox. These environments may include gyms and purpose-built facilities, but more likely will be care homes and other varied community venues.
- Courage and humility: Balancing the knowledge that competent and confident physiotherapists can change the quality of both living and dying, alongside the insight to understand its palpable limitations with those people coming towards the end of life, will be an essential attribute for the practitioner of the future.

The changing world and the current professional and personal challenges for all health and social care workers may cause anxiety, fear and a lack of clarity for the future. However, I believe that physiotherapists are well placed not only to become important players in that future, but also to show the way forward for a range of other professionals who may not be able to access as easily the creativity, vision and potential to begin the essential process of self-examination and scrutiny at this pivotal time in the development of end of life care.

1.3.11 Conclusion

'Rehabilitation must ultimately have as its goal the opening up of new horizons' (Bullington 2009, p. 107).

Physiotherapists working in end of life care in all contexts need to be creative, flexible and well grounded in rigorous therapeutic models. In a climate of more openness to death and dying, patients are often more resilient while surviving their disease progression. Patients are also undergoing active treatment for longer. With high life-quality expectations, they are more proactive in demanding a service to meet their needs. However, a delicate balance exists between the physiotherapist's clinical responsibility and patient choice. **The presence of physiotherapy as a professional group is fortunate in that it is almost invariably seen by the patient as positive. Symptom control addresses the abnormal (that is, the disease). Functional control addresses the loss of the normal, which is more profound.** Other clinicians may focus primarily on symptom control; physiotherapy moves beyond that concept to enhance patient function and activity, and this inspires commitment from both patients and families. Interventions that reflect contemporary lifestyle choices are welcomed. Financial constraints and staff capacity impose a need to work in a 'time-rich' and 'staff-poor' way, but the profession is well-placed in this specialty to contribute greatly to building patient morale. Above all, the chief attribute of the physiotherapist is a pragmatic and 'hands-on' approach, whether at the bedside or in the gymnasium. Personal rewards are huge, as is job satisfaction. The physiotherapist working in end of life care is privileged to travel on this difficult journey with patients, sharing both their good and bad times while remembering that *'these patients are not looking for pity and indulgence … we should look at them with respect and an expectation of courage – and we will see an extraordinary amount of real happiness and even light-heartedness'* (Saunders 2003, p. 3)

REFERENCES

Bullington J. Embodiment and chronic pain: Implications for rehabilitation practice. Health Care Anal 2009;17:100–109.

Cane F, Jennings R, Taylor J. A rehabilitation training programme at the end of life. End of Life Care Journal, 2011;1(1) [online journal]. Available at http://endoflifejournal. stchristophers.org.uk/ clinical-practice-development/a-rehabilitation-training-programme-at-the-end-of-life (last accessed August 2012).

Cheville AL. Rehabilitation of patients with advanced cancer: Cancer rehabilitation in the new millennium. American Cancer Society 2001;92:1,039–1,048.

Chochinov HM, Hack TF, Hassard T, Kristjanson LJ, McClement S, Harlos M. Dignity in the terminally ill: a cross-sectional, cohort study. Lancet 2002;360:2,026–2,030.

Clark D. 'Total pain': Disciplinary power and the body in the world of Cicely Saunders, 1958–1967. Soc Sci Med 1999;49:727–736.

Department of Health, Macmillan Cancer support, NHS Improvement. National Cancer Survivorship Initiative (NCSI) vision. London: The Stationery Office, 2010.

Dietz JH. Rehabilitation of the cancer patient. Med Clin North Am 1969;53:607–624.

Enes S. An exploration of dignity in palliative care. Palliat Med 2003;17:263–269.

Eva G, Wee B. Rehabilitation in end-of-life management. Curr Opin Support Palliat Care 2010;4:158–162.

Hilario AP. Understanding dignity at the end of life: the experience of palliative care patients. In: Steele S, Caswell G (eds). Exploring Issues of Care, Dying, and the End of Life. Oxford: Interdisciplinary Press, 2010: pp. 123–134.

Hopkins KF, Tookman AJ. Rehabilitation and specialist palliative care. Int J Palliat Nurs 2000;6:123–130.

Jacobson N. Dignity and health: a review. Soc Sci Med 2007;64:292–302.

Montagnini M, Lodhi M, Born W. The utilization of physical therapy in a palliative care unit. J Palliat Med 2003;6:11–17.

NICE. Improving supportive and palliative care for adults with cancer. London: National Institute for Clinical Excellence, 2004.

World Health Organization. International Classification of Functioning, Disability and Health (ICF), 2011. Available at http://www.who.int/classifications/icf/en/ (last accessed May 2012).

Platt-Johnson K. Rehabilitation: Imperatives in cancer and palliative care education. In: Foyle L, Hostad J (eds). Innovations in Cancer and Palliative Care Education. Oxford: Radcliffe Publishing, 2007: pp. 236–250.

Saunders C. Care of the dying. Current Medical Abstracts for Practitioners 1963;3:77–82.

Saunders C (ed). St Christopher's in celebration. London: Hodder and Stoughton, 1988.

Saunders C. Foreword. In: Doyle D, Hanks G, MacDonald N (eds). Oxford Textbook of Palliative Medicine. New York: Oxford University Press, 1998: pp. v–ix.

Saunders C. Watch with me: Inspiration for a life in hospice care. Sheffield: Mortal Press, 2003: p. 3.

Seale C, Addington-Hall J. Euthanasia: Why people want to die earlier. Soc Sci Med 1994;39:647–654.

Webster DC, Vaughn K, Webb M, Playter A. Modelling the client's world through brief solution.focused therapy. Issues Ment Health Nurs 1995;16:505–518.

Wells RJ. Rehabilitation: making the most of time. Oncol Nurs Forum 1990;17:503–507.

Wu J, Quill T. Geriatric rehabilitation and palliative care: opportunity for collaboration or oxymoron? Top Geriatr Rehabil 2011;27:29–35.

BIBLIOGRAPHY

ACPOPC Guidelines for Good Practice. Association of Chartered Physiotherapists in Oncology and Palliative Care, Specialist Interest group (SIG), London: Chartered Society of Physiotherapy, 1993.

Chartered Society of Physiotherapy. The role of physiotherapy for people with cancer. Position statement. London: Chartered Society of Physiotherapy, 2003.

Meerabeau L, Wright K (eds). Long-term conditions: Nursing care and management. Oxford: Blackwell Publishing, 2011.

Rankin J, Rob K, Murtagh N, Cooper J, Lewis S (eds). Rehabilitation in cancer care. Oxford: Wiley-Blackwell, 2008.

Saunders C. The care of the dying patient and his family. Contact 1972;38:12–18.

1.4 The right time for physiotherapy: Is there a 'too late' or a 'too early'?

Ylva Dahlin

Patients with incurable diseases may be in continuous need for rehabilitation during their entire life following diagnosis, although the needs may vary over time. The presenting problems can also vary greatly depending on the disease. Some diseases have fast trajectories; for example, if a cancer is diagnosed late. Other diseases have slow trajectories with symptoms manifesting occasionally for many years; for example, COPD.

1.4.1 Early referral to physiotherapist

Physiotherapy early in the disease trajectory can prevent and reduce many problems with serious illness; for example, problems such as deconditioning, fatigue, pain, and oedema. Rehabilitation, including regular exercise, has been shown to be beneficial to people with a multitude of serious diseases. There is a variety of clinical fields where research showed patients with chronic, longstanding and/or palliative diseases improve with activity. For example, Heiwe and Jacobson (2011) found that regular exercise training significantly improved physical fitness, physical functioning, and health-related quality of life in adults with chronic kidney disease. Davies et al. (2010) found that exercise programmes for people with mild to moderate systolic heart failure improved health-related quality of life compared to usual care without the exercise. They also found that there was a reduction in hospital admissions due to systolic heart failure. Puhan et al. (2011) suggest that pulmonary rehabilitation including exercise programmes is a highly effective and safe intervention to reduce hospital admissions and mortality and to improve health-related quality of life in COPD patients who have recently suffered an exacerbation of COPD. Physical activity even appears to reduce the risk of cancer recurrence and overall mortality for patients with colon cancer as well as for colorectal cancer (Meyerhardt et al. 2006a/b).

Researchers with expertise in cancer, fitness, obesity, and exercise training agree that the most important message to cancer patients is to avoid inactivity. Patients should be encouraged to return to normal daily activities as soon as possible after surgery and during adjuvant cancer treatments. Exercise is safe both during and after most types of cancer treatment, including intensive life-threatening treatments such as bone marrow transplant (Schmitz et al. 2010).

1.4.2 Late physiotherapeutic interventions

Physiotherapy is important even late in the disease trajectory. Based on the author's experience and taking into consideration the symptoms and side effects that many patients experience, there is no 'too early', but there is perhaps 'too late'. Without adequate physiotherapeutic interventions, patients' ability to move and exercise deteriorates, which can further reduce fitness and can make their symptoms worse.

Oldervoll (2006) and Paltiel (2009) concluded that physical exercise could improve physical and psychological well-being among patients with incurable cancer. Physical exercise was also feasible and safe for these patients. Clemens et al. (2010) showed good results on physiotherapeutic management of lymphoedema in palliative care patients. Ragnarsson and Thomas (2003) describe how rehabilitation services are frequently requested too late in the care of the cancer patient. They argue that **rehabilitation interventions should be planned and explained to the patient before, during, or immediately following definitive treatment.** Symptoms such as breathlessness, pain and oedema can be alleviated with non-pharmacological interventions, and all palliative care units should have access to a physiotherapist.

1.4.3 The patient journey

The *Nordic Cancer Union* (2004) describes the cancer patient journey in four stages:
- diagnosis and preparation;
- treatment;
- rehabilitation/restoration of health; and
- possible recurrence of cancer and palliation.

Patients with other diseases have different journeys, but parallels can be drawn.

Diagnosis and preparation

At the time of diagnosis many patients are under great stress. During this phase the interventions mostly focus on the provision of information. For many patients it is difficult to take in important information at this time. Nevertheless, the patient must have knowledge of the disease, the procedures for treatment and the side effects of the treatment. A dialogue about what the patient's concerns are physically, psychologically, socially and existentially is important. The most important message from the physiotherapist at this time is to avoid inactivity. Physical activities should be adjusted to the person's individual situation regarding, for example, aerobic fitness, medical comorbidities and psychological state. Individual guidance on and participation in exercise or group activities is a way to facilitate physical activity for the patients, and can greatly improve morale.

Treatment

This is another stressful period for many patients. Side-effects can be severe, including nausea, pain and fatigue. The focus during this phase is on the treatment and how to prevent and reduce these side effects. Physiotherapeutic interventions include, for example, advice on exercise (Schmitz et al. 2010) and postoperative measures such as specific movements to promote joint mobility, pain control and stress management. Most research has focused on exercise and more research is needed concerning, for example, stress management. Clinical experience shows that physiotherapeutic interventions are useful and valuable for patients.

Rehabilitation/restoring health

After the treatment has come to an end, patients can find themselves in a no-man's land. Many patients are supposed to be cured, others will not be cured but will live with their disease and treatments for many years. At this stage the expectation of family and community is that life can go on as before. For the patient the consequences of being a cancer patient are often present for a long time, both mentally and physically.

Experience shows that physiotherapeutic interventions are highly valued by patients at this time. Exercise to restore strength and quality of life is important. For patients who have undergone extensive surgery or received treatments that have altered their physical appearance, exercise can help to improve body image and thereby improve quality of life (Schmitz et al. 2010).

Recurrence/palliation

Since many patients live with cancer and other serious diseases for many years, it becomes ever more difficult to define when the palliative phase starts. Many patients with terminal diseases live active lives, keeping up work and other activities sporadically for a long time. These patients have a great need of support, although these needs may vary over time. This demands great flexibility on the part of the healthcare providers, and there are significant cost implications. In some units a multiprofessional team can work together to provide the services needed, as effective holistic care necessitates referral to other specialities.

1.4.4 Determining the right time for physiotherapy

In palliative care the physiotherapist should, if possible, see the patient on a regular basis to ensure that the level of functioning is as good as possible and that the patient has relevant symptom control. Inadequate pain control and extensive bed rest can lead to unnecessary deterioration and ongoing deconditioning, and the person is at risk of losing important functions too early.

To capture patients' needs and to find the right timing for physiotherapy in palliative care, the ICF (*International Classification of Functioning Disability and Health*) framework can be useful (WHO 2011a/b). The ICF is a framework and classification system that describes functioning and disability in relation to health conditions, body functions and structure, personal factors and environment (➤ Figure 1.7). Describing functioning and disability in this way gives an overall picture of the patient's resources and limitations. The ICF can guide the physiotherapist in joint goal-setting with the patient.

It is important that doctors, nurses and other healthcare providers have adequate knowledge about physiotherapy in palliative care not only to make appropriate but also timely referrals to a physiotherapist. Regular information and educational activities directed towards these professions need to be key components of the job for a physiotherapist in palliative care.

Well-established task forces within the national physiotherapy associations or national palliative care organizations can be valuable resources to help devise effective ways to improve knowledge not only amongst physiotherapists, but also other health care professions.

Self-referral is another way for the patient to define the right time for physiotherapy. But this requires well-informed patients who are able to suggest physiotherapy when they think it will be helpful and relevant. A well-functioning website or information groups have roles to play in achieving this.

Assessments to explore patients' needs for physiotherapy

Regular application of physiotherapeutic assessments of, for example, respiratory, muscular or neurological

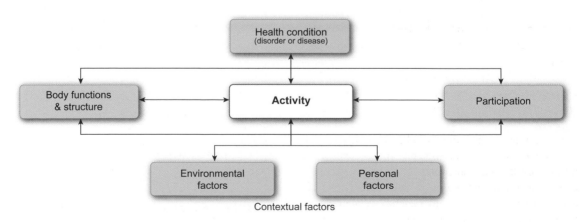

Figure 1.7 ICF [W798/L157]

problems, are of course useful even in end of life care. To capture all dimensions of a person's situation and to find the right time for interventions there is a need for a diverse range of methods of assessing needs in palliative care.

In order to optimize these supportive interventions, Rasmussen et al. (2010) suggest narrative approaches for assessment of symptoms and physical deterioration as a complement to logical scientific methods. Many instruments tend to target distinct problems such as pain, weakness or anxiety. Narrative approaches with open questions asked can open up a range of other views of rehabilitation needs as experienced by patients.

Besides the more traditional route (referral to physiotherapy and first one-to-one subjective assessment), Fyllingen at al. (2009) have implemented the use of computers for self-reporting of symptoms and functioning of patients receiving palliative care. Patients were asked to fill out a questionnaire with a total of 59 questions plus a body map for pain localization on a laptop computer. A majority of the patients included in the study managed to use the computer without assistance.

Patients nowadays often have considerable knowledge of information technology (IT), and the internet is becoming more and more a natural source of knowledge for many. Furthermore, IT infrastructure and electronic patient databases are in use for services in healthcare in many fields and are now extending into the field of palliative care. This is an area that is developing rapidly and has great potential value for enhancing the efficiency of service delivery.

1.4.5 Conclusion

Many patients have a continuous need of, and derive benefit from, rehabilitation and physiotherapy throughout the disease trajectory. But the physiotherapeutic interventions should always be based on the patient's needs, which can vary greatly over time. Physiotherapy should be a natural component of treatment strategies no matter if that treatment is curative or palliative. Too often patients say: *'Why didn't someone tell me about physiotherapy earlier? That would have spared me a lot of suffering.'*

To find the right time for physiotherapy and to meet the needs of the patients, physiotherapists must take action through education to increase the knowledge of physiotherapy among both healthcare providers and patients. Today many patients are not referred to a physiotherapist at all, or are referred later than ideal. Physiotherapy meets so many of the needs that patients in palliative care experience physically, psychologically, socially and existentially, and in order to communicate what role physiotherapy plays in end of life care there is urgency to find and develop relevant methods that can capture both quantitative and qualitative aspects of physiotherapy.

REFERENCES

Clemens KE, Jaspers B, Klaschik E, Nieland P. Evaluation of the clinical effectiveness of physiotherapeutic management of lymphoedema in palliative care patients. Jpn J Clin Oncol 2010;40:1,068–1,072. DOI: 10.1093/jjco/hyq093.

Davies EJ, Moxham T, Rees K, et al. Exercise based rehabilitation for heart failure. Cochrane Database Syst Rev 2001; aktualisierte Fassung 2010;(4):CD003331. Available at http://onlinelibrary.wiley.com/doi/10.1002/14651858.CD003331.pub3/pdf (last accessed May 2012).

Fyllingen EH, Oldervoll LM, Loge JH, et al. Computer-based assessment of symptoms and mobility in palliative care: feasibility and challenges. J Pain Symptom Manage 2009;38:827–836. Available at http://download.journals.elsevierhealth.com/pdfs/journals/0885–3924/PIIS0885392409007465.pdf (last accessed May 2012).

Heiwe S, Jacobson SH. Exercise training for adults with chronic kidney disease. Cochrane Database Syst Rev 2011;(10):CD003236. Available at http://onlinelibrary.wiley.com/doi/10.1002/14651858.CD003236.pub2/pdf (last accessed May 2012).

Meyerhardt JA, Heseltine D, Niedzwiecki D, et al. Impact of physical activity on cancer recurrence and survival in patients with stage III colon cancer: Findings from CALGB 89803. J Clin Oncol 2006a;24:3,535–3,541. Available at http://jco.ascopubs.org/content/24/22/3535.full.pdf (last accessed August 2012).

Meyerhardt JA, Giovannucci EL, Holmes MD, et al. Physical activity and survival after colorectal cancer diagnosis. J Clin Oncol 2006b;24:3,527–3,534. Available at http://jco.ascopubs.org/content/24/22/3527.full (last accessed August 2012).

Nordic Cancer Union. From needs to offers: Rehabilitation of cancer patients. Nordic Cancer Union, 2004. Available at http://www.ncu.nu/pdf_files/From_needs_to_offers.pdf (last accessed August 2012).

Puhan MA, Gimeno-Santos E, Scharplatz M, Troosters T, Walters EH, Steurer J. Pulmonary rehabilitation following exacerbations of chronic obstructive pulmonary disease. Cochrane Database Syst Rev 2011;(10):CD005305. Available at http://onlinelibrary.wiley.com/doi/10.1002/14651858.CD005305.pub3/pdf (last accessed May 2012).

Oldervoll LM, Loge JH, Paltiel H, et al. The effect of a physical exercise program in palliative care: a phase II study. J Pain Symptom Manage 2006;31:421–430. Available at http://download.journals.elsevierhealth.com/pdfs/journals/0885–3924/PIIS0885392406001886.pdf?refuid=S0885–3924(06)00473–8&refissn=0885–3924&mis=.pdf (last accessed August 2012).

Paltiel H, Solvoll E, Loge JH, Kaasa S, Oldervoll L. 'The healthy me appears': palliative cancer patients' experiences of participation in a physical group exercise program. Palliat Support Care 2009;7:459–467.

Ragnarsson KT, Thomas DC. Principles of cancer rehabilitation medicine. In: Bast RC Jr, Kufe DW, Pollock RE, et al. (eds). Cancer Medicine. 6th ed. Hamilton, ON: BC Decker, 2003.

Rasmussen BH, Tishelman C, Lindqvist O. Experiences of living with a deteriorating body in late palliative phases of cancer. Curr Opin Support Palliat Care 2010;4:153–157.

Schmitz KH, Courneya KS, Matthews C, et al. American College of Sports Medicine Roundtable on exercise guidelines for cancer survivors. Med Sci Sports Exerc 2010;42:1,409–,1426. Available at http://journals.lww.com/acsm-msse/Fulltext/2010/07000/American_College_of_Sports_Medicine_Roundtable_on.23.aspx (last accessed August 2012).

World Health Organization, 2011a. Available at http://www.who.int/classifications/icf/en/ (last accessed August 2012)

World Health Organization. Towards a common language for functioning, disability and health (ICF), 2011b. Available at http://www.who.int/classifications/icf/training/icfbeginnersguide.pdf (last accessed August 2012).

1.5 Physiotherapy at end of life: Patients' perspectives

Ylva Dahlin

The role of rehabilitation in palliative care is still relatively unfamiliar to healthcare providers, patients and the public. To improve the quality and the accessibility of rehabilitation in palliative care it is important to take account of patients' experiences and priorities. Many doctors and nurses are unaware of what rehabilitation can do for patients in palliative care concerning symptom control and quality of life. Family members and significant others are sometimes overprotective and do not suggest rehabilitation at this stage. Many patients in palliative care are therefore never referred to rehabilitation services.

Anxiety, fatigue, lack of energy, pain and weakness are frequent symptoms in palliative care patients (Teunissen et al. 2007; Laugsand et al. 2009), and many of the effects of these symptoms are reflected in the patients' comments in this chapter.

1.5.1 Patients' needs and priorities

Quill (2006) investigated what was most important for terminally ill patients to achieve. Four distinct themes emerged:
- Improving quality and meaning: The main aims included regaining independent function, being discharged home, and fulfilling the role of providing support to family and significant others.
- Achieving relief or comfort: The main issues were pain and symptom management and emotional support.

- Influencing the course of the illness progression: Many patients sought to be more involved in key medical decisions. Aims differed, and included either focusing on surviving to achieve specific milestones, or a wishing to die sooner as a way of avoiding prolonged suffering.
- Preparation for dying: This included completing unfinished business, exploring ways to improve the quality of their dying, and aspects of spiritual and/or religious preparation.

Being able to move better and being physically active seem to be important priorities for many patients in palliative care. There is a statistically significant correlation between physical activity and quality of life in patients undergoing palliative chemotherapy. About two thirds of these critically ill patients were interested in participating in training programmes (Oechsle 2011). Research shows that palliative cancer patients are motivated and feel able to take part in physical activity programmes (Lowe 2010).

When exploring what people living with terminal illness considered the areas of priority in their lives, Carter et al. (2004) found that 'taking charge' was a central theme that overshadowed all other themes. Patients' involvement was very important. Understanding patients' perspectives is essential to develop management strategies appropriate to the patients' needs at the end of life.

Dahlin and Heiwe (2009) made a similar discovery when investigating patients' experiences of physiotherapy in palliative cancer care. Patients from two palliative care units in Stockholm, Sweden, were interviewed. Patients in home care and hospital care were included. Reflecting upon physiotherapy, patients described 'participation' as being a prerequisite for satisfaction with physiotherapy on the whole. Participation included issues such as the physiotherapist being a good listener and being open to the patient's suggestions and views. Daily life was often dominated by medical examinations and treatment to which he or she was obliged to adjust. The patients stressed the importance of the physiotherapist seeing the whole picture and taking account of the patient's situation. Two revealing comments follow that illustrate this: *'It's largely about confidence and trust and things like that, so that it isn't an unpleasant experience … it's terribly important that she and I can talk, sort of thing …'* – *'I suppose it's also important for the physiotherapist to be clear about what this person wants and dreams of, so to speak, what you're aiming at …'*

1.5.2 Patients' thoughts on physiotherapy in palliative care

What are patients' expectations and hopes when seeking physiotherapy?

For patients it is often difficult to know what to expect and what to hope for concerning physiotherapy. **Patients mainly have a limited knowledge of what physiotherapy could do for them in the context of palliative care.** Dahlin and Heiwe (2009) showed that some patients felt that they had not received enough information about physiotherapy. Many patients had problems with strength and initiating activity and wanted the physiotherapist to be active in suggesting what should be done. Here are some of their comments: *'I suppose they told us physiotherapy was available. I don't think the information was specially good.'* – *'It's so easy for something like this to get forgotten, more or less, since there are so many other things. You get treatment and doctors' visits and you worry about your future in general.'*

Some patients knew what to ask for, but they felt that they had not been offered enough physiotherapy: *'I got help with surgical stockings, that's about all that I got ... and that crutch. It felt a little thin to me.'* – *'This water gymnastics [aqua aerobics], I mentioned it about six months ago, nothing came of it ...'*

Patients' experiences of physiotherapy

The patients described a wide variety of experiences (➤ Figure 1.8); for example, they described that physiotherapy gave them **hope,** or that meeting a physiotherapist who drew up treatment strategies for them inspired hope. In this context 'hope' meant hope for a time-limited improvement in a limited area, for example pain re-

lief or the ability to manage a certain activity on one's own. They did not mention hope for a cure in this context. Here is an example of what one patient said: *'It's so lovely that someone cares about me and that makes me enormously happy and grateful, and I feel that they believe in me. They're prepared to make an effort for me to get well. That I'll feel better, or whatever ...'*

Patients were also motivated and encouraged by the physiotherapist to **be active.** Fatigue and anxiety often made that difficult. The physiotherapist and patient reflected together on the level of available potential, which patients found very positive: *'You lie there pretty tired out and then it's tremendous to have someone to push you, in fact ...'* – *'When you're not entirely fine and strong, and somewhat depressed, often it's hard to tackle things on your own, actually ...'*

Another important aspect was **independence.** Patients described a fear of being a burden on their social circle, and it was a great relief when they managed to perform some activities on their own. Most often this was a matter of making practical daily life easier; for example, receiving training for a specific technique such as getting out of bed or moving from wheelchair to bed. Here are some quotes from patients in this context: *'It's important to be able to feel free and able to do what you want, even if it's only going down to the shop and buying a paper.'* – *'From my bed to my wheelchair, it was wonderful! I don't need help, I can do it.'*

Patients described that physiotherapy made them feel **more confident.** Many patients had felt insecure about their bodies. They did not know how much they ought to exert themselves when they were seriously ill. Guidance on how and how much they could and should move made them feel secure, as did access to adequate aids; for example, aids to prevent falls. Comments included: *'You're afraid of walking and falling down and things like that ... yes it [the walking frame] spells safety, you can say.'*

Patients valued the physiotherapist, whom they saw as an **expert in the area,** i.e. the physiotherapist is seen as being well informed on the patient's condition and on the condition's medical treatment. Another patient made this insightful remark: *'If I have someone I can rely on, who knows how your body is built up and everything, who says I can manage more, and then you think, I can rely on this. Then I dare to do it too.'*

Relief and well-being was also mentioned as something to which physiotherapy contributed. The patients described various treatment techniques such as acupuncture, TENS (transcutaneous electrical nerve stimulation) and massage, which provide pain relief and relaxation. One patient said: *'It's really lovely to get massage and you can switch off your thoughts for a bit then.'*

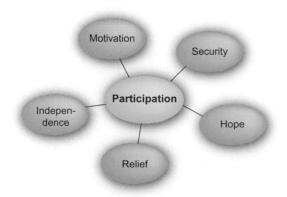

Figure 1.8 A model for patients' experiences of physiotherapy in palliative care [M541/L157]

Physical training gave a feeling of well-being, both physically and mentally. Hydrotherapy was stressed as very positive: the informants felt supple and mobile, and able to disconnect their thoughts from their disease for a while: *'So it [pool training] gives me a lift. I'm happy when I leave the pool, I can tell you.'*

1.5.3 How can we learn from our patients?

Taking account of patients' views and priorities is vital for bringing about improvements in the quality of healthcare in general and of course in palliative care as well. The concept of patient-centred care is developing in many healthcare organizations. It is a model in which health care providers invite patients and families to identify patients' needs and preferences. Healthcare organizations can gather patient feedback in a variety of ways. Questionnaires to patients, family members and significant others can be circulated routinely. Other methods of gathering data and other information are interviews, user groups, forums for comments and complaints, and informal meetings for patients and healthcare providers (Frampton et al. 2008). It is also important to carry out research in this field. Quantitative research methods such as surveys enable the gathering and analysis of a large number of views about certain issues. Qualitative research methods such as focus groups and interviews allow in-depth analysis of views and opinions, which gives further valuable information.

From the patients' points of view the process itself can have a strong meaning for many. **In the context of feeling passive and dependent due to serious illness, being able to contribute something important can give a deep feeling of satisfaction. Physiotherapists should therefore never be afraid to ask.** On the contrary, to further develop physiotherapy in palliative care, physiotherapists must ask their patients how they experience the physiotherapists' interventions. Methods for patient feedback should be integrated in the care programme, both formally and informally. A very effective and unique model of patient feedback is the so-called 'goldfish bowl'.

1.5.4 The goldfish bowl

Jenny Taylor

'If we can come together, not only in our professional capacity, but also in our common vulnerable humanity, there may be no need of words on our part, only of respect and concerned listening' (Saunders 2004).

A teaching method based on active listening (cf. ➤ Chapter 3.1) that has been developed primarily to teach final-year medical students can be readily adapted to serve as a model to inform and educate physiotherapists and associated rehabilitation therapists. The 'goldfish bowl', used in a number of hospices in England from the early 2000s comprises about four to six patients seated in an inner circle facing each other, and 'observers' (health professionals) seated in a wider circle around them (➤ Figure 1.9). A facilitator sits with the patients and asks a selection of open questions, inviting informal response and enabling relaxed discussion (Edmonds/Burman/Sinnott 2004).

The observers can learn much from these sessions. The patients become not only the 'experts', but also collaborative partners in an interprofessional teaching process. In a non-threatening environment, useful insights are gleaned from patients on communication, expectations, fears, hopes, and the impact of life-threatening illness.

Patient preparation and de-briefing for these sessions are both important. Emotions are easily accessed, so the facilitator needs well-developed skills to be competent to moderate the sessions effectively and sensitively. There is potential for much useful data to be gathered, including:

- the overall impact of physiotherapy treatment sessions on the patient;
- a useful perspective on the patient's view of multi-professional working;
- insight to how what is said to patients by clinicians truly impacts on the patient;
- deeper understanding of how personality types influence patient reactions to intervention
- realization that apparently passive patients have a voice too!
- fears and anxieties that physiotherapists may project onto their patients that may not exist;
- insight into the 'control' that physiotherapists may feel they have; is this positive or negative?

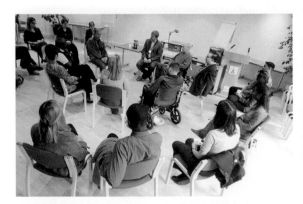

Figure 1.9 The goldfish bowl (© St Christopher's Hospice, London, UK) [T440]

- whether medical information delivered has been too much, too little or about right.

Future models to consider when implementing the 'goldfish bowl' could include combining outpatient/day-care patients with inpatients, and also involving carers. It could also be a very effective teaching module for physiotherapy students on clinical placement in palliative care.

A powerful aspect of the 'goldfish bowl' is the sense that patients really value the opportunity to 'give something back' (Hall/Todd 2007). Patients feel that they can contribute not only to educating the professionals or students but that they are rightly empowered to influence future service provision. The dynamic of the sessions helps to reduce their sense of isolation, while the listening clinicians gain greater empathy and understanding. As Saunders also said: *'We have to learn how to feel with patients without feeling like them if we are to give them a kind of listening and steady support that they need to find their own way through'* (Saunders 2003).

1.5.5 What have we learnt from our patients this far?
Ylva Dahlin

Physiotherapy in palliative care is important from the patients' point of view, since it enables independence, provides relief from distressing symptoms and offers a support system. **The feeling of participating and being in control is a prerequisite for patient satisfaction on the whole.** It is necessary to develop methods for assessing and evaluating qualitative aspects of physiotherapy and functioning. The relevance of measuring various factors – such as hope, independence, motivation, participation and security – in the context of physiotherapy in palliative care seems important.

There is a great need for education in rehabilitation in palliative care. Better communication and coordination within palliative care is also necessary since many patients are not referred to physiotherapy at all. It must be made clear to patients, relatives, and care providers that access to physiotherapy is a part of palliative care services, and that physiotherapy may be used for the prevention and relief of suffering associated with advanced cancer and other end stage diseases.

1.5.6 Three personal testimonies

The following are three case studies of patients: one from Sweden, one from the UK and one from Switzerland. Although very different in character and style, they were all facing the end of their lives. These patients generously gave their time to share thoughts and feelings with an interviewer; all were happy to play their part in developing our understanding.

CASE STUDY

A good physiotherapy experience, but a need for wider education: A formal interview with a patient

Ylva Dahlin and Mrs S. L.

Mrs S. L. was a 60-year-old woman diagnosed with breast cancer four years ago, undergoing palliative treatment.

'Mrs. L, how did you first hear about physiotherapy?'

'I asked a nurse at the oncology department. No one gave me any information in rehabilitation or physiotherapy. I had to ask for it myself.'

'After receiving your course of physiotherapy, what do you feel helped most?'

'Circuit training in the gym helped me to build up my body physically and made me less tired after my first treatment. Lately I have been training in the [swimming] pool, which is wonderful, especially after I had an operation on my hip. I can move a lot better now. The physiotherapist also treated me with acupuncture as I had a lot of pain in my hip. Now I hardly have any pain.'

'What for you was the most significant part of the physiotherapy process?'

'The thought of building up my body made me feel good, since disease and treatment had been breaking it down for a long time. It also gave my daily life a structure. I had to be at the gym at a certain time. I had to get out of bed, get dressed and get there. Sometimes I felt awfully tired but I knew it was good for me so I pulled myself together! It was very motivating to be in a group. I think the circuit class was very good as you don't have to be at the same level of fitness to all be able to train together.

We also had the opportunity to try different activities like Pilates, qi gong and yoga. Different people like different things so that was a good way of helping people to be active.

Talking to other patients was very valuable as well. We could talk about everything since we were in a similar situation. I still see some of these ladies, but now we mostly drink coffee together.'

'What do you feel could have been done better?'

'I think the information on rehabilitation and physiotherapy could have been better. Well, there was none actually, that I can remember. I would have liked something written to take home. You don't always remember everything they say at the hospital.'

CASE STUDY
From apprehension, through confidence to physical achievement: A patient's written impressions

Jenny Taylor and Mr W. H.

Mr W. H. was a patient at St Christopher's Hospice, London, UK, diagnosed with advanced pulmonary fibrosis. He volunteered the following detailed impressions and his subsequent experience of physiotherapy intervention.

'I had hardly ever visited the place [the Hospice] so my impression of it – a rather morbid amalgam of suffering, dying and death – was drawn from my own imaginings and uninformed popular assumptions, rather than first-hand knowledge. It came as a big shock, therefore, when my respiratory consultant at the hospital told me that my diagnosis had no known cure.

The best approach, he said, would be palliative care, including long-term medication and physiotherapy to try to reduce physical suffering. This care would be best provided by the Hospice. Despite my unease, I decided that I owed it to my wife and all the medical team involved in my care to seek this help. I was accepted as a day-care patient, once a week for group activities in which physiotherapy would play a key role. After assessment by a physiotherapist I was invited to attend a circuits group [for gym-based circuit training]. The physiotherapists are not strict disciplinarians, in the manner of old-style school gymnastic teachers, but firm and kind. Also, the absence of over-compensating 'caring' on the part of the physiotherapist combined with respect for the patient as an individual – and it is important to remember, opportunities for humour – add to the unforced dignity of the Hospice.

'The class itself far exceeded my expectations. Given the physical limitations of the patients (there were usually 6–8 of us) I had expected the exercises to be rather tame for someone like me who was used to training in larger, commercially-run establishments, alongside very fit people with a wide range of abilities. The exercises seemed indeed fairly low-key but, more importantly, effective. Also, I had overlooked the fact that my own physical condition had deteriorated considerably after several weeks of inactivity. It was at the end of the first few sessions (when I was actually pleased to find that I had the odd ache or two to remind me where some of my muscles were) that I realized I had done some proper physical work.

'The class starts with a 5-minute seated warm-up of light exercises and stretches to loosen stiff joints and tight muscles, and to ensure they are not injured by unfamiliar exertion. Then follows the circuit training, some involving conventional gym equipment such as a treadmill, small trampoline, exercise bike, weights, and pulleys, and a Wii® fit balance board. This last one is good fun in a group, as well as being excellent for coordination training. Group members are encouraged by the physiotherapist to work to the best of their ability. But, to ensure they don't attempt to do more than they can cope with, they are constantly supervised by trained staff, who manage to integrate time to give members one-to-one instruction. The session ended with more light exercises and stretches to cool down.

'The main problem that I had anticipated – exercising in the company of people, some of whom were visibly very seriously ill – turned out after 2–3 weeks not to be such a problem. My resistance had been, I realized, emotional, not logical, and was largely overcome after a few sessions. After a month or so I found I was actually looking forward to my weekly visits; and my wife, who brought me each week, enjoyed meeting new people who understood. She could relax with a cup of coffee while I went about my activities. After a while we started to see the physiotherapists as friends who would find time to talk to you rather than just be "staff".

'My main objectives in attending were to control my breathing while exerting myself and to regain some of the lost strength and flexibility in my joints and muscles. I feel that I've made progress with these objectives, even though they are not all fully achievable. I still get out of breath fairly quickly and easily become tired. But, on the other hand, my wife says my calf muscles are more defined, I can walk with my oxygen and go out in the car again with her to get some fresh air and enjoy time out of the house.

'Most important of all – and I do not think I am exaggerating – I believe that the physiotherapists at the Hospice have helped to prolong my life and given me a greater quality of life.'

Mr W. H. continued to engage actively with as much physiotherapy as he could tolerate as he slowly deteriorated; always passionate about how much he had benefited and keen to tell any who would listen how much it meant to him to feed back his thoughts and impressions. Over several months he received supportive care at home until he died peacefully in the company of his loving and devoted wife.

CASE STUDY
On the influence of physiotherapists

Brigitte Fiechter Lienert and Mr B.

Mr B., 58 years old, is married with three adult children. He is a general practitioner with additional training in psychosomatics and talk therapy. This personal and professional background enables him to consciously assess, as well as fully comprehend his own medical condition. He is diagnosed as having glioblastoma multiforme grade IV; for some years he has also been suffering from multiple sclerosis. He has been in a wheelchair for several years and has learned to cope, both professionally and privately, with his tetraparesis which is more pronounced on the right than the left. This condition existed prior to the cancer but has now increased in intensity. A neurosurgical procedure was performed a few days ago to resect the brain tumour, and the patient is now receiving chemotherapy and radiotherapy as an inpatient. In parallel, a physiotherapist has initiated a rehabilitation programme.

Mr B. would like a compassionate, holistic and interactive programme of physiotherapy. The physiotherapist asks about his goals and expectations, as well as overriding issues and fears. Not only on account of his professional background, but also through his position as an 'expert patient', Mr B. fears that the physiotherapist may feel pressurised by the idea that he *must* achieve as much as possible. At the same time, he describes his own ambivalence between what needs to be done to improve his functionality, and everything he still wishes to do in the short time he has left. He is fully aware of the short rehabilitative phase of his illness. The challenge in terms of therapy is to fulfil the patient's desires: dialogue, physical mobility and utilising what time is left for people, memories and encounters.

Mr B. raises an interesting topic: What impact do 'physiotherapists' have? It may well be a cliché, Mr B. admits when asked, but during the course of his life he has come to know a number of *very dynamic, athletic and performance-minded* physiotherapists.

A challenge when working with seriously ill and terminally ill individuals is also to reflect on one's own influence. Can the physiotherapist's own physical integrity and the demands he places on the bodies of his patients also be daunting or offensive?

For Mr B., talking *about the* body during the joint therapy session is a very important medium for working *with the* body. Daily mobilisation in his wheelchair and activities for maintaining his independence mean a great deal to Mr B.; however, he does not want to feel pressurised into having to achieve anything just to fulfil the needs that arise from certain 'positive intentions' on the part of the medical team. His family has adjusted to his physical disability and can be used as resources.

The physiotherapy was aligned to the patient's needs, with flexible adaptation to physical awareness, mobilisation and activities of daily living. Skilled dialogue and empathy for the immediate situation were essential during the physiotherapeutic process.

Mr B. was able to hand his practice over to a successor.

REFERENCES

Carter H, MacLeod R, Brander P, McPherson K. Living with a terminal illness: patients' priorities. J Adv Nurs 2004;45: 611–620.

Dahlin Y, Heiwe S. Patients' experiences of physical therapy within palliative cancer care. J Palliat Care 2009;25:12–20.

Frampton S, Guastello S, Brady C, et al. Patient-centered care improvement guide. Camden, ME: Picker Institute, 2008. Available at http://planetree.org/wp-content/up-loads/2012/01/Patient-Centered-Care-Improvement-Guide-10-28-09-Final.pdf (last accessed August 2012).

Edmonds P, Burman R, Sinnott C. The goldfish bowl. Eur J Palliat Care 2004;11:69–71.

Hall E, Todd J. Users as educators: how hospice patients can help in the training of health professionals. In: Jarrett L (ed.). Creative engagement in palliative care: New perspectives on user involvement. Oxford: Radcliffe Publishing, 2004: pp. 116–124.

Laugsand EA, Kaasa S, de Conno F, Hanks G, Klepstad P. Intensity and treatment of symptoms in 3,030 palliative care patients: A cross-sectional survey of the EAPC Research Network. J Opioid Manage 2009;5:11–21.

Lowe SS, Watanabe SM, Baracos VE, Courneya KS. Physical activity interests and preferences in palliative cancer patients. Support Care Cancer 2010;18:1,469–1,475.

Oechsle K, Jensen W, Schmidt T, et al. Physical activity, quality of life, and the interest in physical exercise programs in patients undergoing palliative chemotherapy. Support Care Cancer 2011;19:613–619.

Quill T, Norton S, Shah M, Lam Y, Fridd C, Buckley M. What is most important for you to achieve? An analysis of patient responses when receiving palliative care consultation. J Palliat Med 2006;9:382–388. Available at http://www.liebertonline.com/doi/pdf/10.1089/jpm.2006.9.382 (last accessed May 2012).

Saunders C. Watch with me. Sheffield: Mortal Press, 2003.

Saunders C. Foreword. In: Doyle D, Hanks G, Cherny N, Calman K (eds). Oxford Textbook of Palliative Medicine. 3rd ed. Oxford: Oxford University Press, 2004.

Teunissen SC, Wesker W, Kruitwagen C, et al. Symptom prevalence in patients with incurable cancer: A systematic review. J Pain Symptom Manage 2007;34:94–104. Available at http://download.journals.elsevierhealth.com/pdfs/journals/0885–3924/PIIS0885392407002011.pdf (last accessed May 2012).

1.6 Physiotherapy Students in Palliative Care

Eva Müllauer

Students of physiotherapy are very often confronted during their practical training by the suffering and also the death of patients. Appropriate preparation with a view to dealing with terminally ill patients, and for providing them with therapy, is both desirable and expedient. The following chapter discusses the content and elements of the 'Physiotherapy in Palliative Care' course which are positively welcomed by students. Feedback from participants, as well as comments on the practical placements, are also addressed. Ultimately we examine whether and how physiotherapy students can be motivated to take up the challenging task of palliative care.

Death and dying in physiotherapy practice: the student perspective

Very many students are confronted by the death of a patient during their practical training (Katamay 2003). This can trigger a whole variety of sensations such as sadness, shock, anxiety, confusion and even beyond that to sympathy for the family, amongst others. The intensity of such an experience is described by a female physiotherapy student as follows: *'My patient was no longer responsive and passed away during my therapy (first session). He simply stopped breathing. Initially I couldn't believe it: this can't be real! But then: get somebody quick. The nursing staff had been expecting it – I had absolutely no idea. To start with I was shocked, but after a few minutes I felt sad and began to cry.'* (Katamay 2003, p. 37)

Although, or perhaps because so many emotions are linked with the subject, students of physiotherapy questioned about the need to integrate the topic of 'death and dying' into their training offer very different answers. Two highly contradictory views serve to illustrate this. *'Death is a part of life! The course only needs to briefly touch on the subject!'* (Katamay 2003, p. 47) – *'The subject of death and incurable diseases in physiotherapy is like a poor relation when it comes to training – only very few are able to deal with it and most suppress such experiences … it has to be included in teaching programmes in the future!!'* (Katamay 2003, p. 48)

Whatever the often emotionally charged opinion of an individual student or even a teaching establishment, the reality of everyday physiotherapy demonstrates how important it is for future therapists to be well prepared for such a situation. What should be considered here is the ambivalence in which students find themselves if faced with a teaching course on the subject of palliative care. The topics and content seldom have much in common with the real-life situation of a 20-year-old. In this respect, careful planning and a fearless approach on the part of both lecturer and clinical educator are essential.

Do teaching courses that deal with physiotherapy in the terminally ill, with death, and the role of the physiotherapist in this context as well as the term palliative care, actually change the attitudes and, consequently, the experiences of the students? If this question can be answered with 'yes', then there is quite rightly a need to incorporate such subjects into the basic training programme. Kumar et al. (2011) provide a very clear answer to this question: Students having participated in a specialist palliative care training programme with theoretical input and case studies were found to undergo a significant and positive change in terms of their knowledge, their attitudes, as well as their assumptions and experiences related to palliative care. Nevertheless, there is a need to examine this topic more closely.

Based on necessity as well as the high level of acceptance on the part of students, many institutions have incorporated the subject of 'Physiotherapy in Palliative Care' into their curricula (➤ Chapter 1.2). The following statements, which accompanied the written reflections on the 'Physiotherapy and Palliative Care' teaching course, strengthen this assumption: *'… a report of my reflections on the palliative course is enclosed. I appreciate the fact that it was offered.'* – *'Many thanks for the interesting course: As a result I have grown as a person.'*

Basic framework for the teaching course

Before the course can be structured, the **cognitive, affective and psychomotor study objectives** need to be defined, which in turn are each subject to taxonomy (subcategorisation) (Schewior-Popp 2005). In physiotherapy, practical skills are often acquired by **learning from models:** the teacher who demonstrates a technique becomes a model for the student to follow. This also applies to the practical placement and behaviour towards the patient.

Knowledge from brain research illustrates the methodological possibilities. *'A good teacher narrates. (…) Narratives motivate us, not facts. Narratives can contain facts, but these facts are to the narrative what skeletons are to humans. Anyone who believes that studying means swotting up on facts is completely wrong; details only have meaning when put together as a whole, and it's this whole and this meaning that make the facts interesting. Only if the facts are interesting in this sense will we also remember them'* (Spitzer 2007, p. 35). This implies that when teaching physiotherapy in palliative care **case studies** need to be included. They are the narratives that give the facts meaning, make them interesting and in turn they are learned and retained by students.

Attention, emotion and motivation likewise contribute towards successful study. The role of the teacher in this context should not be underestimated. He draws attention to what needs to be learned, and also influences the emotions by creating a positive study environment. *'Another point (…) on motivation: the teacher's personality is the strongest medium!'* (Spitzer 2007, p. 194). Anyone truly inspired by physiotherapy in palliative care will also be a good teacher and motivator.

Content of the teaching course

Cognitive study objectives

In the cognitive domain it is important to achieve clarity by defining relevant terms such as 'palliative medicine', 'palliative care', 'palliative care unit', 'hospice', etc. The student should be aware of the patient's established diagnoses since he will be seeing the patient regularly outside the palliative care unit or hospice. The objective of physiotherapy in palliative care is to relieve and control symptoms. The students learn to identify both curable and incurable symptoms which can nevertheless be influenced by physiotherapy. The measures for treating the symptoms are identified and discussed. The students will already be familiar with a number of the options from other lessons; a few may be new to them and should also be practised. Pain and breathlessness are symptoms that can be particularly distressing to patients and should be prioritised if there is a lack of resources and not all symptoms can be addressed in full.

The physiotherapy process

In the treatment of palliative care patients, the physiotherapy process is not so very different from that in other disciplines, but there are a certain distinctions (➤ Chapter 2.1). It can/should be orientated to the **ICF model,** with **implementation of the measures in an equally balanced, multiprofessional team.** It is essential to impress upon students that the condition of the patient and therefore the goals can change very rapidly, that this is a 'normal' process and that flexibility is therefore required. It is also important to stress, therefore, that the anticipated deterioration of the disease is no reason for doubting the importance of physiotherapy during the final stages of life. One student describes how she found it difficult to put such an experience into context: *'During the course I had a constant feeling of euphoria and positive vibes, only to then feel down, or alarmed. I find talking about life-threatening illnesses ominous, am sometimes shocked and consequently become anxious. Yet at the same time, seeing what can be done for these patients makes me happy.'*

Physiotherapy goals

It is crucial to convey to students that **objectives on a participatory level** are extremely important to palliative care patients. In patients with lymphoedema of the face and neck, possibly accompanied by a lymphatic fistula, it is not important to reduce the size of the fistula but rather to ensure that the patient's eyes are as wide open as possible after therapy so that they can see their children and grandchildren when they visit. The same value is placed on prompt provision of a wheelchair if the strength in the legs is waning and the risk of falling has increased as a result of sensory disorders. **In palliative medicine, rehabilitation means facilitating participation** – albeit to a lesser extent, perhaps, and without being able to restore functionality completely.

Affective study objectives

In order to agree on such therapeutic goals with the patient and deal with challenging situations, the student must master the skills of **communication, patience, responsibility,** etc. These affective qualities, which enable the physiotherapist to offer the seriously ill patient professional support with an appropriate attitude and approach,

must be learned. At most they can only be introduced during the course of study, e. g. with communication exercises or the teacher explaining 'approaches' in his role as model and mentor. *'To achieve a professional understanding of the quality of the training, it will never suffice to depend on the fact, or refer to the fact that such attitudes and approaches are "somehow" or even "spontaneously" engendered in practice'* (Schewior-Popp 2005, p. 61).

Dealing with the needs of patients for **autonomy and/or therapeutic contact** and the question whether **hands-on or hand-off techniques** are to be applied, are an important part of the teaching course. Time and space should also be dedicated to the subject of 'dying and death'.

Psychomotor study objectives

Psychomotor study objectives can be accomplished, for example, by learning how to stimulate the vestibular system or how to use transfer techniques in seriously ill and pain-troubled patients. The students initially practise such techniques on each other after they have been demonstrated by the teacher. The highest level of naturalisation – i. e. applying the technique in a real situation and on a real patient – can only be facilitated by a real-life work placement (Schewior-Popp 2005).

Methodological implementation (➤ Table 1.2)

Questioning students at the start about their **expectations** and also their **fears or anxieties** concerning the teaching course has proven to be of value. This can be done either by asking students to shout out ideas to be written on a flipchart, or by circulating comment cards. Whichever the method, the results will remain visible on the flipchart or pinboard for all to see until the end of the training course. This procedure provides the teacher with the opportunity to identify the needs in advance and avoid disappointment. Experienced lecturers will set their goals once such a survey has been completed, and can incorporate further topics as the course progresses. Nevertheless, the clear objective must be **first and foremost to broaden one's physiotherapy skills.** Experience has also shown that personal and very private accounts and experiences provided by individual students can, in certain circumstances, be quite overwhelming. Hence the teacher must demonstrate empathy, but for didactic reasons keep it to a minimum.

During the part of the lesson in which dying and death are addressed and students are confronted on a personal level, a more intimate and comfortable setting proves beneficial, e. g. sitting in a circle. Dealing with the

Table 1.2 Proposed methodological structure

Teaching content	Method
Getting started	Reading a text (e. g.: How does a palliative care patient think he is perceived by medical staff?)
Conveying knowledge (terms, definitions, symptoms, measures, …)	Visual presentation (Power Point)
Physiotherapy process	Case studies
Interdisciplinary teamwork	Case studies
Patient needs Attitude towards the patient	Studying audiovisual accounts of actual patient experiences Explore hospice websites for audio/video user feedback
Hands on? – Hands off?	Discussion, case studies
Physiotherapy techniques	Practical exercises
Dying and death	Reading a text (e. g.: Physiotherapist and dying patient) Tranquillity and confrontation with the text through painting, reflecting, … Group discussion of the text and what it invokes (chaired by teacher) Closing text (to brighten and lift the mood) and/or feedback

topic on the one hand provides an opportunity (mostly one-off) to talk about situations during the lesson that have already occurred during the practical placement (death of a patient, treating the seriously ill, reactions of the family or clinical educator to the patient's death). On the other hand, anxieties and perceptions can be expressed if such events have not yet been encountered. This part of the lesson can and should by no means replace or veer in the direction of a specialised seminar on death and dying. Shock and perhaps even tears must be expected, however.

A positive and forward-looking text mostly works well as a means of **closing the subject.** It will break the possibly gloomy mood and allow the session to end on a positive note. This is an aspect which has been confirmed by a student in his reflections on the teaching course: *'I have read "A Life after Birth" to my family. This text gives me a great deal of positive energy.'*

Visiting a palliative care unit or hospice

If possible, students should be given the opportunity to accompany the lecturer on a visit to a hospice or palliative care unit. To experience first hand how a patient is

cared for by a team will round off the positive impression left by the teaching course. *'The visit to the hospice was the perfect ending to the course for me. Talking with the doctor, physiotherapist, nurse and director of the hospice made it immediately clear how they have a completely different attitude towards their work.'*

Practical placement

Whether the practical training is optional or compulsory and involves a practical placement at a specific palliative care institution or clinical unit (internal medicine, geriatrics, neurology, paediatrics, etc.), where often there are also, 'surprisingly', palliative care patients, students should be offered the opportunity of **interprofessional learning** (Morris/Leonard 2007). In such a way they can improve their understanding of their own role within the palliative care team: "All members of the team feel they are equal – and this also applies to the physiotherapy student." They will see themselves developing a flexible approach and must individually adapt their interaction with each patient – as described by the following student in his placement report: *'A palliative care unit demands every skill you have learned so far, pushing you to the limit.'* The team members generally support the students in their learning as part of their practical placement (Morris/Leonard 2007). The student also confirms this in his own words: *'It's the ideal place in which to learn.'*

If no team exists, then the student and mentor are faced with a different challenge. On acute care units communication is often restricted to a minimum, meaning that important information is often missed or received too late by the physiotherapist. So how does a placement work in such a situation?

Ideally, and so as not to strain the student inordinately, an **honest and realistic account of the patient's condition is provided prior to initial contact.** The student is present during therapy and with the consent of the patient will become involved in the therapy as quickly as possible. He will hear about any changes in the patient's condition and whether the terminal or final phase has been reached, and will decide whether he wishes to continue working with the patient. The **clinical educator** will always act as a **motivator and 'confidant'.**

There will be situations, however, in which the unexpected may occur. Here is an example: A physiotherapist enters the room of a patient who he has been treating for several days, accompanied by a student who has not yet met the patient. The therapist was not informed that the patient had reached the final phase, and when asking the patient how he is he receives the simple reply, "terrible." How should the therapist react in such a case, on entering the room with the student and discovering that the patient has reached his terminal phase? If he believes his student to be strong enough, he will adjust the therapy to the patient's condition and then discuss the situation with the student afterwards. If the student has hitherto given the impression of being stressed by difficult situations, it would probably be better to take the student out of the room and then return to the patient. What is important in such a case is to communicate with the patient before, during and after therapy and talk the situation through with the student.

During the practical placement the student experiences the complexity of the physiotherapeutic situation involving the palliative care patient. He also experiences how patients and their families rate the physiotherapy and the therapist's personality: '*I'm very impressed at what my husband can manage with your support. And talking with you is always a tremendous help to him.*' The student therefore learns a great deal at different levels.

Motivation for working in palliative care

'*Since the course I have often wondered whether I can imagine myself working in palliative care. (…) I've found that I really like the idea behind palliative care.*'

If the experiences gained by the student during the course and placement are positive and appreciated, he will also be motivated to try working in this field himself if he feels up to the task: '*I joined the course with the feeling that I am not made for this type of work, and still felt the same at the end. I've taken a lot from it and it has also made me think a lot.*'

Well-designed teaching courses during basic training, enthusiastic teachers and professional clinical educators, make a crucial contribution to such decisions.

REFERENCES

Katamay A. Das Thema Tod und Sterben in der Physiotherapie. Wie gehen Studenten damit um? Diplomarbeit, Akademie für Physiotherapie, Wels, 2003.

Kumar SP, Jim A, Sisodia V. Effects of palliative care training program on knowledge, attitudes, beliefs and experiences among student physiotherapists: A preliminary quasi-experimental study. Indian J Palliat Care 2011;17(1):47–53.

Morris J, Leonard R. Physiotherapy students' experiences of palliative care placements – promoting interprofessional learning and patient-centred approaches. J Interprofessional Care 2007;21(5):569–571.

Schewior-Popp S. Lernsituationen planen und gestalten. Handlungsorientierter Unterricht im Lernfeldkontext. Stuttgart–New York: Thieme, 2005.

Spitzer M. Lernen. Gehirnforschung und die Schule des Lebens. Munich: Elsevier Spektrum Akademischer Verlag, 2007.

2.1 Clinical reasoning

Bronwen Hewitt

Clinical reasoning has been described as *'the complex process undertaken by clinicians to ensure that patients receive both timely and appropriate treatment'* (Wainwright/McGinnis 2009). At its simplest, the clinical reasoning process involves the collation of information by a clinician that then enables him or her to make informed decisions regarding patient care. However, the complexity associated with this process becomes apparent when the different factors that influence the clinical reasoning process are considered. For instance, consider the range of potential information sources available to the clinician. Information may be obtained from the:

- patients' medical records (Childs/Cleland 2006);
- results of diagnostic tests (May et al. 2008);
- theoretical knowledge gained by clinicians during their training and subsequent work experience (Ahmed/Farnie/Dyer 2011; Vogel et al. 2009);
- patients and their family/carers (Ott 2010).

The challenge for the clinician is to determine how best to utilize this diverse range of information in the clinical reasoning process. It is not surprising that the process of clinical reasoning is now considered an essential skill for all clinicians (Ajjawi/Higgs 2008). Furthermore it has also been acknowledged that clinical reasoning is a skill that continues to develop throughout a clinician's professional career (Atkinson/Nixon-Cave 2011; Wainwright/McGinnis 2009; Wainwright et al. 2010).

2.1.1 Clinical reasoning in physiotherapy

Since the 1990s there has been a growing emphasis on the process of clinical reasoning within the physiotherapy profession. This has coincided with the rise in professional autonomy and, subsequently, the accountability of the profession worldwide (Edwards et al. 2004; Wainwright et al. 2010). To date researchers have focused on three aspects of clinical reasoning in physiotherapy. Specifically these are:

- examination of what strategies physiotherapists utilize in the clinical reasoning process (Edwards et al. 2004);
- exploration of the factors that influence the clinical reasoning process in physiotherapy (Smith/Higgs/Ellis 2007);
- examination of how the skill of clinical reasoning is taught and developed within the physiotherapy profession (Ajjawi/Higgs 2008).

From this research it has been established that physiotherapists use a range of different processes to determine a management plan for their patients. **These processes range from the structured hypothetico-deductive reasoning process through to pattern recognition, the use of narrative, collective reasoning and reflection.** A wide range of factors has been identified as influencing the clinical reasoning processes of physiotherapists (➤ Figure 2.1). These include:

- length of time the therapist has been practising (Wainwright et al. 2010; Smith/Higgs/Ellis 2010);
- clinical area in which they work (Greenfield et al. 2008);
- level of collegiate support received (Atkinson/Nixon-Cave 2011, Wainwright/McGinnis 2009);
- individual beliefs held (Wainwright et al. 2011);
- access to and utilization of research literature (Grimmer-Somers et al. 2007);
- the social and political climate within which practice takes place (Edwards/Richardson 2008; Finch et al. 2004).

Researchers have established that it is possible to teach clinical reasoning skills to student physiotherapists (Vogel et al. 2009). However, it has been identified that further work needs to be undertaken to ensure that this necessary skill is then fostered and developed throughout a physiotherapist's career (Ajjawi/Higgs 2008).

2.1.2 Clinical reasoning in physiotherapy in palliative care

Studies have shown that the clinical area in which physiotherapists work shapes, in part, their clinical reasoning process (Greenfield et al. 2008). Specifically, it influences how the therapists obtain relevant clinical information as well as how this information is used to develop management plans for individual patients. There are also other factors – unique to the specific clinical area – that impact on the clinical reasoning process for all clinicians (medical, nursing and allied health) involved. So, when considering the clinical area of end of life/palliative care it is important to identify these influencing factors. Unfortunately, to date, studies have not specifically examined the clinical reasoning process of physiotherapists working in palliative care. Finch et al. (2005) have identified that **physiotherapists experience decision-making regarding end of life care as ethically challenging;** however, this appears to be the extent of the research into this area.

The clinical reasoning process of palliative care clinicians in general however has come under increasing

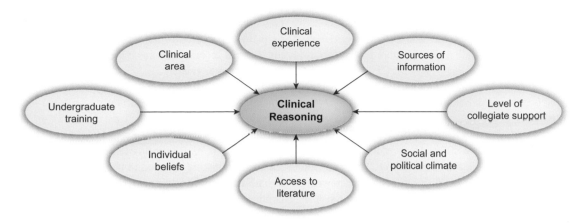

Figure 2.1 Factors influencing the clinical reasoning process [M542/L157]

scrutiny. This has occurred as decisions regarding end of life care – particularly the withdrawing and withholding of treatment – have been debated in both the academic literature and the world media (Mahon 2010a; Olsen/ Swetz/Mueller 2010). As a result, attention has focused on the unique factors in this specialist field that have an impact upon the clinical reasoning of clinicians. To date researchers have examined:

- the relevance of prognostication (Johanson 2009; Murray et al. 2005);
- the importance of involving patients and families (Eliot/Olver 2010; Lee/Kristjanson/Williams 2009; Philip et al. 2009);
- the role of the interdisciplinary team (Mahon 2010b; Ott 2010);
- the role of communication in the clinical reasoning process (Emanuel/Scandrett 2010; Young et al. 2006; Waterworth/Gott 2010).

This chapter explores the clinical reasoning process of physiotherapists working in palliative care. It combines the processes identified as contributing to clinical reasoning of physiotherapists in general with those identified as unique to this clinical context. It is of course impossible to provide a prescription for the clinical reasoning process for each of the multitude of clinical presentations that a physiotherapist could experience working in this area. Instead, utilizing the two case scenarios below, some of the considerations required by a physiotherapist both in **assessment** and in **treatment planning and implementation** are presented. Other areas requiring special consideration – namely, the involvement of patients and their families, the role of hope, goal setting (explored in detail below) and the need for flexibility throughout the clinical reasoning process – are also discussed.

Assessment

The assessment process serves two main purposes for the physiotherapist working in palliative care. The first, and perhaps the most obvious, is to provide the therapist with the information necessary to devise appropriate treatment plans. The second purpose, which is often overlooked, is to engage the physiotherapist with the patient and their family. **It is in these initial interactions that rapport is established and the context of physiotherapy input is defined** (Wainwright et al. 2010). The success of these interactions can also impact on the 'shared decision making process', which is identified as being instrumental to the success of a palliative care approach (Young et al. 2006).

In this section, three aspects of assessment are considered. These are:

- initial assessment;
- re-assessment;
- specialist assessments.

The following discussion alerts readers to the range of considerations that physiotherapists are required to make when working in palliative care.

Initial assessment

Conventionally an initial assessment for physiotherapy consists of a subjective and an objective assessment. The subjective assessment includes information regarding:

- the patient's medical history;
- lifestyle or home situation;
- the patient's emotions, attitudes and goals;
- response to treatment to date;
- any other information relevant to the patient's care or present condition.

In the objective assessment, measurements or observations are made to supplement the information obtained in the subjective assessment. It is from this initial assessment that a physiotherapy treatment plan is formulated.

In palliative care how the initial assessment is conducted is influenced by a number of factors.

Why is the assessment being conducted?

This consideration will dictate what information is collected in both the subjective and objective parts of the assessment. In order to establish why a physiotherapy assessment has either been requested or is required **it is necessary to first understand why the patient has been referred** specifically to palliative care. As the scope of palliative care has expanded over the last few years, patients have been referred to its services much earlier in their disease trajectories. It is therefore remiss to assume that a patient has only been referred to a palliative care service for end of life or terminal care. Before conducting an initial assessment **it is imperative that the physiotherapist understands the stage of the patient's disease as well as taking into consideration current treatment plans.** For instance, consider the following two cases which will guide us through the course of this chapter.

CASE STUDY
Mr A.

Mr A. is a 46-year-old man referred to a community-based physiotherapy programme for 'rehabilitation' following the resection of a large glioblastoma multiforme (Grade 4 astrocytoma) from the right side of his brain. He has limited movement in both his left arm and leg. He has been very drowsy since the surgery, waking for brief periods of time during the day. Married with three small children, his parents and older sister are also heavily involved in his care.

CASE STUDY
Mrs B.

Mrs B. is a 70-year-old woman transferred from an acute hospital to the hospice for 'end-of-life care'. She has end stage heart failure and is at the limit of her therapy. She becomes very short of breath on minimal exertion and has requested that her diuretic medication be reduced as she finds getting to the toilet difficult and is reluctant to use an indwelling catheter. She has stated to her elderly sister that she is 'ready to die'.

In the first case, Mr A. has been referred for a period of post-operative rehabilitation. In this situation the physiotherapist will need to clarify if any further medical treatment – such as palliative radiotherapy or corticosteroid use – is planned. In the second case, whether Mrs B.'s request to reduce her diuretic has been acted upon or not may clarify the overall plan for her care. In both situations the importance for the physiotherapist in identifying the goal of care and ongoing medical management for the patient is evident.

The timing of the initial assessment

This can relate not only to the time of day but also the timing within a particular episode of care. For instance, for Mrs B., attempting to conduct an initial assessment following a period of physical exertion, such as bathing, would be pointless. Similarly, attempting to conduct an initial assessment with Mr A. whilst he is drowsy would also be counterproductive. In both situations, liaison with the patient's family and carers would assist the physiotherapist in establishing an appropriate time to assess the patient. Given the physical condition of both patients, conducting the initial assessment over a number of short sessions could provide more useful information for the physiotherapist. Consideration of when to conduct an assessment during the episode of care is also important. This is often harder to establish and can be dependent on the patient's location of care and/or availability of physiotherapy staff.

Patient and family insight and reactions

Physiotherapists working with patients at end of life have on occasion experienced a mixed reception from patients and their families and carers when attempting to conduct an initial assessment. This can occur due to circumstances that are out of the physiotherapist's control. For instance, it may reflect both the patients' and their family and carers' preconceived ideas of the role of physiotherapy in their current situation. It may also reflect their own fears and, with regard to families and carers, represents their need to protect the patient. These thoughts and feelings can manifest in a number of different ways. In some situations patients may appear withdrawn or may flatly refuse to participate in the assessment process. In others, patients or their families and carers may appear apprehensive of the assessment process and react in a defensive or even hostile manner. Alternatively, some patients and families can appear to attach a disproportionate emphasis on physiotherapy input. In this situation, patients and their families can present as demanding, appear to want to direct or control the physiotherapy assessment or be overly helpful, masking the patient's true condition. **It is important that the physiotherapist recognizes the impact that such thoughts and feelings can have on the assessment process** and identify whether

2

their assessment is being affected by such thoughts or feelings. This may not be obvious at first, and often the signs can be quite subtle. However, unless these feelings and thoughts are addressed, by either the physiotherapist or the team, the assessment process will be flawed.

Physiotherapist attitude and approach

A mixed reaction to an initial assessment can also arise as a result of how the physiotherapist attempts to conduct the assessment. Factors that can influence how a physiotherapist is perceived by the patient and their family and carers include:

- language used by the therapist;
- the therapist's body language;
- any perceived gaps in the therapist's knowledge;
- timing of the assessment.

Care needs to be taken by the physiotherapist to ensure that the patient and their family and carers are comfortable with the assessment process. This will facilitate their participation in the assessment and will potentially provide the physiotherapist with a valuable source of information.

Application of outcome measures

One of the ongoing challenges for physiotherapists working in palliative care is establishing which outcome measures to use as part of the objective assessment of a patient. The clue to determining this is often obtained in the subjective component of the assessment. That is, what does the patient identify as being important to him or her?

CASE STUDY
Mrs B.

Mrs B., for instance, may comment that she wishes to be able to get to the bathroom herself. Therefore, appropriate objective measures for this patient could be the height of the surface from which the patient can stand independently or the distance she can walk. The importance is not necessarily *what* is measured, but *why* it is measured.

⚠ CAUTION

- Adherence to your professional code of conduct is paramount.
- 'No pain, no gain' has no place in palliative care.
- Never assume: always check your facts.
- Patient safety is the ultimate goal.
- Differences of opinion do not necessarily mean that someone is 'wrong'.

Goal setting
Gail Eva

Goal setting is widely recognized as an essential component of rehabilitation. It can be defined as a process of negotiation and discussion in which a patient and health professional(s) decide on the key priorities for the patient and agree on how to work together to accomplish one or more desired objectives within a specified time frame. It is often, however, not a simple and straightforward process, as the literature on goal setting clearly demonstrates (Playford et al. 2009; Wade 2009). In order for goal setting in palliative care rehabilitation to be effective in therapy and useful to patients, we need to take account of a number of issues:
- Why are we setting goals?
- How do we set goals?
- Do goals need to be realistic and achievable?

The purpose of goal setting

Setting goals helps us to accomplish a wide range of things. We can use goal setting both to guide the process of rehabilitation and to assess outcomes. It enables us to:

- understand what is meaningful and important to patients;
- establish shared priorities for how to proceed in rehabilitation;
- assess progress and refine rehabilitation strategies;
- measure outcomes (by evaluating whether a goal is achieved or not achieved);
- motivate patients;
- motivate teams;
- structure and coordinate team activities, identifying otherwise overlooked tasks and actions;
- communicate and promote rehabilitation.

The process of setting goals

In identifying goals with patients, we need to recognize that, **for many people, goal setting is not a natural part of everyday life.** Patients might have difficulty articulating goals, particularly in a palliative care context where the future is often uncertain. Rather than asking patients outright what they want to achieve, it can be useful to take a more indirect approach, asking, for example:

- What are the things you would like to be able to do?
- What kinds of activities have you enjoyed doing in the past?
- What are the things that you need to do?
- Are there things that you particularly want to be able to manage on your own?
- What would you be happy to have help with?

When listening to the responses to these questions, we need to attend carefully to what the person is telling us about themselves and their lives. What is being communicated about things that are important and significant? What is the person saying about their sense of themselves? What can we understand about their hopes and expectations for the future? What do these activities represent to this person? It can be helpful to talk through some of the assumptions that patients make about what is possible and not possible, and what it is essential to do everyday. Having some help with routine tasks, for example, can mean that a person has more energy available to do something that is pleasurable rather than necessary. Where it is not possible for someone to continue to do something they enjoy – cooking a large and complex family meal – it might be possible to find an alternative that has similar significance, such as participating in family activities by baking a cake with a grandchild.

Realistic and achievable goals

Does it matter whether the goals that patients set are realistic and achievable? To answer this question we need to understand two things: the basic paradox at the heart of palliative care rehabilitation, and the difference between a hope and a goal.

A paradox: affirming life while preparing for death   Rehabilitation aims to enhance a person's independence, his or her sense of self-worth and self-efficacy, and his or her ability to participate in society. However, the reality of life-limiting illness is that patients lose function, become more and more reliant on help from others, and they die. The process of goal-setting needs to manage this tension: supporting and affirming joy and pleasure in everyday life, while at the same time, acknowledging and preparing for death (Bye 1998).

Hopes and goals   A goal is clear and specific; it is something that a person has control over, and can work toward achieving; for example, *'Today I'm going to plant some herbs in pots on my kitchen windowsill.'* A hope, by contrast, is something that a person would like, that they do not have complete control over: *'I'd like to be able to go for long walks in the country again,'* or *'I'm looking forward to spending Christmas with my children.'* Hopes can keep alive a sense of optimism, and a perception of oneself as active and sociable, even as the actual activities become more and more difficult.

Case study Goal setting: An illustrative case example
Gail Eva and Ian H.

Ian is a 64-year-old self-employed engineer/inventor. He has advanced bowel cancer with bone secondaries and spinal cord compression. He struggles to walk with a walking frame, and is increasingly reliant on a wheelchair for moving around. Here, he is talking about the things that make life meaningful for him:
'I've had to give up my vegetable garden, which is sad – that was a good break, the winter digging, proper hard work. But now I can't stand and move without a frame. I mean, I could hold on to a fork to steady myself ... but then I wouldn't be able to dig, would I? But I have a few ambitions that I am determined that I will achieve. And the first one – and for me this is the essence of being independent – is to go and hit a golf ball. Proper swing, unaided, followed by a hole.'
On the one hand, Ian understands the practical limitations of his illness: he can't manage his vegetable garden any longer; he does not have enough balance to be able to dig. But this does not stop him from holding on to the idea that, at some point in the future, it will be possible for him to engage in another favourite activity – even though the physical ability required for playing golf exceeds his current capacities by some distance, and he knows and accepts that he has a deteriorating illness. The idea that it could be possible is comforting, and having this aspiration for the future enables him to keep in touch with a sense of himself as a sociable person, as a golfer, and as someone who is active and skilful. **We can see this hope as being connected with positive self-identity, and having little to do with actual achievements.**
However, Ian goes on to describe his intentions for the near future, outlining some very practical plans for an activity that raises concerns about his – and others' – safety: *'My wife and I have always been great caravanners. I realize I won't be able to manage a caravan any more because it's just too heavy to manoeuvre, so I've just bought a second-hand camper van. A couple of friends are helping me to organize some modifications for it, like power steering, and I'm going to put one of those knobs on the steering wheel, like the old*

truck drivers used to have. We'll be able to go away for weekends again.'

This presents a problem: how can we support Ian's enthusiasm, motivation and optimism in a way that is realistic and ensures that he does not do anything reckless? **The first step is to listen to what he is telling us about himself, and about the things that are important and significant to him.** He likes to be active, he enjoys camping and the outdoors, he has helpful friends, and spending time with his wife matters to him. Next, we could discuss ways of matching up his current abilities with an activity or outing that would be satisfying and fulfilling. We could encourage him to start with something enjoyable, but less ambitious: could his wife or a friend drive the camper van to somewhere scenic and local, for a picnic? Ian's goal might be expressed as the wish to have a trip out with his wife in his camper van; therapy goals might include his ability to manage a wheelchair over uneven ground, to get in and out of the van, and to plan his day allowing for rests so that he is able to cope with his fatigue.

Summary

In summary, goal setting can be a valuable part of the rehabilitation process if therapists are able to manage the tension between affirming life and preparing for death. **Goals, by definition, are realistic and achievable. Hopes and dreams need not be. Both are necessary.**

Re-assessment

It is generally recognized that the assessment process is an ongoing one. This ensures that any changes in a patient's condition are identified and that appropriate modifications are made to the physiotherapy treatment plan.

Timing

Careful consideration needs to be given to when this re-assessment occurs as well as what it includes. Neither of these components is easily addressed, especially in this field. Palliative care comprises a patient population in which certain changes can occur quite quickly, and the physiotherapist needs to be proactive to ensure re-assessments are carried out promptly, as and when indicated, to optimize outcomes.

Deteriorating clinical condition

Consider Mrs B. from the second case study.

CASE STUDY
Mrs B.

It is expected that Mrs B.'s condition will deteriorate following the withdrawal of her diuretic medication. In this situation, the physiotherapist needs to monitor closely how this deterioration impacts on her mobility and then revise the treatment plan appropriately. As she is a hospice inpatient, the physiotherapist must liaise with the rest of the staff caring for Mrs B. to ensure not only her safety, but also that of those providing her care.

Change of environment

Another change that can occur quite suddenly is the location of patient care. Faced with a limited prognosis, some family and carers elect to move a patient from an inpatient facility to their home to die. In this case, time is of the essence. In an ideal situation, the option of the patient dying at home would have already been explored with the patient, his or her family and carers as well any formal community care providers. However, this is often not the case and arrangements have to be made quickly. In this situation, the physiotherapist, in conjunction with other team members, will need to consider a number of factors. These include:

- the patient's current level of function;
- the family and carers' capacity to provide hands-on care;
- what equipment is required to ensure patient safety;
- what education the family and carers require to provide appropriate physical care at home.

In both situations above, major responsibility is placed on the physiotherapist to recognize the changing needs of their patients. This is not only as a result of re-assessment of the patient, but possibly more importantly, recognizing when re-assessment needs to occur.

Ongoing review management

Clues to the timing of re-assessment can be found in the patient's underlying diagnosis, the rate of disease progression, changes in medical management and information gleaned through conversations with other team members. Unfortunately the timing of re-assessment is often dictated by the availability of resources; however, it is possible for the physiotherapist to develop strategies with the rest of the team to flag when an urgent re-assessment is required.

Specialist assessment

Physiotherapists working in palliative care have developed a unique range of skills. It is with these skills that they are able to conduct assessments and construct treatment plans that are both sensitive to, and appropriate for, the needs of their patients. Specifically, these skills include the:

- ability to utilize and modify a range of assessment techniques and treatment modalities;
- ability to quickly recognize changes and emergencies in patient condition or circumstances;
- flexibility to respond to a variety of different situations;
- ability to work within a team;
- ability to communicate effectively in a range of different situations.

Simply put, these skills reflect the sensitivity, adaptability and resourcefulness needed to work in this clinical area. Fortunately, due to growing recognition of these specialist skills, palliative care physiotherapists are slowly being utilized more frequently not only within palliative care teams but these transferable skills are being increasingly demanded outside the field.

There are increasing incidences where physiotherapists in other specialist areas are requesting assistance in the management of their patients. Typically this occurs in regards to a specific symptom or disease process, such as lymphoedema (addressed in depth in ➤ Chapter 2.5). However, palliative care physiotherapists can also be consulted by their colleagues for advice on how to approach a difficult situation or to help in understanding the reactions of a patient or their family to a particular treatment approach. This cross referral process within the profession not only assists in patient care, but can also cultivate ongoing professional development.

Palliative care emergencies
Rebecca Jennings

At every assessment, whatever the context or purpose as outlined previously, the physiotherapist must always be aware of potential palliative care emergencies as shown in ➤ Table 2.1.

Treatment planning and implementation
Bronwen Hewitt

The information gained by a physiotherapist through assessment is instrumental in forming a comprehensive

Table 2.1 Palliative care emergencies most relevant to physiotherapists

Emergency	Definition	Signs and symptoms	Treatment
Malignant spinal cord compression (➤ Chapter 2.2)	Neurological complication of advanced cancer caused by an epidural compression of the spinal cord from a tumour or a bony fragment from the collapsed vertebra affected by metastasis. Common in tumours that metastasize to the spinal cord: breast and lung cancer, followed by lymphoma, myeloma, prostate cancer and sarcoma. (Rajer/Kovac 2008)	Spinal pain; muscle weakness; autonomic dysfunction.	Diagnostic confirmation by magnetic resonance imaging (MRI); high dose steroids; radiotherapy; surgery; support and education. (Rosser 2007b)
Superior vena cava obstruction	Compression of the superior vena cava by malignancies that obstruct venous drainage. Common complication of lung cancer and less frequently lymphoma. (Wilson et al. 2007)	Oedema of head, neck and arms; distension of subcutaneous vessels; cyanosis; cough/stridor; dyspnoea.	Radiotherapy/chemotherapy to treat underlying disease; supportive care including positioning. (Rosser 2007b)
Hypercalcaemia	Metabolic disorder associated with cancer caused by release of calcium from bones to increase serum calcium levels (bone metastases are a common feature but not always present). (Rosser 2007a)	Fatigue; anorexia; nausea; vomiting; confusion; decreased consciousness	Aim to correct serum calcium levels; rehydration (oral and IV fluids); bisphosphonate infusion. (Rosser 2007b)
Pulmonary embolism	Consequence of thrombus formation in distal veins which embolizes to the pulmonary vasculature where it occludes blood supply to the lung; depending on size of occlusion can be life threatening (British Medical Journal 2011)	Rapid onset dyspnoea +/– pleuritic chest pain +/– haemoptysis.	Oxygen; anticoagulation. (British Thoracic Society Standards of Care Committee Pulmonary Embolism Guideline Development Group 2003)

treatment plan for a patient. However, there are a number of additional factors to consider when planning and implementing these physiotherapy treatment programmes for a palliative patient. Factors range from the academic to the practical. For instance, it is important that the treatment programme is safe, effective and evidence based. However, it is also important that the treatment programme is achievable for the patient, as well as appropriate for the stage of their disease and goals of care.

✓ GUIDANCE

- Allow adequate time for assessment and treatment.
- Utilize the knowledge, experience and different perspectives of your team and colleagues.
- Establish the focus of the intervention: What is the purpose?
- Be creative: You are limited only by your own imagination.

Other factors to consider include:

- the availability of resources, such as personnel and equipment;
- the treatment environment itself: the hospital/hospice versus a patient's home;
- the timing, frequency and duration of treatment sessions, especially as related to a patient's symptoms;
- the involvement of other team members, for instance in joint treatment sessions;
- the flexibility of the therapist to adjust the treatment plan to accommodate for fluctuations in the patient's condition;
- the expectations of the patient's family and care providers.

The impact that the above factors have on the treatment planning and implementation process can be illustrated through reference to the above introduced case studies.

CASE STUDY
Mr A.

Initial assessment   It is clearly apparent that the astrocytoma patient introduced above wishes to regain his function as quickly as possible. However, assessment by the physiotherapist reveals that although Mr A. is able to move his left arm and leg actively, he is extremely weak and requires assistance with all functional tasks. In particular, transfers are problematic as he is experiencing falls a number of times when attempting to stand up. The physiotherapist observes evidence of spatial neglect as Mr A. requires prompting to attend to the left hand side of his body. He is observed to tire quickly, falling asleep during the assessment. Also the physiotherapist notes that he is rarely left alone, with at least one member of the family present at all times. The physiotherapist watches the different reactions of the family members to Mr A.'s current condition. Specifically, it is noted which family members encourage Mr A.'s desire for independence and which inadvertently impede or undermine his wishes.

Treatment plan   From this initial assessment, a reasonable and realistic treatment plan consists of a weekly session with the physiotherapist and a daily home exercise programme facilitated by the family. The physiotherapist negotiates with Mr A. and his family to limit the practice of transfers and gait retraining to the weekly physiotherapy sessions until his safety has improved. The daily home exercise programme consists of a number of exercises focused on improving strength, function and spatial awareness. Given the patient's wish to spend time with his children, a series of exercises are developed that involve them in the 'rehabilitation' process.

Education   Care must be taken to explain to the family:
- the best times of day to conduct the exercise sessions;
- the number of times each exercise should be repeated;
- appropriate manual strategies for the family and the patient;
- any warning signs that the programme may need to be modified or ceased.

Realistically, this form of multifaceted treatment plan can be successfully implemented with palliative patients across a range of clinical settings.

Reviewing the patient   A re-assessment process will enable the physiotherapist to adjust the treatment plan appropriately to account for any changes in the patient's condition. For instance, in Mr A.'s case, after a number of weeks the physiotherapist notices that he is more alert and able to tolerate longer and more intense therapy sessions. However he is now reporting pain in his left shoulder and requires increased analgesia to manage this pain. After some careful questioning the physiotherapist discovers that Mr A., together with his father, who is frustrated with the perceived slowness of the patient's improvement, have added a series of exercises to the home exercise programme that they have obtained from the internet. In this situation, it may be appropriate for the physiotherapist to suggest that a meeting be convened with the patient, his family and the palliative care team to discuss the patient's progress and further options of treatment.

CASE STUDY
Mrs B.: Complex challenges presented

Turning now to the case of Mrs B., the physiotherapist is faced with an entirely different set of challenges. A treatment plan has been developed, based on the assessment of Mrs B., and focusing on her stated wish to get to the bathroom herself. However the physiotherapist enters the patient's room and is greeted by Mrs B.'s extremely angry sister. It eventually becomes apparent that the sister is frustrated that the physiotherapist appears to be, in her words, *'wearing my sister out'* and ignoring her expressed readiness to die. In this volatile situation the physiotherapist may choose to abandon plans for this particular treatment session and attempt to calmly discuss the treatment plan with the patient and her sister. This discussion might reveal that the patient is providing different pieces of information to the physiotherapist from her sister. Based on this discovery the physiotherapist modifies the initial treatment plan. Alternatively, the discussion may reveal that Mrs B.'s sister is struggling with the patient's decision to limit her diuretic medication. **In this situation, physiotherapy treatment is not the central issue, but rather the sister**'s anticipatory grief is the focus. It could be deduced that Mrs B.'s sister's perspective of the physiotherapy treatment plan may improve if she herself receives appropriate psychosocial support.

Further considerations

There are a number of different factors that impact upon the complexity of the clinical reasoning process of a physiotherapist working in palliative care. Apart from the factors that have already been discussed, there are three additional areas that require special consideration by physiotherapists. These are the:

- facilitation of patient and family/carer involvement in decision making;
- acknowledgement of the role of hope in treatment planning;
- need for flexibility throughout the clinical reasoning process.

Facilitation of patient and family/carer involvement

One of the striking features of palliative care is its ethos of involving patients and their families and carers in decisions surrounding patient care (see also ➤ Chapter 3). Palliative care is not merely something that is done to patients. Rather it is a philosophy of care (Simon 2009). In order **to ensure that these needs are met, the patient, their family and carers need to be engaged in the decision making process.** One of the ways in which a physiotherapist can ensure this is through effective communication. The importance of communication in the clinical reasoning process in the assessment and treatment planning and implementation phase has been illustrated in earlier sections of this chapter. **The involvement of patients, their families and carers in the clinical reasoning process can, of course, be fraught with difficulties and conflict** (Finch et al. 2005; Young et al. 2006); however, the overall benefit to patient care cannot be ignored.

For example, an area that can cause friction within families and the team is location of care. Studies have identified that the majority of patients would prefer to die in their own home (O'Brien/Jack 2010). However, as outlined previously in this chapter, there are a number of practicalities to be considered with this decision. It is not uncommon to find that there are marked differences

in opinion between patients, family members and carers as to location of care. These opinions can also fluctuate during the course of the patient's disease. In this situation, it is important to clarify the current care needs of the patient and from that whether there are appropriate resources available to provide this level of care. **Timely assessment as well as clear, open and frank communication is obviously essential in this process** (➤ Chapter 3.1).

✓ G U I D A N C E
- Self-care is important. Dedicate time for reflection and/or clinical supervision.
- The context of care needs to be considered in both the assessment and treatment planning process.
- **Patient advocacy is a vital aspect of the physiotherapy role.**

The role of hope

One of the dilemmas facing all clinicians working in palliative care is **striking the fine balance between maintaining hope and acknowledging the reality of the patient's situation** (Clayton et al. 2005). While it is important to be honest with a patient, it is also important to recognize that at times disease progression is unpredictable. **The accommodation of honesty, hope and unpredictability into a physiotherapist's clinical reasoning process is not as difficult as it sounds.** Rather it relies on the physiotherapist:

- keeping an open mind;
- exercising tact when confronted with a seemingly impossible request or outlandish question;
- listening to a patient's or family's wishes and incorporating these wishes into the patient's assessment and treatment plan;
- maintaining clear lines of communication with the patient, their family and carers and the rest of the treating team.

The most common situation where physiotherapists may find themselves juggling a patient's hope and their own clinical experience is when attempting to anticipate the outcome of a particular treatment plan.

For instance, consider a patient with metastatic lung cancer who develops compression of his spinal cord at the mid-level of their thoracic spine. Fortunately, the patient receives timely medical input for their cord compression and then subsequently receives encouraging news from both their neurologist and radiation oncologist in regards to his or her recovery. Currently, however, the patient is wheelchair bound and has been referred to physiotherapy to 'facilitate the recovery process'. In this situation, it would not be unexpected for the patient to ask the physiotherapist how quickly he would be walking again.

This question obviously places the physiotherapist in an awkward situation. How the physiotherapist chooses to answer this question can impact on the ongoing rapport with the patient and subsequently the success of the physiotherapy intervention. One approach may be for the physiotherapist to honestly state that he or she does not know when the patient will be walking again. As the ability to walk is obviously important to the patient, it will be a major goal for the physiotherapy sessions. **It is necessary for the physiotherapist to specifically outline, based on his or her assessment, how much recovery needs to occur to enable the patient to walk again.** In conjunction with this, the physiotherapist should ideally outline the specific techniques planned to facilitate the recovery process. In this way, the physiotherapist recognizes the patient's wishes and determines a strategic approach that maintains professional integrity without diminishing the patient's hope (see also 'Goal setting' above).

Flexibility

Throughout this chapter the need for flexibility in the clinical reasoning process has become apparent. From the physiotherapist's perspective this is manifest not only in how the assessment is conducted but also in how the treatment plan is constructed and implemented. However, a degree of flexibility is also required not only by the rest of the treatment team, but also by the patient, their family and carers.

In both case examples **flexibility may be required with regard to how the role of physiotherapy with patients at the end of their lives is perceived.** In some countries physiotherapists are still in the process of establishing themselves as integral members of a palliative care team. As a result physiotherapy input may not even be considered for a patient, or referrals may be made too late to be effective (➤ Chapter 1.4). Alternatively, treatment teams, the patient, their family and carers can become unrealistic in their expectations of physiotherapy. This can be either in their expectations of the outcome of physiotherapy or the frequency and duration of physiotherapy input. How flexibility is promoted is obviously dependent upon the individual situation in which physiotherapists find themselves. However, as identified throughout this chapter, clear communication is paramount. For a clinical example of how flexibility is employed, consider once more the example of Mr A. as introduced above.

CASE STUDY
Mr A.

Specifically, consider the situation where the father of **Mr A.** inadvertently injured his son's shoulder by implementing a series of exercises he obtained from the internet. Some physiotherapists may not have considered the possibility of Mr A.'s father adding his own exercises, so may not reason clinically that this is the source of his shoulder pain. Similarly, some physiotherapists may suggest that his father be discouraged from participating in his son's physiotherapy treatment. However, a more flexible approach to Mr A.'s care would recognize Mr A.'s father's need to be involved in his son's care as well as his resourcefulness in obtaining information. In this case the physiotherapist could provide additional education to his father with regard to his son's care, as well as directing him to more appropriate case-specific resources.

Advocacy for the profession and patient needs

There is a challenge for physiotherapists working in palliative care. Access to physiotherapy services by patients at the end of life sadly remains variable. This can reflect the availability of physiotherapy services to the population as a whole. However it can also reflect the attitude of the palliative care team itself to the role of physiotherapy in end of life care. It is therefore important to reinforce the fact that physiotherapists possess the knowledge and skills to assist patients to *'live as actively as possible until their death'* (WHO 2012). For instance, in both of Mr A.'s and Mrs B.'s cases, physiotherapy input is not only clearly indicated but can undeniably improve the patients' quality of life.

Not only do physiotherapists need to develop and refine the specific skills required to work in this challenging clinical area, but on occasion they need to be able to advocate for their involvement in patient care. Hopefully, as the importance of physiotherapists in end of life care of patients becomes more widely recognized, this advocacy will become less necessary.

2.1.3 Conclusion

This chapter has presented the clinical reasoning process in palliative care through the use of clinical case examples. It has also illustrated the broad range of different factors that a physiotherapist needs to consider when conducting an assessment or when planning and implementing a treatment strategy with a patient at the end of life. **What is apparent is that although the clinical reasoning process can at times be complex, it is not impossible.** If the physiotherapist is prepared to take the time to gather and integrate information from a range of different sources, listen to their patients, and be flexible in their approach then an assessment and treatment plan can be developed that is not only effective and appropriate for the patient but also professionally rewarding for the physiotherapist.

REFERENCES

Ahmed NN, Farnie M, Dyer CB. The effect of geriatric and palliative medicine education on the knowledge and attitudes of internal medicine residents. J Am Geriatr Soc 2011;59:143–147.

Ajjawi R, Higgs J. Learning to reason: a journey of professional socialisation. Adv Health Sci Educ Theory Pract 2008;13:133–150.

Atkinson HL, Nixon-Cave K. A tool for clinical reasoning and reflection using the International Classification of Functioning, Disability and Health (ICF) framework and patient management model. Phys Ther 2011;91:416–430.

British Medical Journal. Best Practice: Pulmonary embolism. 2011. Available at http://bestpractice.bmj.com/best-practice/monograph/116.html (last accessed June 2012). British Thoracic Society Standards of Care Committee Pulmonary Embolism Guideline Development Group. British Thoracic Society guidelines for the management of suspected acute pulmonary embolism. Thorax 2003;58:470–484.

Bye R. When clients are dying: occupational therapists' perspectives. Occup Ther J Res 1998;18:3–24.

Childs JD, Cleland JA. Development and application of clinical prediction rules to improve decision making in physical therapist practice. Phys Ther 2006;86:122–131.

Clayton JM, Butow PN, Arnold RM, Tattersall MHN. Fostering coping and nurturing hope when discussing the future with terminally ill cancer patients and their caregivers. Cancer 2005;103:1,965–1,975.

Edwards I, Richardson B. Clinical reasoning and population health: decision making for an emerging paradigm of health care. Physiother Theory Pract 2008;24:183–193.

Edwards I, Jones M, Carr J, Braunack-Mayer A, Jensen GM. Clinical reasoning strategies in physical therapy. Phys Ther 2004;84:312–335.

Eliott JA, Olver I. Dying cancer patients talk about physician and patient roles in DNR decision making. Health Expect 2011;14:147–158.

Emanuel L, Scandrett KG. Decisions at the end of life: have we come of age? BMC Med 2010;8:57–64.

Finch E, Geddes EL, Larin H. Ethically-based clinical decision-making in physical therapy: process and issues. Physiother Theory Pract 2005;21:147–162.

Greenfield BH, Anderson A, Cox B, Tanner MC. Meaning of caring to 7 novice physical therapists during their first year of clinical practice. Phys Ther 2008;88:1,154–1,166.

Grimmer-Somers K, Lekkas P, Nyland L, Young A, Kumar S. Perspectives on research evidence and clinical practice: a survey of Australian physiotherapists. Physiother Res Int 2007;12:147–161.

Johanson GA. The defined trial period in ethical decision making. J Pain Symptom Manage 2009;38:473–476.

Lee SF, Kristjanson LJ, Williams AM. Professional relationships in palliative care decision making. Support Care Cancer 2009;17:445–450.

Mahon MM. Clinical decision making in palliative care and end of life care. Nurs Clin North Am 2010a;45:345–362.

Mahon MM. Advanced care decision making: Asking the right people the right questions. J Psychosoc Nurs 2010b;48:13–19.

May S, Greasley A, Reeve S, Withers S. Expert therapists use special clinical reasoning processes in the assessment and management of patients with shoulder pain: a qualitative study. Aust J Physiother 2008;54:261–266.

Murray SA, Kendall M, Boyd K, Sheikh A. Illness trajectories and palliative care. BMJ 2005;330(7498):1,007–1,011.

O'Brien M, Jack B. Barriers to dying at home: the impact of poor co-ordination of community service provision for patients with cancer. Health Soc Care Community 2010;18:337–345.

Olsen ML, Swetz KM, Mueller PS. Ethical decision making with end-of-life care: palliative sedation and withholding or withdrawing life-sustaining treatments. Mayo Clin Proc 2010; 85:949–954.

Ott BB. Progress in ethical decision making in the care of the dying. Dimens Crit Care Nurs 2010;29:73–80.

Philip J, Gold M, Schwarz M, Komesaroff P. Patients' views on decision making in advanced cancer. Palliat Support Care 2009;7:181–185.

Playford ED, Siegert R, Levack W, Freeman J. Areas of consensus and controversy about goal setting in rehabilitation: a conference report. Clin Rehab 2009;23:334–344.

Rajer M, Kovac V. Malignant spinal cord compression. Radiol Oncol 2008;42:23–31.

Rosser M. Palliative care emergencies 1: Diagnosis. NursingTimes.net 2007a;103:28. Available at http://www.nursing-times.net/nursing-practice-Clinical-research/palliative-care-emergencies-1-diagnosis/200201.article (last accessed July 2012).

Rosser M. Palliative care emergencies 2: Management. NursingTimes.net, 2007b;103:26. Available at http://www.nursing-times.net/nursing-practice-clinical-research/palliative-care-emergencies-2-management/200215.article (last accessed July 2012).

Simon A. Understanding the key areas of clinical decision making at the end of life. Int J Palliat Nurs 2009;15:264–265.

Smith M, Higgs J, Ellis E. Physiotherapy decision making in acute cardio respiratory care is influenced by factors related to the physiotherapist and the nature and context of the decision: a qualitative study. Austr J Physiother 2007;53: 261–267.

Smith M, Higgs J, Ellis E. Effect of experience on clinical decision making by cardiorespiratory physiotherapists in acute care settings. Physiother Theory Pract 2010;26:89–99.

Vogel KA, Geelhoed M, Grice KO, Murphy D. Do occupational therapy and physical therapy curricula teach critical thinking skills? J Allied Health 2009;38:152–157.

Wade D. Goal setting in rehabilitation: an overview of what, why and how. Clin Rehab 2009;23:291–296.

Wainwright SF, Shepard KF, Harman LB, Stephens J. Factors that influence the clinical decision making of novice and experienced physical therapists. Phys Ther 2011;91:87–101.

Wainwright SF, McGinnis PQ. Factors that influence the clinical decision-making of rehabilitation professionals in long-term care settings. J Allied Health 2009;38:143–151.

Wainwright SF, Shepard KF, Harman LB, Stephens J. Novice and experienced physical therapist clinicians: a comparison of how reflection is used to inform the clinical decision-making process. Phys Ther 2010;90:75–88.

Waterworth S, Gott M. Decision making among older people with advanced heart failure as they transition to dependency and death. Curr Opin Support Palliat Care 2010;4:238–242.

Wilson LD, Detterbeck FC, Yahalom J. Superior vena cava syndrome with malignant causes. N Engl J Med 2007;356:1,862–1,869.

World Health Organization (WHO). Cancer: Palliative Care. 2012. Available at http://www.who.int/cancer/palliative/en/ (last accessed July 2012).

Young B, Moffett JK, Jackson D, McNulty A. Decision-making in community-based paediatric physiotherapy: a qualitative study of children, parents and practitioners. Health Soc Care Community 2006;14:116–124.

2.2 Pain

Jacob van den Broek, Jenny Taylor, Rainer Simader

Pain is one the most difficult symptoms to treat and it can be a real challenge to provide effective symptom control, especially in the terminally ill patient. This is particularly true with regard to the diversity and complexity of different kinds of pain.

About 70 % of all terminally ill tumour patients experience pain at some level (Brescia et al. 1992). Pain arises for a variety of reasons in the palliative care context. Significant causes frequently addressed by physiotherapists include bony metastases, and nerve root pressure by tumour growth. Co-existent pain may emerge due to underlying pathologies, unconnected to the disease process, and secondary pain, for example peripheral neuropathy after chemotherapy. The causes of pain are reported by Grond et al. (1996) as follows:

- 85 % directly attributable to the cancer itself;
- 17 % caused by treatment;
- 9 % due to related pain syndromes or debility;
- 9 % due to concurrent disorder, unrelated to primary disease.

Apart from patients with cancer many other people needing palliative care treatment suffer from pain due to a variety of reasons. Physiotherapists utilize a range of non-pharmacological strategies in the management of pain, many of which are effectively transferable to the end of life/palliative care. Modification of input, flexibility, and an adaptable approach are essential. As families and carers are increasingly involved in supporting patients, consideration to their needs must also be given.

Following a detailed case study, various treatment modalities are explored in this chapter. Physiotherapy offers a broad range of conventional, innovative and alternative treatment strategies in managing patients' pain at the end of life. Physiotherapists should engage in collaborative working alongside other health care professionals in order to help management of this challenging symptom. **Physiotherapists play a powerful role in building confidence in patient groups in a range of health care settings, and this skill can come right to the fore when supporting the vulnerability that so often accompanies pain in the patient at the end of life.**

2.2.1 Case study

Mr A., a 63-year-old man, had been admitted to a high care hospice in the Netherlands. He was an unattached man with an estimated life expectancy of less than three months. He had family and friends, but did not want to burden them, and for that reason he had requested admission. Admission for symptom control of pain and psychosocial support was agreed. His life had totally changed in a very short period, and he needed rest and safety. Mr A. had full insight into his disease.

History   Ten years ago Mr A. had a carcinoma of the tongue. The treatment was tumour resection followed by radiation. He also had concurrent cardiac problems.

Recent diagnosis   He had been diagnosed with an adenocarcinoma, non-small cell left lung cancer, phase IV, with hilar spread. He also had multiple spinal bone metastases in C7, T2 and T10 vertebrae. The initial presenting symptom was thoracic pain on the left side. Prior to admission Mr A. received two courses of palliative chemotherapy. During the chemotherapy there was rapid tumour progression. After chemotherapy the pain increased in his spine and left hip. Further investigation showed new lytic lesions in L1 and L2 and deformation of the L4 body.

Patient's goals   Mr A.'s primary goal was pain reduction. Although optimal pain relief was the priority, he also recognized that due to pain and increasing breathlessness he had difficulties with his functional needs. He asked the physiotherapist to help him with his general mobility, which had deteriorated as he had become weaker and more fatigued. He expressed a wish to be more independent to perform routine activities of daily living (ADL); for example, an initial main goal was to be able to visit the bathroom on his own. Mr A. also wanted to be able to sit longer in his chair by the window to have contact with the outside world. His pain had left him feeling isolated.

To improve his quality of life (QOL), four key questions were asked. These questions were used to establish the role of multidisciplinary therapy input, of which physiotherapy was part:

- What relevant information must be sought before treatment?
- What assessment is appropriate before treatment?
- Which interventions are indicated?
- How should outcomes be evaluated?

Medical history Because of the major influence of pain on the patient's daily functioning, it was vital to have more information about the type, frequency, and nature of the onset of Mr A.'s pain. He reported continual back pain, radiating to both legs and also between the scapulae. The pain became worse during all activities but most particularly on moving his left arm and on deep inspiration. His prescribed pain medication had not achieved an adequate response, and prior to admission his general practitioner had modified both the doses of analgesia and the methods of administration with partial improvement of symptoms; however, a residual level of pain remained.

Assessment Considering Mr A.'s goals, it was necessary to assess his mobility and other functional activities, especially in relation to his experience of pain. This included his resting position, both sitting in his chair and lying in bed. The basic tool used for these assessments was the visual analogue scale (VAS; Wewers/Lowe 1990); the results ranged from VAS 6 to VAS 8. During the mobility test, Mr A. registered continual pain, particularly in his back, and this significantly increased during general activity. Due to this severe pain, Mr A. demonstrated a very unstable walking pattern. Even using a walking frame or rollator, the distance of 8 metres from his bed to the bathroom was challenging for him. Pain disrupted his breathing pattern, which further compromised his activity, especially as he did not pace himself at all. Dyspnoea due to his extensive lung cancer was not only further exacerbated on exertion but also provoked the fear of incident pain in his left chest wall and scapulae. This all caused a vicious cycle of pain and inactivity.

He adopted an antalgic (pain avoidant) position in the chair. Oedema in his legs and ankles was also noted. Mr A. needed maximum assistance to wash and dress; consequently most of his day was spent in bed. He slept quite well when taking optimal pain relief.

In the light of results from the first two questions, the multidisciplinary team (MDT) discussed possible interventions and how to evaluate outcomes.

Intervention (first week of the admission) Mr A.'s pain was not under control and slowly increased (VAS

7–9). Medical review was paramount to establish the nature of his pain, and key to addressing it was close teamwork with regard to both pharmacological and non-pharmacological strategies. The anaesthesiologist reviewed and adjusted the pain medication, and during MDT discussion the physiotherapist and nurses advised the following adjuvant approaches to managing his care:

- warm baths: the patient's choice for promoting comfort, aided by the nurses;
- commencement of physiotherapy: liaising with the attending physician prescribing pain medication before the treatment sessions.

The physiotherapist gave Mr A. specific instructions with regard to energy consumption. The physiotherapist assessed his mobility and monitored his breathing when he walked to the bathroom. Resting points were incorporated en route to address his breathing difficulties. This served to maximize control of his dyspnoea and minimize incipient pain. Instructions were given for managing bed transfers and on how to use his walking frame or rollator. As well as advice given for improving position and comfort when in bed, the physiotherapist instructed the patient in active feet and leg exercises to improve his circulation. To relieve the pain during deep inspiration the physiotherapist instructed Mr A. on how to use the Jacobson relaxation method which also helped to calm his breathing pattern.

Evaluation Due to the rapid progression of the disease in the end of life period, evaluation was a constant ongoing process throughout the treatment. Measurement by VAS was therefore carried out three times a day by nurses and during interventions by the physiotherapist. Due to Mr A.'s ongoing general deterioration and disease progression, his pain was the primary concern, and pharmacological management predominated. Physiotherapy helped Mr A.'s breathing pattern to become more controlled. His confidence grew, and he could manage the walk to the bathroom better than before, less influenced by dyspnoea. As he transferred from bed more easily, he got up and sat out of bed more often. He was able to sit in his chair in different positions and for longer periods and remained more relaxed. These changes greatly improved his quality of life.

Intervention (second week of the admission) Mr A.'s pain had proved very difficult to control (VAS 4–8). Ongoing MDT discussion took place concerning further options. The anaesthesiologist implemented further adjustments of medication and also prescribed a nerve block. The MDT made the decision to trial transcutaneous electrical nerve stimulation (TENS). TENS was proposed as adjuvant pain relief 4–5 times a day specifically for the neuropathic pain in Mr A.'s left hip and leg.

Full instruction in the use of TENS was given to Mr A. by the physiotherapist. Bipolar TENS with a high pulsation frequency was applied for 40 minutes 4–5 times a day to good effect. The physiotherapist also instructed the nurses to continue TENS application during 24-hour care in the hospice. A regular active exercise regime for lower limbs in bed to improve circulation, shown to the patient by the physiotherapist, was also taught to, and reinforced by, the nurses.

Evaluation   Mr A. experienced effective short-term relief of pain after the nerve block. Pain relief was supplemented by a combination of TENS and the Jacobsen relaxation method. However, after a week the patient reported reduced efficacy of the TENS. He became more fatigued, was unable to apply the TENS by himself, and the TENS became less comfortable when being used. Because of Mr A.'s deteriorating condition, both physically and psychologically, the physiotherapist decided that it was inappropriate to continue the application of TENS at that time as any benefit was outweighed by the burden of application for the patient. Constant medical review of pain continued.

Final week   Pain assessment with VAS was no longer appropriate due to the patient's general deterioration. Continued pain evaluation by gaining simple verbal feedback of symptoms and nursing team observations was sought by the medical team at the bedside. All interventions focused on optimal pain relief and patient reassurance. To maintain a comfortable posture in bed and optimal circulation, the physiotherapist and nurses implemented supportive gentle passive physiotherapy techniques, comprising passive movements of the patient's arms, legs and trunk where possible and when tolerated. After three weeks as a hospice inpatient the patient deteriorated further and died.

2.2.2 Pain

The *International Association for the Study of Pain* describes pain with the following definition: *'an unpleasant sensory and emotional experience associated with actual or potential tissue damage, or described in terms of such damage'*. There are many descriptions of various kinds of pain in the literature. The most common forms of pain described, and the most significant encountered in end of life care, are nociceptive and neuropathic pain (Merskey/Bogduk 1994). Perhaps the simplest definition,

which clearly emphasizes the subjective nature of pain, is that of McCaffery who proposed, as early as 1968, the widely accepted definition: *'Pain is whatever the experiencing person says it is, existing whenever the experiencing person says it'* (McCaffery 1968).

This quote suggests how difficult it is to interpret pain. Cicely Saunders first used the term *'total pain'* (➤ Chapter 1.3). 'Total pain' reflects and acknowledges the spiritual, emotional and social suffering of the patient as components of their physical problems. It is an approach to pain that is key to unlocking other problems and issues that point to possible multiple interventions for its resolution. Cicely Saunders described chronic pain as *'not just an event, or a series of events but rather a situation in which the patient is, as it were, held captive'* (Saunders 1970). Especially in terminally ill patients, the major challenge is to use active prophylactic strategies to avoid pain onset; that is, strong analgesia when the onset of pain is predicted, rather than indicated in response to that pain. *'Constant pain needs constant control.'* (Clark 2000). To anticipate the onset of pain and its presentation – as viewed by different disciplines and from different perspectives – is extremely challenging, and the physiotherapist, as part of the multiprofessional team, has an integral role to play.

Pain assessment

Due to the nature of pain, different types of therapy need to be monitored and assessed constantly; repeated and regular follow up by the physiotherapist is therefore important. The physiotherapist must also be proactive in instructing other caregivers; such instruction is important both within the MDT and, where applicable, with families and carers.

Because of the complexity of pain and pain perception, different measurement tools are used to assess it. **Individual interpretation and expression varies, both personally and culturally, and an optimal method of evaluation is particularly difficult to establish.** The visual analogue scale (VAS) and numerical rating scale (NRS) (➤ Figure 2.2), or a combination of these, are the most frequently used tools to measure pain in the palliative care or end of life setting (➤ Chapter 2.9).

VAS/NRS is an easy-to-use method for the assessment of variations in intensity of pain. The clinician asks the patient to mark his or her perception of pain, with the help of descriptors, at a point along a 100 mm line. The physiotherapist records the pain as a number between 0 and 10. Pain assessment using a VAS/NRS for patients with dementia or elements of cognitive impairment is not

2

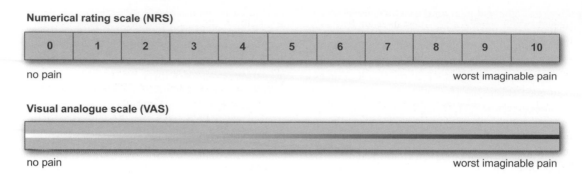

Figure 2.2 Numerical rating scale (Serlin 1995) [L157]

applicable; other assessment tools are available and may be more appropriate for these patients (➤ Chapter 2.6), and also in the case of children (➤ Chapter 2.9). In palliative care these scales can also be used for measuring other elements, e. g. activities of daily living (ADL), quality of life (QOL) or symptoms such as breathlessness or anxiety (➤ Chapter 2.3, ➤ Chapter 2.7). **Relatively non-invasive, the advantage of the VAS/NRS for the assessment of pain is its inherent simplicity in use with this patient group.**

As **pain is a symptom that has a strong impact on a patient's activities of daily living,** an important aspect of any pain review is to assess these parameters. Depending on the patient's goals, functional assessments should be used. For example, in the case of Mr A.'s goal of improving his quality of life by getting out of his bed by himself and going to his chair to sit at the window, these actions were too difficult for him to do not only because of the pain he experienced but also because of his fear of pain onset when commencing activity. By gently exploring, for example, sitting in a chair with supportive armrests, **the presence of pain can be constantly assessed together with the patient 's reaction, the influence of inhibition, and aspects of anxiety and fear when anticipating pain.** The next part of this test could be to trial walking for a short distance, for example: the patient walks at least 3 metres forward, does a half turn and returns to the chair. In this case, a combination of the VAS/NRS and functional assessment tools are very useful to acquire accurate information concerning functional impairment due to pain.

Pharmacological treatment of medical pain
Klaus Reckinger

Many patients faced with a life-threatening illness express the fear, even in the early stages, that they will have to endure uncontrolled pain as their disease progresses. The publication of the **World Health Organisation** (WHO) *Guidelines for the Management of Cancer Pain* in 1986 (revised 1996) has gone some way **to address the fears of patients by educating health professionals to manage pain more effectively.** The recommendations were intended to be straightforward and accessible to health professionals who are non-specialists in pain management. A further requirement was that the guidelines would be valid and practicable worldwide – across different cultures, and in industrial nations as well as developing and emerging countries.

The guidelines were initially limited to cancer pain but over time have also been applied to cover the management of non-cancer pain.

The **key statements** made by these guidelines are still relevant to clinical practice today:

1. oral administration of pain medication (*'by mouth'*);
2. administration according to a fixed time schedule (*'by the clock'*);
3. selection of medication according to a step-by-step regimen (*'by the ladder'*);
4. adaptation to the personal situation (*'for the individual'*);
5. in-depth consideration of all the circumstances (*'attention to detail'*).

Using the oral route the dosage is usually adjustable to daily fluctuations in pain intensity, e. g. exertional pain during the day from bone pain or nocturnal peaks from neuropathic pain.

Once stable background pain relief has been achieved, transdermal patches (transdermal therapeutic systems, or TTS) are a potentially convenient alternative to long-acting oral preparations, especially for patients with dysphagia, and these have, in the author's experience, proved readily acceptable to patients. Transdermal preparations are unsuitable for rapid titration of analgesia and for brief fluctuations in pain intensity.

The duration of effect of any medication is limited. For this reason, it is particularly important to take medicines according to a **fixed schedule** in order to prevent gaps in the therapeutic effect. Studies have revealed that if this is not the case, the pain not only returns but hyperalgesia (heightened sensitivity to pain) may also result (Koppert et al 2001).

Step 1 of the **WHO pain ladder** (➤ Figure 2.3) entails the use of non-opioids such as paracetamol. If the pain is not adequately controlled, a weak opioid (step 2 drug) may be added. If the pain persists despite the maximum dose, the step 2 drug is replaced by a potent step 3 opioid, whilst possibly continuing with the step 1 medication.

Unlike drugs used at steps 1 and 2, there is no "maximum" dose for step 3 opioids. For individual patients, the maximum dose may be limited by intolerable side effects, e. g. sedation. When commencing opioid therapy, an anti-emetic and laxative should be made available (Cascorbi/Sorge/Strumpf 2011).

However standardised the approach, good pain management must suit the **needs of the individual** (*'for the individual'*). When do patients begin their day? What is characteristic of their lifestyle? What psychological and physical stresses are they subjected to? Assessment and management of lifestyle, psycho-social (including treatable psychiatric disorders) and spiritual factors are integral to the management of pain. Inappropriate use of analgesics may occur if inadequate attention is paid to these factors. Adherence to the WHO guidelines has been shown to achieve a clear improvement in the pain management of approximately two-thirds (⅔) of those affected (Felleiter et al. 2005).

Types of pain

Understanding the different types of pain can help target therapy appropriately. The pathophysiology of pain as it informs physiotherapeutic interventions is explored in more detail elsewhere in this chapter.

Nociceptive pain This type of pain, arising for example from soft-tissue or bone, can be treated with paracetamol, non-steroidal anti-inflammatory drugs (NSAIDs) and opioids. Some visceral forms of pain, for example intestinal colic, also respond to anticholinergics such as hyoscine butylbromide (Tytgat 2007). Pain from skeletal muscle can arise due to

spasticity and/or spasms: this type of pain may respond to antispasmodics such as baclofen. Anti-inflammatory agents such as NSAIDs or glucocorticoids are potentially useful if an accompanying **inflammatory reaction** is detectable. The risks of NSAID-associated gastrointestinal, cardiovascular, cerebrovascular and renal toxicities should be weighed against the potential benefits of these drugs (Cascorbi/Sorge/Strumpf 2011).

Likewise, use of long-term glucocorticoids can lead to severe, debilitating side effects which can also be irreversible.

In some diseases, disease-modifying drugs (e. g. cytotoxic chemotherapy agents) may have an analgesic effect.

Neuropathic and other chronic, non-malignant pain Neuropathic pain, defined as the pain arising as a result of actual or potential nerve damage, may respond to opioids, but other useful drugs commonly used include tricyclic antidepressants (e. g. nortriptyline or amitriptyline – noting unlicensed indications) and anticonvulsants (e. g. gabapentin or pregabalin). Duloxetine (a serotonin and noradrenaline uptake inhibitor) is another more recently introduced antidepressant licensed for the management of painful diabetic neuropathy.

In chronic non-malignant pain (such as painful diabetic neuropathy, post herpetic neuralgia, fibromyalgia), these groups of non-opioid drugs should be used ahead of strong opioids because of the risks from long-term chronic opioid administration. In the case of neuropathic pain due to malignancy, it is appropriate to consider strong opioids alongside tricyclics and anticonvulsants. NSAIDs are generally not effective for neuropathic pain.

Mixed pain syndrome Some patients who present with a pattern of mixed nociceptive and neuropathic, non-malignant pain may benefit from tapentadol, a novel agent combining the properties of a μ-opioid receptor agonist and a noradrenaline reuptake inhibitor. As tapentadol has combined opioid and non-opioid properties, it is potentially useful for patients who struggle with tablet burden. However, tapentadol is not usually suitable for patients with cancer pain who may require large doses of strong opioids.

Breakthrough pain in cancer

Breakthrough pain is a common phenomenon (Mercadante et al. 2010). A task group of the *Science Committee of the Association for Palliative Medicine of Great Britain and Ireland* recently defined cancer-related breakthrough pain as *"a transient exacerbation of pain that occurs either spontaneously, or in relation to a specific predictable or unpredictable trigger, despite relatively stable and adequately controlled background pain"* (Davies et al. 2009).

For short-lived episodes of breakthrough pain, the ideal "as required" analgesic will have a rapid onset of action and short duration of effect (Zeppetella/Ribeiro 2006). In UK practice the usual dose of the "as required" analgesic starts at ⅙ of the total daily opioid dosage. However, evidence from studies examining the use of short-acting fentanyl preparations suggests that titration of the "as required" dose should be individualised (Davies et al 2009). The manufacturers of the short-acting fentanyl preparations recommend starting at the lowest strength regardless of the background analgesia.

➤ Table 2.2 lists the products available for treating breakthrough pain.

Physiotherapy and pain

To ensure that the beneficial effects of physiotherapy are optimised, a dose of the patient's usual breakthrough analgesic medication may be required prior to commencing therapy. Good communication between the physiotherapist and the medical team is pivotal. The type and predictability of the breakthrough pain will determine the appropriate medication and route of administration (oral versus sublingual or intranasal) to be used.

Other interventions

In most patients the pain can be treated adequately with the described therapeutic approach. If this is not the case, a **change in the route of administration** may need to be considered. Intravenous and/or epidural/intrathecal administration of drugs may be an approach of choice. In the UK, the subcutaneous route is used more frequently than the intravenous route and PCA (patient-controlled analgesia) is almost never used in the palliative care setting. Implanted intrathecal analgesic pumps are occasionally indicated for palliative care patients with a reasonable prognosis.

The general principles of symptom control also apply to pain management (Reckinger 2011). Consequently, consideration should be given to **treating the underlying process** which is causing the pain before initiating a purely symptomatic form of therapy. Examples of these causes include surgery for tumour debulking or bone fixation, chemotherapy or radiotherapy. The benefits must always be carefully and individually weighed against the potential burdens. Chemotherapeutic agents can decrease the pain for as long as the tumour responds well, but they can also cause pain (e.g. painful polyneuropathies). The analgesic benefits of **palliative radiotherapy,** e.g. for painful bone metastases, are well documented (Doyle/Hanks/MacDonald 1993). The recently published NICE guidelines regarding the use of strong opioids in palliative care (NICE 2012) and EAPC guidelines regarding opioid use for cancer pain (Caraceni et al. 2012) are both useful resources for further understanding of all aspects of the pharmacological management of pain at the end of life.

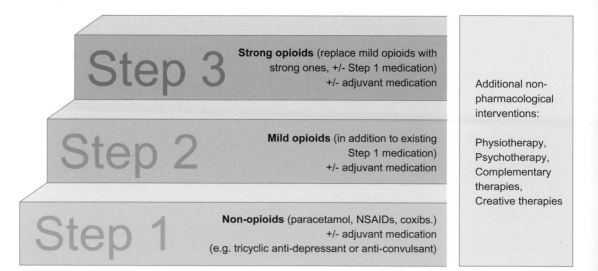

Figure 2.3 WHO „Analgesic Ladder" [W798/L157]

Effective interdisciplinary cooperation in pain management is crucial. Particularly in the time-limited context of palliative care, it is vital that the right discipline is involved. Depending on the clinical setting it may be that the general practitioner is responsible for managing this process. Pain is one of the symptoms that physicians most frequently encounter in palliative care patients, and effective analgesia is the foundation of symptom control.

The physiotherapist must collaborate closely with the general practitioner, medical team or pain specialist and nursing team to ensure optimal pain relief during, for example, pacing and activity training. While it is important to understand that pharmacological management in the form of carefully titrated opioids is pivotal in the treatment of pain, a team approach is key.

As the physiotherapist is so closely involved with patient function during the end of life phase, discussing within the team the possible choices of clinical treatment approaches that might be applicable improves effective management. Furthermore, working closely with the whole team to deliver quick-acting analgesia shortly before a physiotherapy session will provide good support to meet the patient's needs at every stage of treatment.

Table 2.2 Medication for treating breakthrough pain

Substance	Dosage form	Dose strengths available (per unit of administration)
Morphine sulphate immediate release	Film-coated tablets	10 mg/20 mg; 50 mg also in the UK
Morphine sulphate immediate release oral solution	Oral solution	10 mg/5 ml and 20 mg/ml
Morphine sulphate	Injection	10 mg–200 mg (in the UK the strengths are 10, 15, 20, 30 mg per ml)
Oxycodone hydrochloride immediate release	Hard capsules or liquid	Capsules 5 mg/10 mg/20 mg Liquid 1 mg/ml and 10 mg/ml
Oxycodone hydrochloride injection	Injection	10 mg/ml and 50 mg/ml
Hydromorphone	Hard capsules	1.3 mg/2.6 mg
Fentanyl citrate	Lozenges	200 µg–1.600 µg
Fentanyl citrate	Buccal tablets	100 µg–800 µg
Fentanyl citrate	Sublingual tablets	100 µg–800 µg
Fentanyl citrate	Nasal spray	100 µg per spray–400 µg per spray
Fentanyl citrate	Nasal spray	50 µg per spray–200 µg per spray

Non-pharmacological physiotherapeutic interventions

Physiotherapists' contribution to pain management for patients at end of life is to help them to be independent for as long as possible. This is generally very important to patients on various different levels. As pain is so central a symptom, with both physical and psychological foundations in both its origin and development, delivering appropriate training around the pacing of rest and physical activity are important points of interest.

Non-pharmacological symptomatic therapy, once prescribed, can often be self-administered by the patient, and/or can be administered by the patient's family or carers. The choice of which type of treatment will mostly depend on anamnesis; that is, subject to how the patient reports and perceives the pain. For example: What feels good and helps to soothe effectively? Is it warmth, cold, massage, movement, relaxation or diversion? Instruction by professional clinicians is important initially regarding treatment application, and some treatments must only be administered by professionals.

Causes of pain are multifactorial, and challenges faced by patients are unique and personal. Planning the type of treatment involves specific tailoring to each patient's situation and his or her pain experience. Goals are set in the context of possible rapidly changing pain levels, which are often difficult to alleviate and which require constant review. Supportive pain treatment is always best managed by the whole multiprofessional team not only working closely together but also acknowledging the value of different interventions. There are several key specific techniques that physiotherapists can use for pain management. There is evidence that acupuncture, TENS, supportive group therapy, autogenic relaxation and massage therapy may all provide pain relief in cancer pain or in dying patients (Pan et al. 2000).

All interventions must be well coordinated and discussed within the multiprofessional team as multiple concurrent interventions can make it difficult to evaluate effectiveness and outcomes. A range of treatment modalities and techniques are discussed here, with particular focus on how standard physiotherapeutic pain approaches can be modified for the end of life setting.

Physical training

It is widely accepted by clinicians that a welcome benefit of exercise therapy can be a positive effect on pain (Ferrell et al. 1997; Wells 1994; Williamson/Schultz 1995), and it has been suggested that brief periods of exercise may activate the descending pain inhibition pathways (Souvlis/Wright 1997). As diseases progress patients are often generally deconditioned, not only due to pain, but also due to fatigue, increasing weakness, breathlessness and associated anxiety. Inhibition of movement can in turn cause 'guarding', or protective behaviour. Goals of physical training regarding pain control are not only to help patients to manage their pain creatively in a supportive therapeutic environment but, in so doing, to improve posture, mobility, strength, flexibility and circulation; all of these aspects play a part in pain reduction. **The decreased activity levels inherent in patients with pain tend to be accompanied by an anticipatory fear of more pain, as well as an increased perception of pain.** Debate is ongoing that encouraging patients to exercise with cognitive approaches discourages pain-avoidant behaviour, while ensuring that strategies used in the palliative care field must carefully balance physiology and psycho-therapeutics (Merskey 1999).

Exercise therapy, carefully and sensitively introduced, both constantly modified and closely monitored, can help to break the vicious cycle significantly by improving functional movement and activity in general. This in turn results in a simultaneously positive psychological effect, and much enhanced confidence and well-being. The physiotherapist is perfectly placed to note subtle but significant changes in reported pain on movement, and the onset of a new pain must always be treated seriously as a potential palliative care emergency; for example, incipient spinal cord compression.

This physical training, either in the form of individual support or group therapy, can focus on the prevention of pain-provoking tension while performing ADLs. Liaison with an Occupational Therapist is helpful to incorporate advice on life-style adaptations, equipment to improve autonomy and increase independence, and strategies to lessen pain-avoidant behaviour. Supports, splints and orthoses to mitigate pain on activity should be considered, as long as they are realistically assessed in the end of life context and are not too restrictive or cumbersome in use.

Massage and manipulation

The literature shows that massage produces a reduction of pain and anxiety and enhances feelings of relaxation (Pan et al. 2000). The effective mechanism of massage is a decrease in transmission of afferent pain signals, via the mechano-receptors influenced by touch. Increased efferent activity then reinforces pain suppression. At the end of life, patients may present with localized pain or generalized tension or stress; both of these can be indications for the application of massage. There are different kinds of massage techniques that can be implemented.

Gentle stretches and manipulation can influence areas of the anatomy that have been guarded due to pain and consequently become stiff and less functional. The following symptoms may be partially eased with an appropriate hands-on approach: protective spasm and hypertonicity; also, adhesions or contractures arising from invasive surgery, for example major debulking or amputation.

Specific soft-tissue manipulation massage therapies for pain are applied by physiotherapists to myofascial trigger points using a variety of techniques predominantly applied to the painful area. Careful clinical reasoning is however crucial where deep soft tissue pressure or manipulation is concerned in the palliative care setting to ensure the application used is appropriate to the underlying disease process.

Concerning more generalized body massage techniques – for example, effleurage – it is advisable to establish close cooperation and liaison with the complementary therapy team where available and appropriate. The use of aromatherapy oils can further enhance the relaxation and pain-relieving effect. Many palliative care institutions also offer a massage programme for carers; this has been found to be hugely beneficial to their stress and life quality.

⚠ **C A U T I O N**

- Avoid massage directly over tumour sites, areas of recent skin irradiation, dermatitis or vascular impairment.
- Is painful swelling due to lymphoedema, dependant oedema or other causes? If so, bear in mind that lymphoedema massage is a specialist technique and conventional massage techniques are not appropriate for its management (➤ Chapter 2.5).
- Ensure massage for pain is addressed by the appropriate professional through multiprofessional team discussion.
- Severe and painful disfiguring disease may not always preclude manual therapies; touch can contribute to assisting physical and psychological adjustment and integration.

Hot and cold therapy

Warmth

Warmth works by decreasing the transmission of pain signals and has a local effect following muscle relaxation and increased blood circulation. Warmth can also be effective in addressing tension and stress-related pain through inducing relaxation. Best applied in the palliative care setting by thermostatically controlled electrical pads, which can be switched on and off, heat can be applied frequently and safely during the day or night by nurses or carers. Other devices include hot gel or water packs, and medical devices that can be heated in a microwave; when using these techniques, the application should be discontinued when the temperature of the hot pack reverts to below body temperature. Levels of cognitive awareness are important factors to consider at the end of life. These will include confusion, dementia, and decreasing levels of consciousness whether due to sedation or disease progression. An ability to move away from the source of therapy and/or alert staff to any discomfort is of particular significance in the palliative-care setting. Most practical are devices that the patients and/or carers are able to manage themselves after instruction, as this reduces dependency on medical staff. Contraindications must be carefully assessed, and precautions followed; for example, applying paraffin wax should only be done by a physiotherapist (Pan et al. 2000).

Cold

Cryotherapy has a local anaesthetic effect by decreasing blood circulation and inhibiting inflammatory symptoms. It can be used for deep pain, inflammatory, joint and local pain, and is especially appropriate for patients who perceive the sensation of cold as pain relief. Cold can be applied by means of a cold pack or cubed ice. To comply with the usual guidelines of no direct contact of the cold pack or cube ice with the skin, layering with a soft towel is often most comfortable for the palliative care patient. All applications can be carried out by nurses and other caregivers after meticulous instruction by the physiotherapist (Graeff et al. 2010).

⚠ **CAUTION**

Due to high friability of skin at end of life, warmth and cold treatments must be supervised more closely than with other patients. Always ensure extra precautions are taken to provide a barrier between hot/cold source and the patient's skin. Avoid application to areas of:
- recent irradiation;
- dermatitis;
- fungating wounds;
- skin breakdown;
- allodynia;
- decreased blood supply and Raynaud's syndrome;
- lymphatic oedema.

Transcutaneous Electrical Nerve Stimulation

Transcutaneous Electrical Nerve Stimulation (TENS) is a method of electrotherapy that is the most known and applied non-pharmacological treatment modality for pain in palliative/end of life settings. As well as addressing disease-related local, visceral or neuropathic pain,

TENS can also be implemented for pain that may arise in the end of life context from other underlying causes, such as osteoarthritis or previous soft tissue injuries. Evidence of efficacy remains inconclusive (Robb et al. 2008), and research is ongoing (Pan et al. 2000); nevertheless many patients give very positive feedback. The mechanism of the analgesia produced by TENS is explained by the gate-control theory proposed by Melzack and Wall (1965). TENS is usually applied to the skin using two or more electrodes. A typical battery-operated TENS unit is able to modulate pulse width, frequency and intensity. Generally TENS for these patients is applied at high frequency (>50 Hz) with a low intensity below motor contraction (sensory intensity) or low frequency (<10 Hz) with a high intensity, sometimes referred to as acupuncture-like (Filshie/Thompson 2000; Pan et al. 2000). To maintain effective pain relief, possible accommodation can be overcome by a flexible approach to the use of 'continuous', 'modulated' or 'burst' modes as appropriate.

The optimal placements of electrodes on 'trigger points' may correspond with acupuncture analgesia points. TENS can be used as an adjuvant approach, mostly 3–5 times a day by patients themselves, following application instruction by the physiotherapist. This kind of therapy contributes to the independence of the patient because of its portability, self-management aspect; as a key modality it is part of a comprehensive multifaceted approach to pain control. An additional benefit of this treatment modality is that the patient can exert control over the use of TENS. **This adds a valuable empowerment aspect to pain management when patients so often are demoralized by helplessness.** Along with the other pain therapy applications, TENS can be applied by caregivers after instructions from the physiotherapist or specific pain team. Care must be taken to be aware of areas of less sensitivity and also inflammation (Graeff et al. 2010).

✓ **GUIDANCE**
Transcutaneous Electrical Nerve Stimulation (TENS)

- Pain takes a sense of control away from the patient; TENS helps to give control back.
- Patient routines and activities are not disrupted by treatment application.
- Removal of fear of 'overdose' or 'dependence' reduces patient anxiety.

Acupuncture

Acupuncture is increasingly becoming a component of complementary/alternative therapies in many cancer and palliative care settings. In 13 countries an average of 30 % usage has been reported (Ernst/Cassileth 1998). The exact mechanism remains unclear, but it is thought to modulate pain via the release of the body's own opioids (endorphins). Acupuncture needles are applied to stimulate sensory nerves in the skin and muscles and to transmit signals to the spinal cord and midbrain. Alternatively, acupressure using finger or hand pressure can be applied over acupoints stimulating the same energy pathways.

Most effective for musculoskeletal pain, acupuncture is however also helpful for neuropathic pain when needles are applied within the appropriate anatomical segment (Filshie 2000). At end of life, acupuncture can address the needs of certain patients who are excessively sensitive to normal doses of analgesia (Thompson/Filshie 1998), and acupuncture has been found to be very relaxing for patients who feel angry, are in denial, or are finding it difficult to come to terms with their disease (Filshie, unpublished observations).

Clinicians, usually either physiotherapists or complementary therapists, need to have had specific accredited training, and it is important to be aware that treatments are time-consuming. In a study of a retrospective audit of 339 patients with cancer it was found that the more advanced the disease, the shorter lasting was the response (Filshie 1990). Significant contraindications include bleeding and auto-immune system disorders, skin infections and localized disease, lymphoedema, valvular heart disease, and anxious, frightened or needle-phobic patients.

Relaxation techniques

An additional non-pharmacological strategy to manage pain is relaxation. Relaxation methods are based on muscle relaxant and tension reduction techniques. Often used in conjunction with imagery techniques, relaxation techniques may be particularly appropriate for reducing intractable pain in dying patients; whether alone or in combination with acupuncture or TENS (Pan et al. 2000).

As a treatment method it is indicated in cases where patients complain of pain in relation to continuous increased muscle tension particularly associated with mental stress and anxiety.

The following basic types of relaxation methods may be applicable at end of life:

Progressive muscle relaxation (Jacobson Method): The patient is instructed to consciously and systematically tighten specific muscle groups in sequence, followed by gradual release.

Simple physiological relaxation (Mitchell Method): The patient is instructed to tense opposing agonist muscles to produce contrasting release of tension in antagonist muscle groups.

Autogenic Training (Schultz Method): The patient is simply physically passive, and follows instructions to concentrate on body self-awareness, leading to a feeling of warmth, heaviness, calm breathing and total relaxation.

The physiotherapist should implement all methods in a quiet, undisturbed area, always ensuring maximum comfort and support for the patient. Breathing awareness can be incorporated throughout all treatment sessions, and relaxation methods can be combined with visualization exercises and meditation. In the palliative care setting group sessions can work well, maybe with the incorporation of appropriate music; consideration should also be given to advice and support to carers to help to reinforce techniques learnt for use at home. CDs with relaxation/exercises are available to enable patients to apply the technique by themselves when they want or need to, which gives patients self-management strategies away from the therapeutic context.

✓ GUIDANCE
Relaxation

- Relaxation techniques are particularly useful for intractable pain in the dying patient as they are non-invasive and are seen as supportive by families and carers.
- Instruction in relaxation can improve sleep patterns for patients disturbed by pain symptoms (Graeff et al. 2010).
- A simply devised self-help leaflet on relaxation strategies can assist both patients and families in alleviating both their fears around pain and its negative effects on QOL.

Complementary therapy

Understanding the total pain concept is paramount when addressing patients' needs. In their assessments and regular contacts physiotherapists must be alert to other causes of the symptom 'pain', which are possibly non-physical and/or should be additionally treated by other members of the MDT. Complementary therapy also plays an important role in palliative pain management. Depending on the underlying cause of pain and interest of the patient, the following is a selection of options which, amongst other therapies, may be indicated: art therapy, music therapy, other creative therapy approaches, aromatherapy, hypnotherapy, reflexology, etc. These options may be used not only for pain management but also for other symptoms such as dyspnoea, fatigue and anxiety. By working through complex emotions and stress, patients often experience feelings of comfort and improved well-being (Gambles/Crooke/ Wilkinson 2002; Pan et al. 2000). Basic knowledge of different complementary methods is important to be able to suggest these interventions to patients and to refer patients to appropriate team members.

2.2.3 Spinal cord compression
Kristina Coe

Definition and incidence

Metastatic spinal cord compression (MSCC) is a rare oncological emergency producing considerable devastation to function, quality of life and life expectancy (Stubberfield/Bilsky 2007). It is defined as *compression of the dural sac and its contents (spinal cord and/or cauda equina) by an extradural tumour mass. The minimum radiological evidence is indentation of the theca at the level of clinical features'* (Laperriere in Pease/Harris/Finlay 2004).

There are an estimated 4,000 MSCC cases per annum in the UK (NICE 2008), which relates to 5 %–10 % of the cancer population (Tang et al. 2007) and occurs most commonly in the fifth to seventh decades of life (Harel/Angelov 2010; Levack et al. 2002).

MSCC is considered a late evolutionary effect of primary disease (Levack et al. 2002), and as patients are surviving longer with advances in treatment, the incidence is predicted to rise (NICE 2008). Empirically MSCC patients have a poor prognostic outcome. Only 20 % achieve 12-month survival, with the majority living an average of 3–4 months (Allan et al. 2009; Harel/Angelov 2010; Stubberfield/Bilsky 2007; ➤ Figure 2.4).

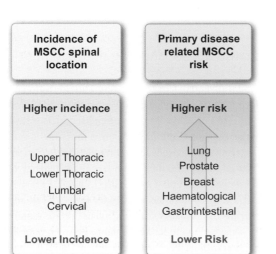

Figure 2.4 MSCC: Risk and incidence of location [M543/L157]

Presentation and red flags

Presentation to or transfer into physiotherapy management occurs across acute, community (home) and specialist care settings with **94 % complaining of back pain as their primary symptom** (Levack et al. 2002). This can make identification difficult when only 1 in every 5,000 general back pain patients have MSCC (NICE 2008), and 25 % of these will not have a known cancer diagnosis (Levack et al. 2002).

Multiple studies cite consistent delays in diagnosis of MSCC, secondary to poor awareness of the warning signs and symptoms of serious spinal pathology (red flags) and awaiting definitive (late) signs before suspecting MSCC and referring for imaging (Allan et al. 2009; Husband/Grant/Romaniuk 2001; Levack et al. 2002; McLinton/Hutchinson 2006; ➤ Figure 2.5). Levack et al. (2002) report diagnostic delays of up to 3 months, with the majority of patients referred beyond the time for *'treatment to be of any value'*, because **those with paraplegia for more than 48 hours are unlikely to regain active movement through surgery or radiotherapy.** (Patchell et al. 2005; The Christie NHS Foundation Trust 2011)

Due to their knowledge of red flags and detailed clinical assessments, physiotherapists are well equipped to identify not only early and changing symptoms, but also those signs sitting outside the standard clinical picture of back pain. If survivorship, or indeed quality of life in the palliative phase is to improve, suspicion and diagnostic imaging needs to occur before the 'late signs' have developed. Consequently **future physiotherapy practice must promote education of red flags** to all health professionals and patients at every stage in order to achieve early prophylactic intervention instead of the current late palliative management, which is failing patients (Levack et al. 2002).

Suspicion and identification

It is imperative that physiotherapists are involved from the outset, regardless of clinical setting, to facilitate early detection, urgent referral onto the MSCC care pathway (➤ Figure 2.6) and to ensure preservation of spinal integrity.

⚠ **CAUTION**

'Following suspicion of MSCC and in the presence of mechanical pain and neurological signs suggestive of spinal instability, patients should be nursed flat and log rolled as soon as possible. This is to allow preservation of neurology and function until bony and neurological stability can be ensured' (NICE 2008, p. xiii).

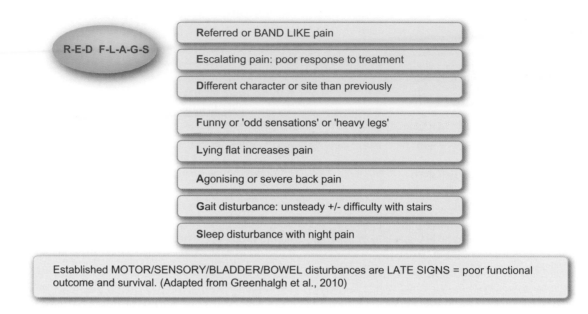

R-E-D F-L-A-G-S

Referred or BAND LIKE pain

Escalating pain: poor response to treatment

Different character or site than previously

Funny or 'odd sensations' or 'heavy legs'

Lying flat increases pain

Agonising or severe back pain

Gait disturbance: unsteady +/- difficulty with stairs

Sleep disturbance with night pain

Established MOTOR/SENSORY/BLADDER/BOWEL disturbances are LATE SIGNS = poor functional outcome and survival. (Adapted from Greenhalgh et al., 2010)

Figure 2.5 Early warning signs of MSCC [W825/L157]

Imaging

Magnetic resonance imaging (MRI) offers superior imaging against less costly x-rays and computerized tomography (CT) scans (Husband/Grant/Romaniuk 2001). Use of pain and sensory levels to guide imaging area are unreliable (Levack et al. 2002) as approximately 20 % of patients will have MSCC at least 4 levels higher than that reported, and 25 % of patients have multilevel involvement (Husband/Grant/Romaniuk 2001). As a result **whole spine MRI within 24 hours is the recommended gold standard** (NICE 2008) to avoid false negatives.

Spinal stability

There is much uncertainty around spinal stability as imaging only provides a 'snapshot' in time and cannot unequivocally confirm its existence (Pease/Harris/Finlay 2004). Clinical features offer the most reliable indicator, and therefore decisions regarding its presence and management should always be discussed between the radiologist, oncologist and physiotherapist (NICE 2008; The Christie 2011). **Addressing stability, even in the palliative phase, may save some from further disability, which has substantial implications to both quality and length of life.** Furthermore, even when treatment is not indicated or patient choice prevails, adherence to flat bed rest may prove unnecessarily detrimental to quality

of life; again discussion with the MDT, palliative team and the patient should guide management (NICE 2008; The Christie 2011; ➤ Figure 2.6).

Mobilization and rehabilitation

Once definitive treatment is agreed on and commenced, graduated mobilization protocols with regular subjective and objective re-assessment is recommended in order to promote early movement, whilst monitoring and minimizing any deterioration in neurology (➤ Figure 2.6).

Discharge and/or ongoing management

Rehabilitation and discharge planning should commence on diagnosis and ideally be coordinated by a named lead person (GMCCN 2011). There is often pressure for rapid discharge, but it is complex and convoluted due to multiple barriers, which can lead to unrealistic expectations, unachievable goals and delays if not managed effectively (Stubberfield/Bilsky 2007; ➤ Figure 2.7).

Determining appropriate settings for ongoing care support during the palliative and end of life phase requires careful consideration to strike a balance between optimizing function without adverse encroachment into remaining life. **It is a challenging period with patients mourning the life they once had whilst coming to terms with an**

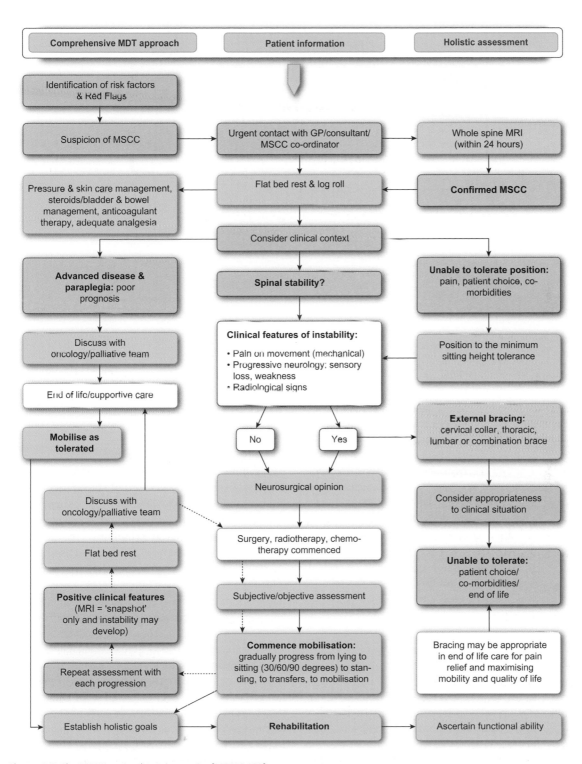

Figure 2.6 The MSCC care pathway in practice [M543/L157]

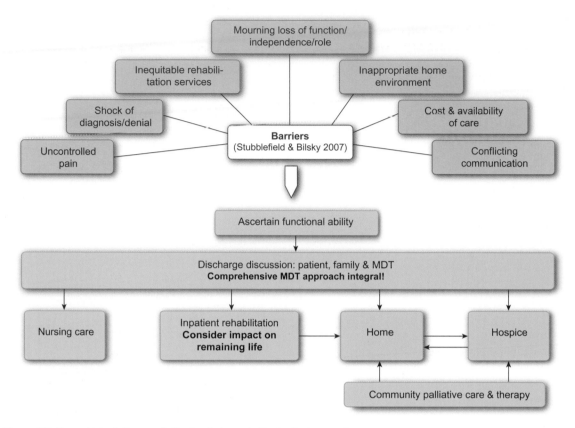

Figure 2.7 The multiple challenges of effective discharge facilitation [M543/L157]

uncertain future, the treatment side effects and their home environment no longer being compatible with their new level of function (Stubberfield/Bilsky 2007). However, physiotherapists can facilitate education, guide early rehabilitation and integrate MDT communication successfully, thereby aiding the patient (and family) to overcome these challenges and to manage symptoms more effectively. In essence, it is these key attributes that promote the best journey for patients and their family and enable quality of life.

2.2.4 Conclusion
Jacob van den Broek, Jenny Taylor, Rainer Simader

Fear can be prevalent where there is pain at end of life. Physical pain as a component of 'total pain', presents a situation fraught with challenges but ripe with possibilities. Experience of pain reduces functional ability and often, with that, a perception of any ability to overcome physical difficulties. Antalgic behaviour makes it difficult to develop the appropriate strategies to perform even the simplest daily tasks. **Because of the multiple influences of situations and disease symptoms,**

pain should, where possible, be managed preemptively. The goal of the MDT is to analyze the impact of these different influences. **The intensity of a patient's pain will be influenced by his or her individual emotional response to the physical symptoms** (Souvlis/Wright 1997). The physiotherapist's principle role is to look at alternative ways of solving functional dilemmas; moving aside from trying to correct impairment, it will be more important to focus on adaptive strategies (Robb/Ewer-Smith 2008). The physiotherapist can combine a variety of strategies and applications for a broad and total treatment, while applying good psychosocial skills that are crucial to managing patients' vulnerability. Families and carers can be very distressed around issues of pain, and this can, in turn, be demoralizing for the multiprofessional team. **The pragmatic approach of the physiotherapist is often seen as an empowering and stabilizing presence within the medical team.**

Combining techniques can have an additional advantage in influencing specific goals. To maintain general well-being at an optimal level, it is necessary to manage pain with therapy as early as possible in the disease trajectory and also preventatively (➤ Chapter 1.4). Offering the possibility of an alternative non-pharmacological symptomatic and therapeutic approach, physiotherapists can support the patient at an earlier stage. They have a key role in symptom control of pain alongside other specialties, and we must maintain the skills to cross-refer when necessary and appropriate. However it can be a significant challenge to offer patients a personalized training package not only to maintain their functional status, but also to prevent, decrease or even just stabilize pain. Pharmacology remains the mainstay of pain management.

2.2.5 Reflective questions

- When assessing a patient's pain, are there aspects of symptoms presented that indicate underlying secondary disease or an unrelated pathology?
- How can you introduce self-management strategies and carer/family support in any pain treatment programme?
- What other multiprofessional approaches should you consider to reduce the impact of pain on a patient's function and ability to cope?
- What confidence-building strategies can you implement as a physiotherapist to address pain in the dying patient?

REFERENCES

Allan L, Baker L, Eljamel S, et al. Suspected malignant cord compression – improving time to diagnosis via a 'hotline': a prospective audit. Br J Cancer 2009;100:1,867–1,872.

Brescia FJ, Portenoy RK, Ryan M, et al. Pain, opioid use, and survival in hospitalized patients with advanced cancer. J Clin Oncol 1992;10:149–155.

Caraceni A, Hanks G, Kaasa S, et al.; European Palliative Care Research Collaborative (EPCRC); European Association for Palliative Care (EAPC). Use of opioid analgesics in the treatment of cancer pain: evidence-based recommendations from the EAPC. Lancet Oncol 2012;13(2):e58–68. Review.

Cascorbi I, Sorge J, Strumpf M. Analgetika und Coanalgetika: Anwendung, gesetzliche Grundlagen und Probleme. In: Baron R, Koppert W, Strumpf M, Willweber-Strumpf A (eds). Praktische Schmerztherapie. 2nd ed. Berlin–Heidelberg–New York: Springer, 2011: pp. 229–270.

Clark D. From margins to centre: a review of the history of palliative care in cancer. Lancet Oncol 2007;8:430–438. Available at: www.thelancet.com/journals/lanonc/article/PI-IS1470-2045(07)70138-9/fulltext (last accessed August 2012).

Davies AN, Dickman A, Reid C, Stevens AM, Zeppetella G. The management of cancer-related breakthrough pain: recommendations of a task group of the Science Committee of the Association for Palliative Medicine of Great Britain and Ireland. Eur J Pain 2009;13(4):331–338.

Doyle D, Hanks GWC, MacDonald N. Oxford Textbook of Palliative Medicine. 2nd ed. New York: Oxford University Press, 1999: pp. 249–281.

Ernst E, Cassileth B. The prevalence of complementary/alternative medicine in cancer: a systematic review. Cancer 1998;83:777–782.

Felleiter P, Gustorff B, Lierz P, Hornykewycz S, Kress HG. Einsatz der WHO-Leitlinien für die Tumorschmerztherapie vor Zuweisung in eine Schmerzklinik. Der Schmerz 2005;19(4):265–271.

Ferrell BA, Josephson KR, Pollan AM, Loy S, Ferrell BR. A randomized trial of walking versus physical methods for chronic pain management. Aging Clin Exp Res 1997;9:99–105.

Filshie J. Acupuncture for malignant pain. Acupunct Med 1990;8:38–39.

Filshie J. Acupuncture in palliative care. Eur J Palliat Care 2000;7:41–44.

Filshie J, Thompson JW. Acupuncture and TENS. In: Simpson K, Budd K (eds). Cancer Pain management. Oxford: Oxford University Press, 2000: pp. 188–200.

Gambles M, Crooke M, Wilkinson S. Evaluation of a hospice based reflexology service: a qualitative audit of patient perceptions. Eur J Oncol Nurs 2002;6:37–44.

Graeff A de, Van Bommel J, Van Deijck R, et al. Palliatieve zorg. Richtlijnen voor de praktijk. Utrecht: Vereniging van Integrale Kankercentra, 2010: pp. 537–540.

Greater Manchester and Cheshire Cancer Network (GMCCN). GMCCN-metastatic spinal cord compression rehabilitation pathway, 2011. Available at: http://www.gmccn.nhs.uk/portal_repository/files/MetastaticSpinalCordCompressionCarepathwayNamedLeads.doc (last accessed August 2012).

Greenhalgh S, Turnpenney, Richards L, Self J. Metastatic spinal cord compression (MSCC) key red flags. Briefing paper: The use of red flags to identify serious spinal pathology, 2010. Available at: http://www.gmccn.nhs.uk/portal_repository/files/TheuseofRedFlagstoidentifyseriousspinalpathology-briefingpaper.pdf (last accessed August 2012).

Grond S, Zech D, Diefenbach C, Radbruch L, Lehmann KA. Assessment of cancer pain: a prospective evaluation in 2,266 cancer patients referred to a pain service. Pain 1996;64:107–114.

Harel R, Angelov L. Spine metastases: current treatments and future directions. Eur J Cancer 2010;46:2,696–2,707.

Husband DJ, Grant KA, Romaniuk CS. MRI in the diagnosis and treatment of suspected malignant spinal cord compression. Br J Radiol 2001;74:15–23.

Koppert W, Dern SK, Sittl R, Albrecht S, Schüttler J, Schmelz M. A new model of electrically evoked pain and hyperalgesia in human skin. Anesthesiology 2001;95(2):395–402.

Levack P, Graham J, Collie D, et al. Don't wait for a sensory level – listen to the symptoms: a prospective audit of the delays in diagnosis of malignant cord compression. Clin Oncol 2002;14:472–480.

McCaffery M. Nursing practice theories related to cognition, bodily pain, and man-environment interactions. Los Angeles: University of California at LA, 1968.

McLinton A, Hutchinson C. Malignant spinal cord compression: a retrospective audit of clinical practice at a UK regional cancer centre. Br J Cancer 2006;94:486–491.

Melzack R, Wall PD. Pain mechanisms: a new theory. Science 1965;150:971–979.

Mercadante S, Zagonel V, Breda E, et al. Breakthrough pain in oncology: a longitudinal study. J Pain Symptom Manag 2010;40(2):183–190.

Merskey H, Bogduk N. Pain terms: a current list with definitions and notes on usage. In: Mersky H, Bogduk N (eds). Classification of Chronic Pain. 2nd ed. Seattle, MI: International Association for the Study of Pain Task Force on Taxonomy (IASP) Press, 1994: pp. 209–214.

Merskey H. Pain and psychological medicine. In: Wall PD, Melzack R (eds). Textbook of Pain. 4th edition. Edinburgh: Churchill Livingstone 1999: pp. 940–941.

National Cancer Action Team (NCAT). Rehabilitation care pathway metastatic spinal cord compression, 2010. Available at: http://www.gmccn.nhs.uk/hp/portal_repository/files/SymptomSpecificPathways.pdf (last accessed August 2012).

National Institute for Health and Clinical Excellence (NICE). Metastatic spinal cord compression: diagnosis and management of patients at risk of or with metastatic spinal cord compression. Full guideline. Cardiff: National Collaborating Centre for Cancer, 2008.

NICE Clinical Guideline 140. Opioids in palliative care: safe and effective prescribing of strong opioids for pain in palliative care of adults. Issued May 2012. Available at: http://guidance.nice.org.uk/cg140 (last accessed August 2012).

Pan CX, Morrison RS, Ness J, Fugh-Berman A, Leipzig M. Complementary and alternative medicine in the management of pain, dyspnoea, and nausea and vomiting near the end of life: a systematic review. J Pain Symptom Manage 2000;20:374–387.

Patchell RA, Tibbs PA, Regine WF, et al. Direct decompressive surgical resection in the treatment of spinal cord compression caused by metastatic cancer: a randomised trial. Lancet 2005;366:643–648.

Pease NJ, Harris RJ, Finlay IG. Development and audit of a care pathway for the management of patients with suspected malignant spinal cord compression. Physiotherapy 2004;90:27–34.

Reckinger K. Schmerztherapie bei Palliativpatienten. In: Baron R, Koppert W, Strumpf M, Willweber-Strumpf A (eds). Praktische Schmerztherapie. 2nd ed. Berlin–Heidelberg–New York: Springer, 2011: pp. 413–422.

Robb K, Bennett M, Johnson M, Simpson K, Oxberry S. Transcutaneous electric nerve stimulation (TENS) for cancer pain in adults. Cochrane Database Syst Rev 2008(3):1–5.

Robb K, Ewer-Smith C. Cancer pain. In: Rankin J, Robb K, Murtagh N, Cooper J, Lewis S (eds). Rehabilitation in Cancer Care. Chichester: Wiley-Blackwell, 2008: pp. 280–302.

Saunders C. Nature and management of terminal pain. In: Shotter EF (ed). Matters of Life and Death. London: Dartman, Longman and Todd, 1970: pp. 15–26.

Serlin C, Mendoza T, Nakamura Y, Edwards K, Cleeland C. When is cancer pain mild, moderate or severe? Grading pain severity by its interference with function. Pain 1995;61:277–284.

Souvlis T, Wright A. The tolerance effect: Its relevance to analgesia produced by physiotherapy interventions. Phys Ther Rev 1997;2:227–237.

Stubberfield MD, Bilsky MH. Barriers to rehabilitation of the neurological spine cancer patient. J Spin Oncol 2007;95:419–426.

Tang V, Harvey D, Park D'Orsay J, Jiang S, Rathbone MP. Prognostic indicators in metastatic spinal cord compression: using functional independence measure and Tokuhashi scale to optimise rehabilitation planning. Spin Cord 2007;45:671–677.

The Christie NHS Foundation Trust. Guidelines for the management of malignant spinal cord compression, 2011. Available at: www.Christie.nhs.uk/the-foundation-trust/treatments-and-clinical-services/spinal-cord-compression.aspx (last accessed: August 2012).

Thompson JW, Filshie J. Transcutaneous electrical nerve stimulation (TENS) and acupuncture. In: Doyle D, Hanks G, MacDonald N (eds). Oxford Textbook of Palliative Medicine. Oxford: Oxford University Press, 1998: pp. 421–437.

Tytgat GN. Hyoscine butylbromide: a review of its use in the treatment of abdominal cramping and pain. Drugs 2007;67(9):1,343–1,357. Review.

Wells P. Movement education and limitation of movement. In: Wall PD, Melzack R (eds). Textbook of Pain. 3rd ed. Edinburgh: Churchill Livingstone, 1994: pp. 741–750.

Wewers ME, Lowe NK. A critical review of visual analogue scales in the measurement of clinical phenomena. Res Nurs Health 1990;13:227–236.

Williamson G, Schultz R. Activity restriction mediates the association between pain and depressed affect: a study of younger and older cancer patients. Psychol Aging 1995;10:369–378.

World Health Organization (WHO). Cancer Pain Relief. 2nd ed. Geneva: World Health Organisation, 1996. Available at: http://whqlibdoc.who.int/publications/9241544821.pdf (last accessed: August 2012).

Zeppetella G, Ribeiro MD. Opioids for the management of breakthrough (episodic) pain in cancer patients. Cochrane Database Syst Rev. 2006;(1):CD004311.

BIBLIOGRAPHY

Filshie J, White A. Complementary therapies for cancer pain. In: Sykes N, Fallon M (eds). Clinical pain management. London: Edward Arnold, 2002.

Kilbride L, Cox M, Kennedy CM, Hwa Lee S, Grant R. Metastatic spinal cord compression: A review of practice and care. J Clin Nurs 2010;19:1,767–1,783.

Robinson AJ, Lynn Snyder-Mackler. Clinical Electrophysiology: Electrotherapy and Electrophysiologic Testing. 3rd ed. Baltimore, MD: Lippincott Williams & Wilkins, 2007.

Twycross R. Cancer pain syndromes. In: Sykes N, Fallon M, Patt R (eds). Clinical Pain Management: Cancer Pain. London: Arnold, 2003: p. 3.

World Health Organization (WHO). Cancer pain and relief. Technical reports series 804. Geneva: World Health Organization, 1990.

2.3 Respiratory symptoms: dyspnoea/breathlessness from airway obstruction and impaired oxygen capacity

Eva Müllauer

Dyspnoea on exertion is one of the initial symptoms of airway obstruction and impaired oxygen capacity. This chapter primarily addresses the causes, i. e. how to treat what is causing the dyspnoea, in many pulmonological patients. If they are not treated sufficiently, a serious shortness of breath and anxiety can result. This complex system is discussed in detail in ➤ Chapter 2.4 below.

In the introductory case study, a female patient exhibits both symptoms along with their sequelae, all of which are very pronounced. The triggers are then listed, the treatment approaches described and the topic of 'cough' examined. Ultimately, the measures are discussed which are perceived as helpful irrespective of the underlying diagnosis in the terminal phase.

A number of patients who are affected are not found in palliative care units or hospices, but in a hospital where they have been admitted for acute exacerbation and where they are receiving care in the palliative stage of their disease. The case study also aims to illustrate how, for ethical reasons, a curative approach must also be taken with acute events, even during the preterminal or terminal phase.

2.3.1 Case study

Initial assessment   Mrs S. is 65 years old and has been admitted by the department of respiratory and lung diseases due to exacerbation of her chronic obstructive pulmonary disease (COPD). The unit's physiotherapist has been instructed to undertake inhalation training and clearance of secretion. Mrs S. is dependent on long term oxygen therapy (LTOT).

At the first assessment, the therapist finds the patient half-sitting in bed. The first impression is that she is remarkably calm, despite finding it very difficult to breathe in and out. She is responsive, but at times seems absent and very tired. Mrs S. is receiving 2 litres of oxygen per minute via nasal cannula. She frequently rolls her eyes and repeatedly attempts to breathe out with pursed lips. The therapist introduces himself and explains that he is aware of the hazardous situation due to her evident lack of breath and will try to help her. He tests the situation by initially touching the patient's shoulder to see if she can tolerate physical contact or feels threatened. He then takes her hand and assures her that he can see the effort it is taking to breathe. The therapist is calm and confident, and explains to Mrs S. that he is going to place his other hand on her chest in order to feel whether there is a problem with secretion. The sternum and ribs of the patient protrude, and respiratory movements are detectable at the upper thoracic level. The therapist can see that the sagittal thorax diameter is considerably enlarged. Secretions are neither audible nor palpable at this point.

Functional problem in the acute setting   The pronounced pulmonary disease has greatly impaired the vital function of breathing, both in terms of inspiration and – to a greater extent – expiration. Active movement and speech are almost impossible. Mrs S. exhibits severe speech and resting dyspnoea. Nevertheless, she attempts to maintain the conditioned behaviour: breathing in through the nose to benefit from the oxygen, breathing out through pursed lips to counteract the obstruction.

Physiotherapeutic goals in the acute setting:
1. Gain the patient's confidence and convey assurance in order to prevent onset of panic.
2. Reduce the airway obstruction in order to relieve the dyspnoea.

Physiotherapeutic strategy in the acute setting   To reduce the dyspnoea, the therapist prepares for the prescribed inhalation with a bronchodilating drug using a nebuliser and attached PEP (positive expiratory pressure) device to prevent the airways from collapsing. The therapist should expect frequent intervals to ensue during the inhalation process due to the patient's need for oxygen, hence an additional oxygen line is connected to the PEP attachment (➤ Figure 2.8). This ensures that Mrs S. is supplied with oxygen both during the inhalation procedure as well as when breathing in through the nose when taking a break. The therapist explains to the patient that he wishes to consult the doctor before carrying out the planned procedure and that he will return in a few minutes. He makes sure that the patient is positioned comfortably and encourages her to breathe out through pursed lips as often as possible.

After consulting the ward doctor, the blood gases are measured and inhalation is prepared by the therapist. To avoid any stress, he uses continuous nebulisation instead of an interval nebuliser in which depression of the interrupter button has to be coordinated with the patient's respiration, which in the patient's present condition could not be achieved independently. Mrs S. takes a few breaths from the mouthpiece, breathing through the nebuliser and also through the attached PEP device. When taking a break, she breathes through the nasal cannula and mouth. Since having to constantly breathe out through pursed lips was initially too strenuous, the patient breathes with the mouth slightly open, while emitting a *'whee, whee, whee'* sound. This phonetic sequence has a similar effect to an oscillating PEP system and reduces respiratory resistance. Since Mrs S. is weak from the breathing exercise, the therapist holds the handpiece of the nebuliser during the entire 30-minute inhalation procedure, including the intervals. The effect of the medication is relatively rapid thanks to the excellent compliance of the patient.

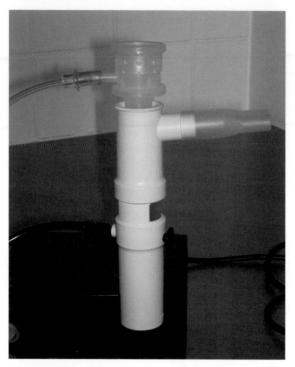

Figure 2.8 LL nebuliser with PEP attachment and oxygen line [M544]

On completing inhalation, the respiratory rate has dropped and breathing appears to be slightly less laboured. As there is a danger of the carbon dioxide content of the blood being very high, the therapist prepares the patient for the possible use of non-invasive ventilation using a full face mask (➤ Figure 2.10). He explains the nature and function of the mask and stresses the support that will be provided by the mask both during inspiration and expiration. Subsequently the patient is transferred to the monitoring station with a carbon dioxide level of 84 mm Hg (normal value: <44 mm Hg), receiving non-invasive ventilation from a face mask in BIPAP (bilevel positive airway pressure) mode.

Further procedures   The patient is found to be much improved the next day. Her blood carbon dioxide level has dropped to below 60 mm Hg and the resting or speech dyspnoea has disappeared. The patient reports that she feels much better. The first thing she says to the therapist is: *'You were such a great help yesterday! You were very reassuring and made me feel very safe! I'm feeling much better.'* To stabilise the situation, Mrs S. needs to regularly inhale bronchodilatory medications as well as undergo regular PEP therapy. This will reduce the airway obstruction on the one hand, and help to stabilise or even reduce the emphysema on the other. In turn, the respiratory effort will be reduced and quality

of life improved. PEP therapy is also an adjuvant means of clearing secretions. Further goals for the therapist are to explain how to carefully handle the prescribed oxygen, as well as strengthen the muscles and provide functional training at the request of the patient, who says: *'My whole body is so weak.'* The doctor proposes continuation of the non-invasive BIPAP ventilation at night. This should help not only to better control the carbon dioxide levels in the patient's blood, but also relieve the diaphragm and thus prevent diaphragmatic fatigue.

Ongoing management   The scheduled measures are performed for a few days, though the patient continues to weaken despite all the efforts made, reaching the terminal stage of her illness. The therapist adjusts his approach accordingly and omits the PEP therapy since it is proving too strenuous for Mrs S. The strengthening exercises are also discontinued. The inhalation procedure is continued with the assistance of the therapist or nursing staff until two days before the patient's death. Mrs S. was also given leg or hand massages with an essential oil of her choice. No further episodes of acute congestion or dyspnoea occurred before the patient died.

⚠ **CAUTION**

Patients in acute respiratory situations often feel constrained! On first examining the patient, give them sufficient space and refrain from repositioning them as would be necessary for auscultation, for instance. Establish whether the patient is able to cope with hands-on techniques in such a situation.

2.3.2 Airway obstruction in the palliative care setting

Airway obstruction in the palliative care context can have various causes, only some of which can be influenced to a certain extent by physiotherapeutic interventions – hence physiotherapy cannot always primarily alleviate the symptoms. In the case of a tumour constricting the airways, for example, surgery or radiotherapy is the first line of action, where possible. However, radiation can cause tracheal stenosis or even tracheo-oesophageal fistulae to develop. In turn these lead to obstruction of the airways and also, in the case of a fistula, to aspiration difficulties. The symptoms can usually be relieved by insertion of a stent. In such cases, physiotherapy can be of valuable support, helping to alleviate the patient's breathlessness by means of saving energy, pacing and relaxation techniques.

The domain of respiratory physiotherapy broadly covers the management of airflow reduction due to increased airway resistance, and/or enhancing pulmonary compliance. Physiotherapeutic measures can help considerably in relieving the symptoms associated with these problems. Conditions that typically entail a reduction in airflow as well as secretory obstruction of the airways are **COPD, cystic fibrosis (CF)** or **panbronchiolitis.** Whereas CF is characterised by abnormally tenacious sputum, inflammation is the dominant component of COPD, leading primarily to destruction of the small airways and thus to airway obstruction (Hogg 2004). In the case of panbronchiolitis, which is mostly seen in Asia, inflammation is likewise the overriding factor that leads to airway obstruction (Visscher/Myers 2006).

Assessment and physiotherapeutic examination

The **clinical pattern** exhibited by the patient often masks the true extent of the disease due to adaptation processes that occur when dealing with a chronic condition. It is therefore helpful and wise to revert to **objective parameters** that can be examined with the help of a lung X-ray, blood gas analysis and pulmonary function tests. These parameters provide the therapist with information on the issues of secretion, the degree of airway obstruction, the existence of pulmonary emphysema and the presence and extent of any respiratory insufficiency. Such data can be used for designing a suitable therapeutic programme.

If the patient has been admitted in an acute respiratory condition, or is not on a respiratory ward, results of tests may not be readily available, and the therapist will need to rely primarily on his **physiotherapeutic assessment findings** (➤ Table 2.3).

⚠ **C A U T I O N**

If the patient is found to be in an **acute respiratory state** only a very limited number of physiotherapeutic assessments can be performed. The therapist will therefore have to rely mainly on **visual findings** and select his approach on that basis.

Physiotherapy for airway obstruction

Important methods for treating airway obstruction are the **inhalation** of bronchodilating and anti-inflammatory medications, **PEP therapy** and patient **training** with

Table 2.3 Physiotherapeutic examination

Assessment	What to assess
Visual findings	Posture and position of the patient, signs of hypoxaemia, shape of the chest, thoracic symmetry, use of accessory breathing muscles, respiratory and heart rate, respiratory pattern, airway position, breathing rhythm, paradoxical movements, respiratory sounds
Palpation	Skin temperature, secretory vibrations, position of trachea, shape of chest wall, pain triggered by touch
Patient questioning	Shortness of breath (when? triggered by? what helps? dyspnoea scale!); cough (when? productive? appearance of mucus? how much mucus?); pain (when? triggered by? what helps?)
Auscultation	Secretions? reduced air entry?

a view to crisis management and conserving energy in their activities of daily living. If a secretion problem is causing the airway obstruction, inhalations – also for stimulating secretion – and measures for **mucus clearance and expectoration** can likewise be applied.

Inhalation therapy

Inhalation therapy is a suitable means of **relieving the symptoms of exertional dyspnoea** as well as **speech and resting dyspnoea** (a manifestation of airway obstruction) if the given conditions are advanced. There is adequate evidence to suggest that bronchodilating and anti-inflammatory, inhalational drugs have a positive effect on COPD (Albert/Calverley 2008) and CF (Hess 2007). The efficacy of expectorant inhalations in CF has not yet been adequately proven (Hess 2007). In the opinion of the author, however, the effect in many patients is positive, loosening the secretions from the mucous membrane and facilitating turbulence and expectoration.

In palliative care patients, the method of administration of the drug to be inhaled is particularly important. Whereas **powder inhalations** require a certain degree of inspiratory strength on the part of the patient in order to be effective, this is not the case with **metered dose aerosols** or **moist inhalations** (Laube et al. 2011). The latter two differ in terms of inhalation time, namely a few seconds and roughly 15 minutes per active ingredient, respectively. An appropriate method of administration must be chosen to suit the patient's condition and dexterity. As far as possible, therapy should entail moist inhalation.

The devices used here can be combined with PEP systems and thus prevent dynamic hyperinflation with the deeper breaths during inhalation. At the same time, exhalation against resistance will mobilise the secretions. The inhaled aerosol (particles of active ingredient dissolved in liquid) moistens the airways, which in turn helps to transport the mucus. The less the patient drinks, the more important this becomes. Most hand-held devices can also be connected to an oxygen line during inhalation, meaning that patients who require oxygen do not have to take a break during the inhalation procedure. Pacing may be necessary due to the reduced general health of a patient, however, as described in the case study.

PEP therapy

PEP therapy permits the patient to **breathe out longer and more easily,** since the applied stenoses produce a positive expiratory pressure that stabilises the airways and patency on forced expiration. The smaller the stenosis, the greater the effect in the small airways which are no longer supported by cartilage. This is an appropriate method for **reducing resistance** and, in the case of increased compliance, **preventing the airways from collapsing.** This technique is one of the components of physiotherapy for COPD within the framework of respiratory rehabilitation (Clini/Ambrosino 2008). Evidence of its efficacy has also been seen in the treatment of CF (Placidi et al. 2006, Lester/Flume 2009). The simplest form of PEP is pursed lips, with which a pressure of approx. 7 mbar can be achieved. This will alleviate the breathing in the event of advanced or acute airway obstruction. For therapy to be more efficient, pressures of 20 to 100 mbar need to be applied, which in the case of acute dyspnoea is not possible.

A pressure gauge can be used with PEP systems to indicate the pressure developed, helping in the selection of the appropriate stenosis. Varying sizes of stenosis mean that different sections of the airways can be reached and the pressure as well as flow velocity can be regulated. This permits targeted movement of secretions. Therapy can be administered by the patients themselves in various starting positions or with the manual support of the therapist (using chest compressions). Preference should be given to continuous PEP systems over oscillating PEP systems (Flutter, Acapella® etc.) if the condition is very advanced. Oscillating systems can cause bleeding in the bronchial system, a common complication in CF (Flume 2009).

Non-invasive ventilation

Non-invasive ventilation (NIV) is likewise a means for **mobilising the secretion in CF patients** (Windisch

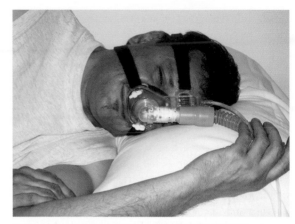

Figure 2.9 CF patient on NIV via nasal mask [M544]

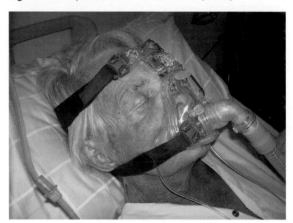

Figure 2.10 COPD patient on NIV via full face mask [M544]

et al. 2010). Such therapy can on the one hand help the diaphragm to recover, and on the other hand allow sufficient air to reach the mucus so that it can be mobilised more easily (➤ Figure 2.9, ➤ Figure 2.10). A number of CF patients suffer from diaphragmatic weakness on account of pronounced pulmonary hyperinflation and permanently increased respiratory effort.

NIV should be offered to those affected as soon as possible. This enables the use of smaller nasal masks and acclimatisation to the device before the situation becomes life-threatening, as unfortunately happened in the case study.

NIV does not offer any major improvement in patients whose COPD is stable (Kolodziej et al. 2007). In the event of **acute exacerbation of COPD (AECOPD)**, however, NIV is superior to standard pharmacological therapy (Clini/Ambrosino 2008) and is increasing in use (Chandra et al. 2012). The physiotherapist should prepare the patient for the ventilation procedure and face mask in order to increase compliance (see Case Study). If no physiotherapist is available, this can usually be carried out by the nursing staff. Palliative NIV is a means of relieving the symptoms in patients with **end-stage COPD.** It reduces dyspnoea even if hypercapnic respiratory failure has not occurred (Cuomo et al. 2004). NIV is a suitable palliative measure if the patient and/or family have decided against life-prolonging measures and would prefer comfort and quality of life (Curtis et al. 2007).

Further techniques for mucus clearance

Further approaches for counteracting airway obstruction through mucus clearance are to **position** the patient appropriately as well as to use the **Active Cycle of Breathing Technique (ACBT)** or **autogenic drainage.** Positioning is also a successful method, even in the very advanced stages of a disease. Movements elicited in the bronchial system by inspiration and expiration work like shear forces and more or less 'mechanically' turn the secretions into liquid. In such a way, the mucus can be transported more easily by the cilia. Using gravitational effects, mobilisation is greatest in an adult patient lying on his side. To get the mucus moving, therefore, it is beneficial to alternate the patient's position between left and right (Schenker 2000).

ACBT and autogenic drainage require the concentration of the patient and stable airways in order to clear the mucus from all areas of the lungs (Lester/Flume 2009). In order for autogenic drainage to be effective, it is necessary to briefly hold the breath after inhaling through the open glottis (Agostini/Knowles 2007) – something which is seldom possible in patients who are already short of breath due to airway obstruction. Hence, in the opinion of the author, neither technique can be applied to full effect in palliative care patients.

Cough generally develops towards the end of secretion mobilisation, effecting clearance of the mucus. This is a complicated process triggered by a reflex that serves to protect the airways. The cough depends on an **intact respiratory pump** with all its components: the respiratory centre in the brain stem, central and peripheral nerves, bony thorax and respiratory muscles.

Obstructive ventilatory disorders such as COPD and CF impair the respiratory pump. One of the triggers is a rigid thorax (from massive hyperinflation of the lungs due to airway obstruction), the other a weakness in the respiratory muscles. The muscles become fatigued due to the constant imbalance between exertion and pump capacity (Oczenski/Werba/Andel 2000). The outcome of a weak cough is secretion congestion which in turn leads to obstruction of the airways, as well as the development of atelectases and subsequent hypoxaemia and hypercapnia.

There are various physiotherapeutic techniques for supporting the patient appropriately when a **weak cough** develops. Such techniques should be practised early on by patients with COPD and CF. It is important to begin by **training the respiratory muscles** as soon as the maximum inspiratory pressure (MIP) drops to below 60 mm Hg. Learning to **huff** (forced exhalation with open glottis) as part of the autogenic drainage and ACBT procedures can be useful as a 'cough substitute'. A mild form of '**air stacking**', whereby the patient breathes in several times without breathing out in between in order to get as much air as possible into the lungs and behind the mucus, can help to increase the pulmonary volume and render the cough more efficient. **Passive measures** such as the epigastric push, manual chest compression by the therapist when coughing and stabilisation of the abdominal wall using a belt, can all be supportive in the cough process.

Mechanical cough aids such as CoughAssist® or Pegaso Cough® have proven beneficial in patients with a high transverse lesion or neuromuscular disease (Windisch et al. 2010). They are less suitable in obstructive diseases, however (Winck et al. 2004). The CoughAssist® package leaflet lists emphysema as a contraindication. Complications such as circulatory problems or pneumothorax have been observed in obstructive diseases.

Aspiration is also to be viewed critically since when too deep or repeated too often it can lead to inflammatory changes and thus to the intensified development of secretions. If large quantities of secretions cannot be coughed up from the trachea or pharynx, then the patient must be suctioned in order to prevent agonising suffocation.

2.3.3 Impaired oxygen capacity in the palliative care setting

The following section addresses the role of physiotherapy in chronic respiratory hypoxaemia. For better understanding, an explanation is first provided of the important terms and normal values.

Arterial **oxygen saturation** (SaO_2) in the blood ranges from 95 % to 98 % and indicates the amount of haemoglobin that has been saturated with oxygen. SaO_2 depends on the **partial oxygen pressure** (paO_2) which, when measured in the arterial blood, is between 70 and 105 mm Hg and decreases with age (Oczenski/Werba/Andel 2000). The **oxygen content** in arterial blood is determined from the haemoglobin concentration and SaO_2. The paO_2 concentration is reduced in the presence of primary arterial hypoxia. In the palliative care setting, it is often caused by severe pulmonary dysfunction (**chronic respiratory hypoxaemia**). This should be distinguished from **anaemic hypoxia,** as seen in cancer patients, which is caused by a drop in the concentration of functional haemoglobin (Thews/Vaupel 2005). The patients concerned may be found to have normal levels of SaO_2, but the paO_2 concentration will be reduced.

Severe pulmonary dysfunction, which can lead to chronic respiratory hypoxaemia, occurs both with obstructive ventilatory disorders such as COPD or CF and with restrictive ventilatory disorders such as pulmonary fibrosis. Chest deformities and neuromuscular diseases can likewise result in arterial hypoxaemia (Aigner et al. 2001). Whilst it tends to progress slowly in the presence of obstructive ventilatory disorders, it can advance quite rapidly in the case of pulmonary fibrosis. The **cardinal symptom is always dyspnoea,** which initially appears as exertional dyspnoea. **Training is invariably an expedient intervention if hypoxaemia has not developed** (Clini/Ambrosino 2008, Spruit et al. 2009). **Long-term oxygen therapy** (**LTOT**) at least brings temporary relief and improves quality of life in the case of chronic hypoxaemia.

Long-term oxygen therapy (LTOT)

Studies by the NOTT (*Nocturnal Oxygen Therapy Trial*) Group and MRC (*Medical Research Council*) Working Party resulted in the introduction of **criteria and guidelines for LTOT** in almost every industrial nation (Rous 2008). Its prescription is now clearly regulated as a result, with reimbursement of the costs depending on the country concerned. Whilst there is evidence to back the use of long-term oxygen therapy in COPD with a view to quality of life (Corrado/Renda/Bertini 2010), this cannot be confirmed in CF (Elphick/Mallory 2011). From experience, the author can confirm that both patients with CF and those with pulmonary fibrosis benefit from such treatment since they can lead a more active life due to (re)gained mobility.

The criteria for LTOT help in determining the quantity of oxygen that should be delivered to a patient when at rest, on exertion and during the night. Which oxygen system (liquid oxygen or oxygen concentrator) is used and the method with which the oxygen should be applied (by **mask** or **cannula**) should ideally be determined by the physiotherapist in discussion with the patient. Essential to this decision is the quantity of oxygen to be administered per minute, since there are fewer oxygen devices that can deliver more than 6 L/min. A further criterion that influences the choice of device is the

airway most suitable for the patient. **Mobile devices** which are very light and can also be used when lying down are particularly suitable for palliative care patients (➤ Figure 2.11), but these only function properly if administered via the nose.

If a patient with dyspnoea prefers to breathe through the mouth, it is best to use an oxygen mask. The **Oxy-Mask™**, entailing an open oxygen delivery system, is ideal. The openings in the mask mean that liquids can be consumed through a straw, secretions can be mobilised with a PEP system, and suctioning is also possible in an emergency without having to interrupt the oxygen supply.

If the patient needs large quantities of oxygen, use of an oxygen mask should also be considered in order to relieve the nasal mucosa. Patients often tend to be dismissive of such an approach, however. If the patient insists on a nasal mask, care should be taken to ensure that it can deliver the required flow rate. Conventional nasal masks are designed to achieve a flow rate of up to 4 L/min. Patients with pulmonary fibrosis in particular often require 12 to 15 L/min on exertion, however. To this end there are special nasal masks and portable oxygen devices that should additionally be fitted with an appliance for humidifying the oxygen in order to protect the nasal mucosa.

When handling the oxygen, the physiotherapist generally assumes an advisory and educational role. The patient will only benefit if a system suitable to his requirements is prescribed and he and/or the family have a good

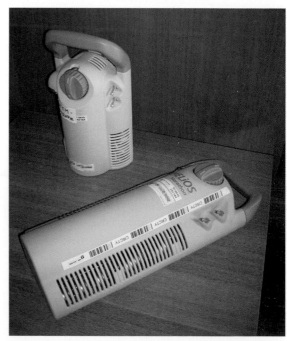

Figure 2.11 Helios™ Marathon and Helios™ 300 [M544]

command of the system. If the treatment is appropriate, the patient will be capable of pursuing activities of daily living without or with much less marked dyspnoea, and thus will experience an improvement in his quality of life.

> ⚠ **CAUTION**
> - Patients who smoke *and* have cognitive impairments may not be left unattended during LTOT. The oxygen must be switched off and the device removed when smoking.
> - Patients with hypercapnia must be advised not to independently increase the prescribed dose of oxygen, since they could fall into a CO_2 coma as a result.

Terminal phase physiotherapy

The measures discussed in ➤ Chapter 2. 4 are also used – albeit with limitations (adjusted relaxation techniques) – in patients with airway obstruction and impaired oxygen capacity during the terminal phase. In the author's experience, use of a fan to relieve breathlessness (Bausewein et al. 2010a) tends to be welcomed by patients with pulmonary fibrosis more than those with obstructive symptoms. Aromatherapy massages for alleviating anxiety and depression (Wilkinson et al. 2007) are beneficial not only in cancer patients, but also for patients with COPD, CF or PF.

> √ **GUIDANCE**
> Patients with advanced pulmonary diseases benefit most in a setting in which both specialist respiratory physiotherapists, doctors and nursing staff, as well as professionals trained in palliative care, are present.

2.3.4 Medication for breathlessness and associated symptoms
Claudia Bausewein

Symptomatic pharmacological therapy for breathlessness must always be viewed as an adjunct in combination with non-pharmacological measures and, above all, should only be used once all the treatable causes of the breathlessness (e.g. obstruction, left ventricular insufficiency, pleural effusion) have been adequately dealt with. Treatment for all chronic and advanced diseases (cancer, COPD, pulmonary fibrosis, etc.) should be symptomatic. This does not include acute conditions of respiratory distress, such as asthma or hyperventilation.

Medication should basically be given orally for as long as possible (tablets, liquids, sublingual, buccal, etc.).

Only if the patient can no longer swallow is parenteral (and above all subcutaneous) administration indicated.

Opioids

Opioids are the first-line choice when treating breathlessness in patients with malignant and non-malignant diseases. There is sound evidence to substantiate the use of oral and parenteral opioids, but not inhalational agents (Jennings et al. 2001). Opioids such as morphine are started at a low dose and titrated slowly according to their effect. A short-acting opioid with a duration of effect of approx. 4 hours is usually used to begin with (e.g. morphine drip) and is then switched, once the effective dose is reached, to a slow-acting, slow-release product for long-term management along with emergency medication. A dose titration study found that symptoms were alleviated satisfactorily in 70% of patients on 10 mg morphine/24 h (Currow et al. 2011). If the patient is already receiving opioids for pain management the dose may be increased or a different substance class chosen, though there is no evidence to back such an approach. There is also a lack of evidence concerning which opioid works best in the treatment of breathlessness. It is also unclear whether switching to a different opioid will be effective in the event that a patient does not respond to an opioid. Fast-acting opioids, e.g. fentanyl, will possibly become important to episodes of breathlessness in the future. Their use at present is based primarily on clinical experience, however, since to date there is a lack of alternative evidence.

Opioids have different side effects which must be taken into account and treated, as necessary (➤ Table 2.4).

Benzodiazepines

Benzodiazepines are often used in palliative care to treat breathlessness, especially if there is a pronounced element of anxiety. There is insufficient evidence, however,

Table 2.4 Opioid side effects and possible measures

Opioid side effect	Measures
Constipation	Prophylactic laxatives
Nausea	Antiemetics
Disorientation	Dose reduction, possible opioid rotation
Sedation	Dose reduction, possible opioid rotation
Respiratory depression	Provided that titration (gradual increase) of the opioids is aligned to the dyspnoea, respiratory depression will not occur.

to suggest that their use is beneficial in alleviating breathlessness (Simon et al. 2010). The anxiolytic component in benzodiazepines possibly plays a supportive role in the treatment of anxiety or panic – situations that are often encountered with dyspnoea. Benzodiazepines should be combined with opioids and should not be given alone (Simon et al. 2010). In addition to lorazepam, which has a good anxiolytic effect and is also available as tablets for dissolving in the mouth, diazepam (due to its prolonged duration of effect) and midazolam can be administered subcutaneously. Benzodiazepines with a shorter duration of effect (e. g. lorazepam and midazolam) can also be used as emergency medication, whereas those with a long duration of effect (e. g. diazepam) should be given at a fixed dosage.

Other medications for treatment of dyspnoea

In pulmonology in particular, low-strength neuroleptic agents such as promethazine and levomepromazine are used instead of benzodiazepines for sedation. Such use is based more on clinical experience than on study data, since the latter do not suffice to enable safety analysis (Simon/Bausewein 2009). Steroids are occasionally used in patients with carcinomatous lymphangiosis on the assumption that the peritumour oedema in the lymph tracts can be reduced. The available study data are very sparse, however. Steroids are only effective if used for several days.

Oxygen

Oxygen is often used as a reflex when treating breathlessness, without giving it much further thought. Pharmacological and non-pharmacological treatment, administered by a physiotherapist for example, is always preferable. Oxygen is often required when symptomatic therapy is being administered.

Oxygen saturation is an important criterion when deciding whether oxygen is indicated. To date, oxygen has not been found to offer any advantages over ambient air in non-hypoxic patients (O_2 saturation >90 %) (Abernethy et al. 2010). A large multicentre study did in fact report that symptoms were initially alleviated after administering oxygen or ambient air, but there was no difference between the two groups. The airflow is perhaps more likely to be responsible for the effect than the oxygen itself. Airflow can be produced much more easily and with less side effects by a table or hand-held fan (Abernethy et al. 2010, Galbraith et al. 2010).

Oxygen may be indicated in hypoxic patients; trial therapy should ensue in the individual case, however, in order to ascertain whether the patient gains any benefit. Evidence that the long-term administration of oxygen ($\geq$15 h per day) is beneficial to quality of life and survival has only been found in patients with COPD and hypoxia (Corrado/Renda/Bertini 2010). Caution is advised in the event of hypercapnia, however, since the respiratory output is reduced when correcting hypoxia. Oxygen should be viewed as a drug and may not be indiscriminately increased or decreased, but instead be adapted individually to each patient.

The advantages and disadvantages of oxygen must always be considered whenever it is prescribed. The administration of oxygen has a psychological effect (that 'something is being done') on both patient and carer, and certainly also has a placebo effect. In addition it is readily available, especially in hospital environments, meaning that its administration is often inadequately questioned. In parallel, patients can develop a psychological dependency on the 'tube' and become more difficult to discharge because oxygen administration in the outpatient setting, though possible, is very complex. The main side effect of which patients complain is dry mouth and nasal mucosa which to some extent may also bleed.

Medication for treatment of rattles

Rattles are a common symptom in the terminal phase. Though they can be very disturbing to those in the vicinity, it is not clear whether they cause patients suffering and, above all, whether patients suffer from breathlessness as a result.

Aside from reducing fluids and positioning, the bronchial secretion that causes the rattles can be attenuated by medication. In such a case, anticholinergic agents can be used in particular, such as butylscopolamine or glycopyrronium (Bausewein 2005). It is important that they are introduced early, because existing mucus cannot be influenced by such therapy.

2.3.5 Summary
Eva Müllauer

A diagnosis of COPD, CF or PF is often the basis for airway obstruction and impaired oxygen capacity. The patients will often have reached a very advanced stage of their disease and will be receiving care in an emergency hospital rather than at a palliative care unit or hospice if lung transplantation is not, or no longer possible. The need for palliative care is just as high in these patients as in cancer patients, however. Due to the complexity of the disease, it appears wise to continue caring for CF patients during the palliative phase at specialised CF units. Ideally, a palliative care team will administer support in line with the Palliative Care Guidelines and Pathways (Bourke et al. 2009). COPD patients suffer from the same symptoms as patients with lung cancer, though sometimes they may be more intense. Nevertheless they are provided with palliative care to a lesser degree (Gore/Brophy/Greenstone 2000; Bausewein et al. 2010b). Physiotherapists make a valuable contribution towards improved understanding of the disease and an integrated approach to therapy, as well as facilitating the smooth transition from management of a chronic disease to palliative care in the terminal phase (Michaud-Young/Rocker 2009). If patients wish to die at home, it is up to the team and also the physiotherapists to provide the necessary equipment and assistance for such care so that the situation can be managed by the family and any significant carers.

2.3.6 Reflective questions

- What is my level of expertise and which other skills should I acquire in order to adequately treat patients with airway obstruction in the acute and chronic phases of dyspnoea?
- If I think of my last patient who suffered from acute breathlessness – what could I have done differently?
- Where in my files can I find the LTOT guidelines?
- How could I optimise the multiprofessional care of patients with airway obstruction and impaired oxygen capacity in my working environment?
- Would it be useful to organise advanced training for my team on the subject of oxygen and respiratory apparatus?

REFERENCES

Abernethy AP, McDonald CF, Frith PA, et al. Effect of palliative oxygen versus room air in relief of breathlessness in patients with refractory dyspnoea: a double-blind, randomised controlled trial. Lancet 2010;376:784–793.

Agostini P, Knowles N. Autogenic drainage: the technique, physiological basis and evidence. Physiotherapy 2007;93:157–163.

Aigner K, Burghuber OC, Hartl S, et al. Verordnung von Sauerstofflangzeittherapie und mechanischen Atemhilfen. Richtlinien der Österreichischen Gesellschaft für Lungenerkrankungen und Tuberkulose (ÖGLUT). Atemw Lungenkrkh 2001;27(2):66–73.

Albert P, Calverley PM. Drugs (including oxygen) in severe COPD. Eur Respir J 2008;31:1,114–1,124.

Bausewein C. Symptome in der Terminalphase. Onkologe 2005;11:420–426.

Bausewein C, Booth S, Gysels M, Kühnbach R, Higginson IJ. Effectiveness of a hand-held fan for breathlessness: a randomised phase II trial. BMC Palliative Care 2010a;9:22.

Bausewein C, Booth S, Gysels M, Kühnbach R, Haberland B, Higginsons IJ. Understanding breathlessness: cross-sectional comparison of symptom burden and palliative care needs in chronic obstructive pulmonary disease and cancer. J Palliat Med 2010b;13(9):1,109–1,118.

Bourke SJ, Doe SJ, Gascoigne AD, Heslop K. An integrated model of provision of palliative care to patients with cystic fibrosis. Palliat Med 2009;23:512–517.

Chandra D, Stamm JA, Taylor B, et al. Outcomes of noninvasive ventilation for acute exacerbation of chronic obstructive pulmonary disease in the United States, 1998–2008. Am J Respir Crit Care Med 2012;185(2):152–159.

Clini EM, Ambrosino N. Nonpharmacological treatment and relief of symptoms in COPD. Eur Respir J 2008;32:218–228.

Corrado R, Renda T, Bertini S. Long-term oxygen therapy in COPD: evidences and open questions of current indications. Monaldi Arch Chest Dis 2010;73:34–43.

Cuomo A, Delmastro M, Ceriana P, et al. Noninvasive mechanical ventilation as a palliative treatment of acute respiratory failure in patients with end-stage solid cancer. Palliat Med 2004;18(7):602–610.

Currow DC, McDonald C, Oaten S, et al. Once-daily opioids for chronic dyspnea: a dose increment and pharmacovigilance study. J Pain Symptom Manag 2011;42:388–399.

Curtis JR, Cook DJ, Sinuff T, et al. Noninvasive positive pressure ventilation in critical and palliative care settings: understanding the goals of therapy. Crit Care Med 2007;35(3):932–939.

Elphick HE, Mallory G. Oxygen therapy for cystic fibrosis (review). The Cochrane Library 2011, Issue 3.

Flume PA. Pulmonary complications of cystic fibrosis. Respir Care 2009;54(5):618–627.

Galbraith S, Fagan P, Perkins P, Lynch A, Booth S. Does the use of a handheld fan improve intractable breathlessness? J Pain Symptom Manag 2010;39(5):831–838.

Gore JM, Brophy CJ, Greenstone MA. How well do we care for patients with end stage chronic obstructive pulmonary disease (COPD)? A comparison of palliative care and quality of life in COPD and lung cancer. Thorax 2000;55:1,000–1,006.

Hess DR. Airway clearance: physiology, pharmacology, techniques, and practice. Respir Care 2007;52(10):1,392–1,396.

Hogg JC. Pathophysiology of airflow limitation in chronic obstructive pulmonary disease. Lancet 2004;364:709–721.

Jennings AL, Davies AN, Higgins JP, Broadley K. Opioids for the palliation of breathlessness in terminal illness (review). Cochrane Database Syst Rev 2001(4): CD002066.

Kolodziej MA, Jensen L, Rowe B, Sin D. Systematic review of noninvasive positive pressure ventilation in severe stable COPD. Eur Respir J 2007;30:293–306.

Laube BL, Janssens HM, de Jongh FHC, et al. What the pulmonary specialist should know about the new inhalation therapies. Eur Respir J 2011;37:1,308–1,331.

Lester MK, Flume PA. Airway-clearance therapy guidelines and implementation. Respir Care 2009;54(6):733–750/751–753.

Michaud-Young J, Rocker GM. Facilitating palliative care in advanced COPD: a unique leadership opportunity for respiratory therapists. Can J Respir Ther 2009;45(4):27–29.

Oczenski W, Werba A, Andel H. Atmen – Atemhilfen: Atemphysiologie und Beatmungstechnik. 4. A. Berlin–Wien: Wiley-Blackwell, 2000.

Placidi G, Cornacchia M, Polese G, Zanolla L, Assael BM, Braggion C. Chest physiotherapy with positive airway pressure: a pilot study of short-term effects on sputum clearance in

2

patients with cystic fibrosis and severe airway obstruction. Respir Care 2006;51(10):1,145–1,153.

Rous RG. Long-term oxygen therapy: Are we prescribing appropriately? Int J Chron Obstruct Pulmon Dis 2008;3(2):231–237.

Schenker MA. Analytische Atemphysiotherapie. Untersuchung, Analyse und Behandlung in der Atemphysiotherapie. Bern: Edition Phi, 2000.

Simon ST, Bausewein C. Management of refractory breathlessness in patients with advanced cancer. Wien Med Wochenschr 2009;159:591–598.

Simon ST, Higginson IJ, Booth S, Harding R, Bausewein C. Benzodiazepines for the relief of breathlessness in advanced malignant and non-malignant diseases in adults. Cochrane Database Syst Rev 2010: CD007354.

Spruit MA, Janssen D, Franssen F, Wouters E. Rehabilitation and palliative care in lung fibrosis. Respirology 2009;14:781–787.

Thews G, Vaupel P. Vegetative Physiologie. 5th ed. Heidelberg: Springer Medizin, 2005.

Visscher DW, Myers JL. Bronchiolitis: the pathologist's perspective. Proc Am Thorac Soc 2006;3:41–47.

Wilkinson SM, Love SB, Westcombe AM, et al. Effectiveness of aromatherapy massage in the management of anxiety and depression in patients with cancer: a multicenter randomized controlled trial. J Clin Oncol 2007;25:532–539.

Winck JC, Goncalves MR, Lourenco C, Viana P, Lameida J, Bach JR. Effects of mechanical insufflation-exsufflation on respiratory parameters for patients with chronic airway secretion encumbrance. Chest 2004;126:774–780.

Windisch W, Walterspacher S, Karsten S, Geiseler J, Sitter H. S2-Guidelines for non-invasive and invasive mechanical ventilation for treatment of chronic respiratory failure. Pneumologie 2010;64(10):640–652.

2.4 Breathlessness and fear

Jenny Taylor

Breathlessness engenders fear, and as associated symptoms they present together as one of the most difficult challenges for physiotherapists caring for patients at the end of life. Breathlessness is described as a *'subjective experience of difficult, laboured or uncomfortable breathing'* (Zhao/Yates 2008, p. 693). The management of respiratory symptoms is a core skill of physiotherapists worldwide. In end of life care, respiratory and functional skills of the physiotherapist play a key role in a multiprofessional team approach, and are applied to good effect in palliating breathlessness and anxiety. Problems presented however will also be emotional and existential. The patient's clinical picture is often unstable, and the burden of symptoms extends to activity avoidance and consequent social isolation (Ek/Ternestedt 2008). Anxiety and panic can be very significant, but often hidden, components of the symptoms presented by patients referred for treatment. A range of strategies has been shown to markedly contribute to improved function and quality of life (Bausewein et al. 2008; Hately et al. 2003; Hoyal et al. 2002). In this chapter an overview of non-pharmacological physiotherapeutic strategies that can be implemented at end of life together with treatment models and contexts will be discussed; space precludes addressing diagnosis-specific issues. The following case study will help to illustrate many of the factors affecting the severely breathless patient, the various approaches to treatment, and the role of the physiotherapist in working with patients to improve management of these complex and distressing symptoms.

In this chapter aspects of context, presentation and physiotherapeutic approach to the breathless, fearful patient are addressed. Breathing control, coping strategies, anxiety management, and the pacing of functional activities are discussed together with innovative approaches to empower the patient through building confidence and independence. Optimizing management throughout the disease trajectory is achieved by a shifting balance of pharmacological and non-pharmacological approaches, and best practice uses a multiprofessional holistic approach. The aim is to keep control in the patient's hands (Corner et al. 1996; Hately et al. 2001), and at the heart of a whole team approach is understanding the patient (Krishnasamy et al. 2001; Luker et al. 2000).

2.4.1 Case study

John is a 68-year-old male, retired high-level civil servant (government executive) referred to physiotherapy by the Hospice Home Care Team for breathlessness and panic management. He is married and has long-term spinal problems. They have no children.

Diagnosis   Idiopathic pulmonary fibrosis, discovered after routine tests for episodic memory loss.

Past medical history
- angioplasty and coronary stent 12 years previously;
- long-term history of depression and associated panic attacks.

Recent history   Acute admission to hospital with deteriorating lung function, severe breathlessness and persistent cough. Discharged home on 2 litres of continuous oxygen, for 10 hours daily, and reducing steroids.

Assessment   John was breathless after a short walk to the physiotherapy department. He was accompanied by his wife, who was often tearful. Fiercely protective of her, John worried about the strain on her and also for her future. He tended to be dismissive of his symptoms, masked his respiratory compromise, and continued his customary preparation of meals and housework at home. His wife reported his erratic breathing rate at night. John said his sleep was undisturbed, however, but did acknowledge he slept much of the day. He reported using oxygen for 15 hours daily. John was very positive about physiotherapy input and open about his potential to panic; but he was depressed since his enforced recent resignation from gym membership.

On examination   His posture was tense, with elevated shoulders and he presented with constant peripheral fidgeting movements. His basal chest expansion was very limited, his chest was clear, and a rapid respiratory rate was exacerbated by conversation. His exercise tolerance had reduced to 300 metres. Oxygen saturation was measured with a pulse oximeter: at rest it registered 89%, on minimal exertion 87%, after recovery time 91% (within 2 minutes). John's main functional problem was climbing stairs, which provoked severe breathlessness and regular onset of panic. Although strongly intellectual in approach he also had a tendency to be introverted and found difficulty with self expression. He was reluctant to take prescribed morphine and anxiolytic, due to a misplaced fear of addiction.

Planned intervention   Weekly 1-hour session when attending Hospice Day Care.
Content:
- anatomy and physiology of respiration explained;
- relaxation strategies for posture and shoulder girdle;
- thoracic mobility exercises with breathing control, seated;
- breathing control from sitting to standing to walking;
- progressive step climbing incorporating breathing control;
- static bicycle exercise to increase tone in major lower limb muscles;
- pacing and coping techniques when mobilizing independently;
- planned rests with breathing control;
- mechanism of panic explored and strategies for the patient and his wife to manage;
- supplied with user leaflets on breathing, panic, pacing and coping advice;
- reassurance about pharmacological/non-pharmacological interaction;
- liaison with nurse.

Initial progress   After three individual sessions, improved oxygen saturation on exertion and confidence in pacing was noted. His oxygen saturation on exertion was 87%; after implementing breathing control strategy this rose to 98% (within 1 minute). John was introduced to a weekly circuits group with nine modalities for power/range lower/upper limbs, stamina and balance. These included: treadmill, trampoline, interactive technology balance board, reclining bicycle, reciprocal arm pulleys, hand weights, stairs. A home exercise programme was supplied. At a multiprofessional team meeting to discuss John's symptom management, additional intervention was planned as shown in ➤ Table 2.5.

Continued therapy   John continued with regular physiotherapy sessions for his breathing control and

Table 2.5 Multiprofessional input

Input	Professional	Goal
Fatigue and breathlessness management course (attended by John and wife)	• Cognitive behavioural therapist • Physiotherapist • Dietitian • Occupational therapist • Complementary therapist	• Avoiding negative thinking traps • Exercise with breathing control • Nutrition advice to combat fatigue • Energy saving tips and equipment • Relaxation and sleep advice
Singing and percussion (for John)	Music therapist	Enhance breathing control, reduce inhibition and empower self-expression and confidence
Spiritual care (for John and wife, together and separately)	Chaplain/pastor	Exploring faith, grief and loss issues, and planning funeral
Psychosocial support (for John and wife, together and separately)	Social worker	Partnership, financial welfare, adjustment and support issues
Aromatherapy massage (for wife)	Complementary therapist	Pampering, and relief of stress
In-depth medical discussion (with John and wife)	Consultant doctor	Reassurance about dying process and its management, after John admitted to feeling fearful that he would die 'gasping for breath'

particularly lower limb strength and function. Sessions continued during three admissions to the hospice inpatient unit (for two chest infections, and one planned respite for John's wife).

Goals met:
- The patient managed to exercise without his oxygen as he became less anxious.
- Oxygen saturation levels reverted quicker after exertion, using breathing control techniques.
- The patient rarely experienced panic feelings since receiving physiotherapy advice about breathing control strategies.
- Following hospital respiratory clinic review, the patient's oxygen was reduced from 2 l/min to 1 l/min.

Mobility:
- A wheelchair was loaned to enable John and his wife to go out to socialize more.
- A walking stick was supplied for John to use to pace his slow walking and breathing.
- The patient was able to climb stairs slowly and steadily (previously he had to stop every third step).
- The patient was no longer going to bed during the day, and his mood was very much improved.

Patient outcome

Both John and his wife described the Hospice programme as a *'lifeline'*, and John's motivation to attend was very high. Although still occasionally forgetful due to hypoxia, his wife said: *'he looks completely different after physiotherapy; brighter and more dynamic. He walks with a straighter back, feels uplifted and a "man" again'*.

As John's disease progressed, he sustained several falls as he became weaker. Nursed with support at home, he no longer struggled with his breathing. At the time of writing, John takes his regular medication, and feels well supported by the Hospice Home Care team. His worries for his wife's future coping have receded, and they both feel *'safe'*.

2.4.2 Context of breathlessness at end of life

Breathlessness (also known as dyspnoea) is a complex multifactorial symptom, which has been variously defined as an uncomfortable awareness of breathing (Gift 1990), more specifically as the subjective sensation of breathlessness that occurs when the demand for oxygen is greater than the body's ability to supply it (Regnard/Ahmedzai 1990) and when there is 'air hunger' (Simon et al. 1990). Like pain, it is subjective in nature. Past studies have shown that up to 75 % of patients with advanced cancer suffer from breathlessness (Ripamonti/Bruera 1997), and it affects over 50 % with end-stage AIDS, chronic obstructive airways disease (COPD), and heart and renal disease (Solano/Gomes/Higginson 2006). In a study of 923 cancer outpatients by Dudgeon et al. (2001a), 46 % were breathless, but only 4 % had lung cancer, and 5.4 % lung secondaries. Moreover, it has been described as amongst the top 10 most frequently occurring symptoms (Hately et al. 2003). On this background of complex presentation, a palliative care physiotherapist frequently observes that disease burden does not appear to correlate directly with the severity of breathlessness reported. Despite much investigation, the sensation of breathlessness is still not fully understood (O'Donnell et al. 2007). However, the fact that physical emotional and existential components of the symptom are inextricably bound together is now widely accepted, and a key approach is to help to reduce the perception of breathlessness by improving self management. The causes of breathlessness are wide-ranging (➤ Table 2.6), and the physiotherapist should be aware of co-existent pathologies often present in this patient group. Close liaison with members of the medical team is crucial, as some aspects of end of life breathlessness may be reversible. These may include chest infection, effusions, and anaemia, amongst others (NHS Lothian 2009). Pharmacological measures, including opiates and anxiolytics, make a significant contribution to the alleviation of symptoms. Nebulizers, for bronchodilatation or secretion clearance, oxygen provision, and NIPPV (non-invasive positive pressure ventilation) all may have a role to play. Chest clearance strategies have been addressed fully in a previous chapter (➤ Chapter 2.3).

The challenge of outcome measures in end of life breathlessness

In the current climate of survivorship the indications for physiotherapy intervention are broadening. As well as managing patients with progressive breathing difficulties in the acute terminal phase of their disease, physiotherapy is of significant benefit for many respiratory conditions with longer disease trajectories, and presenting with transient episodes of breathlessness. Evidence shows that early identification of respiratory problems and their impact on patients' everyday life is key to optimal management (Currow et al. 2009). Use of outcome

Table 2.6 Causes of breathlessness at end of life (adapted from Dudgeon/Rosenthal 1996)

Direct tumour related	Secondary
• Primary or metastatic pulmonary disease • Airway obstruction by tumour • Cancer of pleura • Pleural effusion • Pericardial effusion • Ascites • Microemboli • Superior vena cava obstruction • Lymphangitic carcinomatosis • Hepatomegaly • Phrenic nerve paralysis	• Cachexia • Anaemia • Pneumonia • Pulmonary aspiration • Pulmonary embolus • Neurologic paraneoplastic syndrome • Electrolyte abnormalities

Caused by cancer treatments	Non-cancer end-stage disease
• Surgery • Radiotherapy • Chemotherapy induced pulmonary disease • Chemotherapy induced cardiomyopathy	• Chronic obstructive airways disease (COPD) • Asthma • Congestive cardiac failure (CCF) • Interstitial lung disease • Neuromuscular disorders • Pulmonary vascular disease

Contributory
• Anxiety • Chest wall deformity • Obesity • Pneumothorax

measures – e.g. visual analogue scales (VAS), Borg modified scale, and others – is well researched and reviewed (Bausewein et al. 2007; Dorman et al. 2007); however, application is variable in this field. A consensus exists that finds measurement tools tend to focus on objective functional health and not on the patient's subjective 'uniqueness' (Carr/Higginson 2001). In the author's opinion, problems of appropriateness, response shift and issues of patient compliance conspire to make their use questionable at end of life.

Presenting features of the breathless patient

The extent of a patient's symptoms may not be immediately evident on initial presentation. Symptoms range from breathlessness on exertion, for example walking up slopes or climbing stairs, to difficulty even when speaking, eating or drinking. Some physical and behavioural features are commonly presented (see Cautions) Accessory muscle use increases fatigue and this, in turn, will increase

oxygen consumption. Pursed lip breathing is a characteristic feature for many patients managing long-standing progressive disease (Dechman/Wilson 2004). Thought to work by slowing the respiratory rate, raising the intra-airway pressure and decreasing small airway lung collapse, it nevertheless increases the intercostal muscle work of breathing. Its habitual nature is difficult for the physiotherapist to influence, or for the patient to correct; relaxation techniques may help. **But beyond visible signs, it is the hidden nature of the symptom that can impact greatly on patient/family/carer stress.** Frightening acute episodes induce feelings of helplessness and powerlessness. It is the *'heavy psychological burden that is so influential in restricting freedom'* (Bailey 1995, p. 186).

Refractory breathlessness in the terminal phase (that is where underlying causes have been addressed but the symptom is poorly controlled) is difficult for both patient and physiotherapist. Agitation and restlessness can cause much distress for patient, family and medical/nursing staff; seamless team-working is pivotal.

⚠ CAUTION

Breathlessness *is what the patient says it is,* not how the physiotherapist assesses it.
• Physical alerts: elevated shoulders, excessive use of accessory muscles of respiration (especially sternocleidomastoid and scalene muscles recruited to elevate the rib cage), neck tension, increased respiratory rate, hypoxia, peripheral cyanosis, frequent sighing, excessive yawning.
• Lifestyle alerts: anxiety, activity avoidance, breath holding on functional activity, sleep disturbance, poor concentration, irritability, poor appetite, reduced confidence and social isolation.

✓ GUIDANCE

Teach simple anatomy and physiology of breathing:
• Where are the lungs?
• How do they work?
• What is the diaphragm?
• How does inspiration and expiration work?
• How does breathing work when asleep?
• What happens when we exercise?
• Is breathlessness normal?
Address fears and restrictions in activity; be **realistic and honest** when goal-setting.
Breathing techniques need to be as **simple** and **non-challenging** as possible.

2.4.3 Effective physiotherapy strategies for managing breathlessness

Key to managing this complex symptom is mastery; that is, the patient's inherent ability to implement strategies to self-manage and cope. Confidence is enhanced by encouragement and positive reinforcement from an insightful physiotherapist, able to draw out the patient's inner resources and resilience. The initial assessment involves careful listening to the patient to instil trust and confidence.

Breathing control strategies

Breathing is a reflex and is central to life; existential distress is compounded for the patient by the rarely understood fact that respiration is essentially carbon-dioxide driven. Patients instinctively breathe in more deeply in an attempt to satisfy their air hunger. Explaining simply, but thoroughly, the anatomy and physiology of breathing is, in the author's experience, revelatory and of huge value to the patient. With supportive instruction, much relief is achieved by assisting the patient to extend the expiratory phase. This is best demonstrated by simple lateral costal hands-on contact as the physiotherapist breathes out slowly synchronized with the patient. This enables the patient to then feel the rib cage recoil immediately following the expiratory phase.

Techniques to improve trunk and rib cage mobility

Postural rigidity has a physical and psychological element due to deconditioned trunk and thoracic muscles, fear of exertion and gradually reducing functional activity. Relaxation techniques help to reduce tension (➤ Table 2.7). The focus is initially around the jaw, face, arms, shoulders and spine and then progresses to mobilizing, incorporating natural rhythmic movements.

The role of gentle exercise

Carefully modified exercises are best devised collaboratively with the patient. Patients' thoracic movements are often markedly reduced due to intercostal muscle weakness, deconditioning or pain.

Mechano-receptors in the intercostal muscles and diaphragm play a major role in communicating with higher centres controlling respiration; it is therefore important to engage these muscles to maximize their efficiency. Trunk exercises (➤ Table 2.7) have a dual effect of maximizing lung capacity and gently restoring often long-standing inhibited movement. By mobilizing the thorax, together with full-range arm and shoulder exercises, which have a supplemental impact on the rib cage,

Table 2.7 Exercises for trunk, rib cage and relaxation in breathlessness

Seated exercises for trunk and rib cage	Relaxation techniques for breathlessness
• Shoulder girdle elevation and retraction • Trunk/thoracic side-to-side rotation • Fingers on shoulders and full elbow circling • Trunk/thoracic side flexion • Bilateral arm elevation with stretch • Trunk forward flexion with breathing control	• Gentle stroking from jaw to neck and down arms • Lift shoulders, breathe in, then relax, sigh out • Breathe in 2, 3; then out 2, 3, 4, 5; relax ... • Focus on dropping shoulders before any activity • Make tight fists, hold, then relax hands and sigh • Lying flat, count slowly down from 10 to 1 • Relax each limb in turn, 10, 9, 8, 7, buttocks 6, abdomen 5, shoulders 4, neck 3, head 2, and face 1

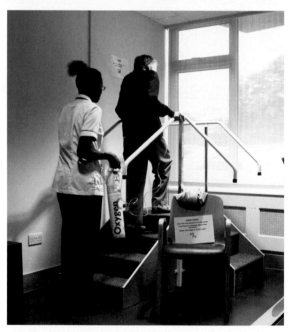

Figure 2.12 Supervised stair climbing with patient on continuous oxygen (© St Christopher's Hospice, London, UK) [T440]

a pectoral stretch is exerted that improves respiratory muscle capacity and resilience.

Aerobic exercise training has been shown to help breathing control (Nici et al. 2006), and if gently introduced incorporating careful pacing, it will push the boundaries of activity and enhance coping. A trial by Hochstetter et al. (Hochstetter/Lewis/Soares-Smith 2005) found that patients were able to incorporate stair-climbing techniques to positively impact breathlessness perception (➤ Figure 2.12).

Table 2.8 Supportive breathing control strategies for breathlessness and anxiety management (© St Christopher's Hospice, London, UK)

Strategy	Application	Rationale
Fan	Room, table or hand-held, directed across the face	This stimulates branches of the trigeminal nerve that react to mechanical and thermal stimuli and reduce perception of breathlessness (Galbraith et al. 2010; Schwartzstein et al. 1987).
Cold compress	Soft cloth wrung out with ice cold water produces cooling effect on the face	This is thought to lower heart rate, and conserve oxygen by mimicking aspects of the dive reflex (research ongoing).
Positioning	Upright or semi-reclined trunk position in chair or bed; head, arms and lumbar curve supported with pillows	Good anatomical support opens out the rib cage to allow greater diaphragm descent, and maximizes thoracic capacity.
Relaxation	Quiet undisturbed space, warm and comfortable; massage/aromatherapy; relaxation CDs, meditation, and hypnotherapy	Relaxation is induced via afferent impulses to the central nervous system; reduced tension and stress help to slow the heart rate and calm respiratory rate.
Reassurance and presence	Call bell, hands-on contact, planned family phone contact, community nursing team visits and support	Open discussion with patient, family and carers via medical team explores ways to meet anxieties in personalized way.
Acupressure	Sedation of lung meridian, anterior aspect of shoulder to thumb; stroking axilla to thumbnail; 60 sec pressure applied to thumbnail/wrist crease on little finger side of forearm, then slow release	Promotes endorphin response to encourage relaxation and relieve breathlessness; 70 % of patients reported relief that was short-lived, but with no side effects (Lewith et al. 2004).
TENS	Electrodes applied each side of T3 vertebral bodies; burst mode for 20 minutes	When applied to acupoints, effectiveness is commensurate with acupressure; no side effects and patient controlled.
Singing	individual or group intervention, led or self-directed	Helps lung function, breathing control, and builds confidence and morale (Lord et al. 2010).

The physiotherapist observes the patient's breathing rate throughout exertion, and works within the patient's comfort level. Monitoring oxygen saturation levels with a finger oximeter during exercise can be a revelation for some patients as it reassures by objectively showing the result of effective breathing control. The acutely breathless bedridden patient benefits from a range of approaches (➤ Table 2.8), but in the terminal phase pharmacological intervention gradually outweighs the non-pharmacological.

Referral to other professionals accesses further useful resources throughout the disease trajectory to help manage both breathlessness and anxiety (cf. ➤ Table 2.5). For the more able patient, group exercise in a supportive environment works well for breathlessness management (➤ Figure 2.13).

This can gently improve strength and activity to reach short-term goals within the restrictions imposed by diminishing lung function (Ambrosino/Strambi 2004; Gigliotti et al. 2003). Pacing and coping advice can be incorporated into patient and carer groups where opportunities exist to share experiences and helpful tips with other patients. This lifts morale and eases carer stress.

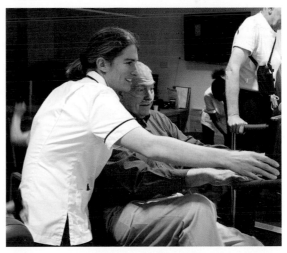

Figure 2.13 Achieving beyond expectations in a group setting (© St Christopher's Hospice, London, UK) [T440]

⚠ **C A U T I O N**
- Avoid focus on abdominal/diaphragmatic breathing and attempted correction of pursed lip breathing.
- Although **touch** can be reassuring and relaxing for the breathless patient, **know your patient!** Closeness can induce psychological discomfort through perceived invasion of personal space. It is a very individual preference.

2

• The physiotherapist sets activity goals *with* the patient, and not *for* the patient. This avoids crisis episodes, possible demoralization and a vicious circle of exertional failure.

✓ G U I D A N C E
• Acknowledge limitations.
• Explore simpler ways of carrying out tasks.
• Enlist help from others.
• Perform simple home exercises; for example: grip a door frame on each side and lean forward to gently open out the rib cage and expand the chest (Hough 1997).
• Avoid closed-in spaces.
• Avoid very hot showers/baths.
• Keep rooms well ventilated, especially at night.
• Sitting/lying by a window with an open view enhances perception of air availability.
• Utilize equipment and modifications that reduce exertion (refer to occupational therapist):
  – riser-recliner chair;
  – raised toilet seat;
  – walking stick or frame;
  – wheelchair for distances;
  – shoe horn and hosiery applicator;
  – long-handled pick-up device.

Patients often acknowledge that even the simplest of everyday activities is compromised by their breathlessness. This is not only frightening, but it can also be embarrassing. To be able to address these realities, with the fears associated, can bring reassurance and relief. While a range of strategies to adapt and pace should be part of the physiotherapist's repertoire, it is useful to seek new tips from the patients, as **they often discover for themselves their own most effective tried and tested techniques** (➤ Table 2.9).

Table 2.9 Adaptive and pacing strategies for breathless management

Adaptive strategies for breathlessness management	Pacing strategies for breathlessness management
• Dress/undress sitting down as far as practicable. • Avoid shoes with laces to tie. • Use a shower seat. • Put on a towelling robe immediately after taking a shower. • Use electric toothbrush rather than manual. • Pause every 2–3 steps when climbing stairs.	• Eat and drink slowly with frequent pauses; swallowing demands breath holding. • Speak in short sentences, and enlist family support to allow adequate time for conversation. • On exertion, pause as respiratory rate increases; use extended expiration breathing control strategy until rate settles. Resume activity.

✓ G U I D A N C E
"You are the car and your breathing is the petrol?"
'When the petrol gauge in a car registers 'low' would you drive very fast to the petrol station to fill up quickly? How would you drive, and why?'
This has proved to be a very useful analogy that the author has used to teach patients how to pace and manage activity within the constraints of their respiratory capacity

2.4.4 Context of anxiety and panic in the breathless patient

Research has shown that anxiety and panic are correlates of breathlessness (Dudgeon et al. 2001b). The drive to breathe arises from a neural network in the brain stem. Afferent sources of breathing sensation emanate from receptors in the upper airways, lungs and chest wall as well as the autonomic centres in both brain stem and motor cortex (O'Donnell et al. 2007). The sensory receptors in the diaphragm and skeletal muscles respond by ensuring a fine balance is maintained between oxygen need and demand (Mahler et al. 1996). When this balance is disrupted, cognitive awareness induces fear. Areas of the insula and amygdala associated with anxiety, emotion, memory and behaviour are activated and responses associated with the limbic system trigger corresponding reactions to those arising from harmful stimuli and threat (Gilman/Banzett 2009; O'Donnell et al. 2007). This in turn results in activity avoidance, anxiety and – in extreme cases – overwhelming panic. The anxiety that is such a feature of respiratory compromise can in itself elicit breathless episodes (Bailey 2004; Bruera 2000), and these may be disproportionate to the level of disease (Mahler et al. 1996). In a small audit (unpublished) conducted in 2004 at St Christopher's Hospice, London, UK it was discovered that of 34 patients referred for breathlessness management the symptoms of breathlessness, anxiety and panic were differently perceived by patient, referrer and physiotherapist. The physiotherapist discovered that episodes of panic were revealed in 62% of this patient group and as many as 88% of the patients admitted anxiety. Both symptoms were higher than initially recognized at the time of referral, anxiety significantly more so (➤ Figure 2.14). This audit revealed the importance of gently exploring anxiety and panic issues with all breathless patients at initial assessment, as these very distressing symptoms very likely remain unaddressed without the intervention of the skilled physiotherapist.

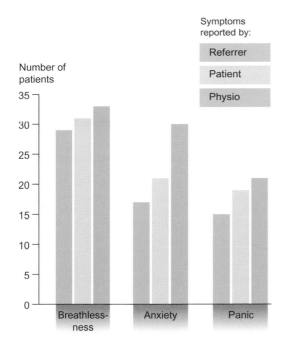

Symptoms reported by:

Referrer

Patient

Physio

Figure 2.14 Audit (unpublished) of 34 patients referred to physiotherapy for breathlessness management [M541/L157]

Key features of the breathless patient presenting with anxiety and panic

Patients often conceal this aspect of breathlessness. It is associated with a range of physical, behavioural and intensely emotional features (see above Cautions). Gentle encouragement is needed from the physiotherapist, with other members of the clinical team, to enable a patient to gradually express his or her deepest fears. Patients use powerful and vivid descriptors to express the profound terror experienced: *'Imagine standing on the extreme edge of a cliff, and feeling that someone behind you is going to suddenly push you off: that is how I feel when I panic'* (Mr G. T., a patient with metastatic lung cancer).

Carers often carry a particularly heavy burden of anxiety with little respite. They observe irritability, exacerbation of pre-existent phobias and anxiety around acute episodes, which provoke anticipatory panic. This results in a vicious circle of decreasing activity levels and loss of autonomy for the patient (Howard et al. 2009).

2.4.5 A physiotherapy approach to managing anxiety and panic in the context of breathlessness

Key to managing this distressing aspect of breathlessness is 'normalizing' the symptom. Sensitive exploration of patients' feelings can be linked to a physiological explanation

to help make sense of this reflex response to threat. The mechanism of panic embodies a universal safety device for all humankind, and is not intrinsically life-threatening. Helping the patient to understand this, how to anticipate patterns of behaviour, and then modify his or her responses can result in much improved mastery. Simple breathing exercises help to make the link between escalating respiratory rates and consequent reflex physiological responses. Patients will often hyperventilate, and excess oxygen will then depress the drive to breathe. A breathlessness poem

---

Breathlessness poem

Be still – be calm
Drop the shoulders
Slowly sigh out – and – out
Hear the sigh – Haaaaah – soft and quiet
Feel control returning
Peaceful and safe

J. M. Taylor 2005

(see above) devised by the author is based on simplicity of expression with minimal words. This proves helpful for both patient and family members as the phrases are easily memorized, and can be recited step by step.

When progress is made with mastering panic feelings, activity is gradually increased to carefully provoke breathlessness and then implement pacing and coping techniques. Gradually anxiety diminishes and the 'panic memory' may be reconstructed. Positive distraction has a strong role to play. Creative therapies (including art and music) can add to the multiprofessional repertoire of support (again see ➤ Table 2.5). **Patients who are anxious will often be deconditioned, as apprehension can paralyse activity.** A group that incorporates gentle exercise as an adjunct to addressing breathlessness and panic provides an opportunity for shifting focus away from the panic, through sharing concerns and mutual support, towards realizing that they are not alone with their existential distress (Brenes 2003). Carers too can benefit from a wider support system and can access help and advice from other health professionals and each other. Further considerations on group work in palliative care are included in ➤ Chapter 2.6.

Education for professionals and families

An important role for the physiotherapist is education to increase awareness and understanding of the many strategies that can alleviate both breathlessness and the associated fear. This is best implemented both inter-professionally and also with carers and families. The nurse at the bedside plays a key role in supporting the terminally breathless patient. With enhanced knowledge of some simple non-pharmacological techniques that he or she can confidently use, best practice is improved (Taylor 2007). Advising and educating families and carers helps to empower them to continue to support the patient. Constant exposure to the particularly distressing aspects of these symptoms can be very demoralizing, and anxiety in a relative will compound anxiety in the patient.

2.4.6 Conclusion

Breathlessness is probably one of the most difficult symptoms encountered by health professionals caring for patients at the end of life. Attention must be paid to close clinical supervision and the provision of support structures for the physiotherapist. Physical, emotional and spiritual distress is inextricably interwoven and strikes at the very heart of existence. A multiprofessional holistic approach should carefully balance pharmacological and non-pharmacological interventions, and work towards building confidence, autonomy and independence (Gallo-Silver/Pollack 2000). Enabling these very frightened patients to talk openly about feelings for their future can be challenging, but there is much that the physiotherapist can do to bring reassurance and hope. If patients can be empowered to regain control over their breathlessness symptoms, both physical and psychological, their quality of life will be maximized and their horizons expanded. The physiotherapist is a key professional to work with these vulnerable and frightened patients and has the necessary skills to instil a sense of dignity, resilience and coping, which should sit at the centre of good palliative care.

2.4.7 Reflective questions

- In your workplace, which treatment strategies can you implement to manage the breathless patient? What difficulties do you anticipate?
- How can you work inter-professionally to help ensure a consistent approach is adopted?
- Thinking of the context of your work as a physiotherapist, how will you develop an understanding of the anxious, fearful, breathless patient?
- What opportunities are there for you to develop services for both patients and their families/carers and offer resources for them to manage these symptoms together?

REFERENCES

Ambrosino N, Strambi S. New strategies to improve exercise tolerance in chronic obstructive airways disease. Eur Resp J 2004;24:313–322.

Bailey C. Nursing as therapy in the management of breathlessness in lung cancer. Eur J Palliat Care 1995;4:184–190.

Bailey PH. The dyspnea-anxiety-dyspnea cycle: COPD patients' stories of breathlessness: 'It's scary when you can't breathe'. Qual Health Res 2004;14:760–778.

Bausewein C, Booth S, Gysels M, Higginson IJ. Non-pharmacological interventions for breathlessness in advanced stages of malignant and non-malignant diseases. Cochrane Database Syst Rev 2008;(2):CD005623.

Bausewein C, Farquhar M, Booth S, Gysels M, Higginson IJ. Measurement of breathlessness in advanced disease: a systematic review. Respir Med 2007;101:399–410.

Brenes G. Anxiety and chronic obstructive airways disease: Prevalence, impact and treatment. Psychosom Med 2003;65:963–970.

Bruera E, Schmitz B, Pither J, Neumann CM, Hanson J. The frequency and correlates of dyspnea in patients with advanced cancer. J Pain Symptom Manage 2000;19:357–362.

Carr AJ, Higginson IJ. Measuring quality of life: Are quality of life measures patient-centred? BMJ 2001;322:1,357–1,360.

Corner J, Plant H, A'Hern R, Bailey C. Non-pharmacological intervention for breathlessness in lung cancer. Palliat Med 1996;10:299–305.

Currow DC, Plummer JL, Crockett A, Abernethy AP. A community population survey of prevalence and severity of dyspnea in adults. J Pain Symptom Manage 2009;38:533–545.

Dechman G, Wilson CR. Evidence underlying breathing retraining in people with stable chronic obstructive airways disease. Phys Ther 2004;84:1,189–1,197.

Dorman S, Byrne A, Edwards A. Which measurement scales should we use to measure breathlessness in palliative care? A systematic review. Palliat Med 2007;21:177–191.

Dudgeon DJ, Rosenthal S. Management of dyspnea and cough in patients with cancer. Hematol Oncol Clin North Am 1996;10:157–171.

Dudgeon D, Kristianson L, Sloan J, Lertzman M, Clement K. Dyspnea in cancer patients: prevalence and associated factors. J Pain Symptom Manage 2001a;21:95–102.

Dudgeon D, Lertzman M, Askew G. Physiological changes and clinical correlations of dyspnea in cancer outpatients. J Pain Symptom Manage 2001b;21:373–379.

Ek K, Ternestedt B. Living with chronic obstructive airways disease at the end of life: a phenomenological study. J Adv Nurs 2008;62:470–478.

Galbraith S, Fagan P, Perkins P, Lynch A, Booth S. Does a hand-held fan improve chronic dyspnea? A randomized, controlled, crossover trial. J Pain Symptom Manage 2010;39:831–838.

Gallo-Silver L, Pollack B. Behavioural interventions for lung cancer related breathlessness. Cancer Pract 2000;8:268–273.

Gift A. A dyspnoea assessment guide. Crit Care Nurse 1990;9:79–87.

Gigliotti F, Coli C, Bianchi R, Romagnoli I, Ianini B, Binazzi B. Exercise training improves exertional dyspnea in patients with chronic obstructive airways disease. Chest 2003;123:1,794–1,802.

Gilman SA, Banzett RB. Physiologic changes and clinical correlates of advanced dyspnea. Curr Opin Support Palliat Care 2009;3:93–97.

Hately J, Scott A, Laurence V, Baker R, Thomas P. A palliative care approach for breathlessness in cancer: a clinical evaluation. Help the Hospice: London; 2001.

Hately J, Laurence V, Scott A, Baker R, Thomas P. Breathlessness clinics within specialist palliative care settings can improve the quality of life and functional capacity of patients with lung cancer. Palliat Med 2003;17:410–417.

Hochstetter JK, Lewis J, Soares-Smith L. An investigation into the immediate impact of breathlessness management on the breathless patient: randomised controlled trial Physiotherapy 2005;91:178–185.

Hough A. Physiotherapy in respiratory care. 3rd ed. London: Stanley Thornes Ltd; 1997.

Howard C, Hallas CN, Wray J, Carby M. The relationship between illness perceptions and panic in chronic obstructive pulmonary disease. Behav Res Ther 2009;47:71–76.

Hoyal C, Grant J, Chamberlain F, Cox R, Campbell T. Improving the management of breathlessness using a clinical effectiveness programme. Int J Palliat Nurs 2002;8:78–87.

Krishnasamy M, Corner J, Bredin M, Plant H, Bailey C. Cancer nursing practice development: understanding breathlessness. J Clin Nurs 2001;10:103–108.

Lewith GT, Prescott P, Davis CL. Can a standardised acupuncture technique palliate disabling breathlessness: a single-blind, placebo-controlled crossover study. Chest 2004;125:1,783–1,790.

Lord VM, Cave P, Hume VJ, et al. Singing teaching as a therapy for chronic respiratory disease – a randomised controlled trial and qualitative evaluation. BMC Pulm Med 2010;10:41.

Luker K, Austin L, Caress A, Hallett CE. The importance of 'know the patient': community nurses' constructions of quality in providing palliative care. J Adv Nurs 2000;31:775–782.

Mahler DA, Harver A, Lentine T, Scott JA, Beck K, Schwartzstein RM. Descriptors of breathlessness in cardiorespiratory diseases. Am J Respir Crit Care Med 1996;154:1,357–1,363.

NHS Lothian. Palliative Care Guidelines: Breathlessness. NHS Lothian, 2009 [online]. Available at: www.palliativecare-guidelines.scot.nhs.uk/documents/breathlessnessfinal.pdf (last accessed August 2012).

Nici L, Donner C, Wonters E, Zuwallack R, Ambrosino N, Bourbeau J. American Thoracic Society/European Respiratory Society statement on pulmonary rehabilitation. Am J Respir Crit Care Med 2006;173:1,390–1,413.

O'Donnell DE, Banzett RB, Carrieri-Kohlman V, et al. Pathophysiology of dyspnea in chronic obstructive pulmonary disease: a roundtable. Proc Am Thorac Soc 2007;4:145–168.

Regnard C, Ahmedzai S. Dyspnea in advanced non-malignant disease: a flow diagram. Palliat Med 1991;5:56–60.

Ripamonti C, Bruera E. Dyspnea: pathophysiology and assessment. J Pain Symptom Manage 1997;13:220–232.

Schwartzstein RM, Lahive K, Pope A, Weinberger SE, Weiss JW. Cold facial stimulation reduces breathlessness induced in normal subjects. Am Rev Respir Dis 1987;136:58–61.

Solano JP, Gomes B, Higginson IJ. A comparison of symptoms prevalent in far advanced cancer, AIDS, heart disease, chronic obstructive pulmonary disease, and renal disease. J Pain Symptom Manage 2006;31:58–69.

Simon PM, Schwartzstein RM, Weiss JW, Fencl V, Teghtsoonian M, Weinberger SE. Distinguishable types of dyspnea in patients with shortness of breath. Am Rev Respir Dis 1990;142:1,009–1,014.

Taylor J. The non-pharmacological management of breathlessness. End of Life Care 2007;1:20–27.

Zhao I, Yates P. Non-pharmacological interventions for breathlessness management in patients with lung cancer: a systematic review. Palliat Med 2008;22:683–701.

Zigmond AS, Snaith RP. The Hospital Anxiety and Depression Scale. Acta Psychiat Scand 1983;67:361–70.

2.5 Lymphoedema
Peter Nieland

Lymphoedema is a commonly observed, physically and psychologically very distressing symptom in those who are critically ill and dying. There are no conclusive statistical data on the incidence with which lymphoedema actually occurs in the palliative care setting, however. In Germany, the figure is assumed to be between 1.5‰ and 1.6 % of all palliative care patients (Miller/Knetsch 2007), which appears to be very low and should be subjected to further statistical scrutiny. Within the context of the physiotherapeutic management of palliative care patients lymphoedema is a constant challenge due to the potentially rapid increase in oedema, tissue induration, increased organ failure, multi-morbidity and immobility. This chapter addresses the cause, outcomes and therapeutic strategies specific to the palliative care setting.

2.5.1 Case study

Mr S., 61 years old, has an inoperable, progressive, metastatic carcinoma of the hypopharynx; he suffers from severe cancer pain, dyspnoea and swallowing difficulties, and has lost a lot of weight. After two operations to reduce the tumour he was given a tracheostomy, which has reduced his cancer-related dyspnoea. Because of the residual tumour and surgery to the cervical spine, the patient has developed sensory impairment in both hands and extensive oedema of the head. The oedema is a tremendous emotional strain to Mr S., making him feel disfigured. Additionally, general muscle weakness and severe muscle tension in the upper trunk are limiting his activities of daily living and quality of life. Prior to his illness, Mr S. was physically very active, in addition to holding down a demanding management job at an international company.

Palliative management
- Step III opioids combined with a step I analgesia (➤ Chapter 2.2) to reduce the cancer pain;
- PEG tube for feeding and dispensing of an anticonvulsant for irritable bowel;

- complex physical decongestive therapy (PDT) for the lymphoedematous regions of the head, neck and throat to make him more recognisable to family, friends and colleagues;
- respiratory therapy for relieving the dyspnoea;
- back massages to relieve the painful muscle tension;
- movement therapy to maintain and potentially improve trunk strength and coordination for as long as possible.

Primary physiotherapeutic goal agreed with the patient   On initial assessment it is clear that Mr S's. main problem is the profound stress he suffers due to the visible facial oedema and the associated embarrassment on the part of his wife, family and those around him. The fact that the oedema and the tumour site cannot be concealed and are causing visible disfigurement is so difficult to bear, that even the physically palpable tension around the tumour as well as other symptoms have become secondary to his distress. Mr S. would like the facial oedema to be

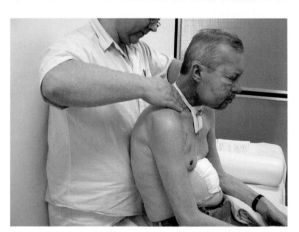

Figure 2.15 Manual lymph drainage, seated, starting position 1 [0597]

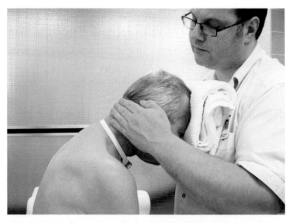

Figure 2.16 Manual lymph drainage, seated, starting position 2 [0597]

reduced, especially in the area of the cheeks and mouth, in order that he looks better and *'more like his former self'*. A further goal is to reduce the oedematous tension local to the tumour which has already begun to grow again.

Physiotherapeutic strategy   In starting position 1 (➤ Figure 2.15) the patient sits leaning with his back against the therapist, as he feels much more relaxed in this position than when recumbent, as is customary in standard manual lymph drainage. (Lying down, he cannot get enough air through the tracheostomy). In starting position 2 (➤ Figure 2.16) Mr S. leans with his head against the therapist, enabling him to relieve the very strained muscles in his neck. This starting position also helps him to relax during therapy. Therapy begins with retrograde massage action, using stationary circles, to the terminus (under the clavicle) and profundus (side of the neck) region lateral to the tracheostomy, directed towards the right and left axillae. From the axillae the lymphangiomotor function is activated across the neck and the entire head and face. This treatment starts distally to proximally in order to facilitate free-flowing lymph. After activating all the dorsal lymph tracts of the head and throat, stationary circles of minimal pressure are applied, moving progressively from the face in the direction of the neck and from there towards the back of the throat and into the right and left axillae. As this approach alone is not sufficient to clear the resultant inflowing volume of lymph, the lymphatic system in the lower quadrant of the body also requires activation at the right and left groin. As a result, lymph is released via the cisterna chyli and thoracic duct into the superior vena cava. To facilitate this second additional route of drainage, the patient is positioned on his back with the upper body optimally elevated.

Ongoing management   Mr S. spends a total of 12 weeks in physiotherapy: the first three weeks as an inpatient with daily treatment for 45 minutes, and the subsequent nine weeks as an outpatient, attending 3 times a week for 45-minute sessions. Lymph drainage is performed each time and is combined, if appropriate and his condition permits, with respiratory therapy, massage and exercise therapy. At some appointments the patient's wife receives massages for relaxation and stress reduction in parallel to her husband's therapy.

Result of primary goal   Mr S. describes his subjective experience and the outcome of treatment for his oedema in the correspondence below:

Dear Mr Nieland, now that the first series of the proposed manual lymph drainage sessions is complete, I would like to write you a brief account, as I am aware that applying this therapy 'when seated' is a hotly debated subject amongst therapists and is often dismissed or only carried out reluctantly. In my own case I must and can only confirm/claim the opposite! Due to my tracheal tube with speech cannula and the very restricted amount of air I am able to breathe in as a result, drainage is not possible when I lie on my stomach or back. I also mostly sleep in a sitting position. Hence your therapy when I am seated with my head leaning forward, or with my back leaning against you, is just what I need and is very comfortable! In fact it is so good that my breathing is completely calm, almost to the point of sleeping, and I find the whole therapy perfectly relaxing. As far as I am concerned the sessions could be longer, though I'm then likely to fall asleep. The outcome of the treatments is also entirely positive! The lymph fluid does in fact continue to flow so that I have to mop it up, but the tumour site is certainly nowhere near as hard and swollen as before the treatments.

Hoping that the treatments continue to prove successful, with best wishes, S.

Secondary goals The needs-centred, carefully judged combination of oedema and respiratory therapy for dyspnoea, relaxation massages to the back and active exercises for maintaining strength and mobility contribute considerably, as described by the patient, towards alleviating the additional physical problems mentioned above, delivering a positive therapeutic outcome.

However, the overall condition of the patient deteriorated over the course of the following weeks due to the continued growth of the tumour in his neck. Metastases also appeared in the lungs and skeletal system. As Mr S. continued to weaken, the plan was for physiotherapy to be carried out by colleagues making home visits, as patient need indicated. This did not transpire, however, as Mr S. died at home two weeks later in the presence of his family.

2.5.2 Lymphatic system and potential disorders

The primary function of the lymphatic system is to remove interstitial fluid via the lymph capillaries into the **lymph collectors** (lymph collecting vessels), which are divided into three subcategories:

- subcutaneous or prefascial lymphatic vessels that drain the skin and subcutaneous tissue;
- subfascial lymphatic vessels that drain the deeper structures: joints, synovial membranes, nerves, muscles;
- visceral lymphatic vessels that drain the deep lying structures of the blood vessels and organs.

Large molecular substances are removed (e.g. cell debris, proteins or waste products) and the **immune defences** of the lymphocytes and macrophages play an important role (Földi 2011; Schingale 2011; Lawenda et al 2009).

Oedema is the pathological accumulation of fluid in the interstitial and extravasal space that leads to tissue swelling (Degenhardt 1991), and is both visible and palpable (Földi/Földi 2009). A distinction is made between primary and secondary lymphoedema; both types may be encountered in palliative care.

Primary lymphoedema

Primary lymphoedema can present at any time, but although according to Herpetz (2010) it occurs at a rate of 34 % in palliative care, it is generally much less common than the secondary form (Schingale 2011).

Causes

The causes for primary lymphoedema are:
- hereditary developmental disorders of the lymphatic system:
  - aplasia: congenital defect of the initial lymphatic vessels with collateral circulation;
  - hypoplasia: under-development of the lymphatic vessels;
  - hyperplasia: over-development of the lymphatic vessels combined with lymphangiectasia;
- inguinal lymph node fibrosis, the cause of which is not yet known (Herpertz 2010).

Physical signs of primary lymphoedema (lower limbs)

- Increased swelling in the extremities of the legs spreading towards the trunk;
- frequent oedema on the dorsa of the feet, often accompanied by early swelling in the area of the ankles, around the Achilles tendon and malleoli;
- development of deep folds at the anterior ankle crease;
- positive Stemmer's sign.

These key signs are defined and expanded in more depth later.

Secondary lymphoedema

In palliative care, secondary lymphoedema is seen primarily as **lymphostatic oedema** with malignant tumours infiltrating and destroying the lymph tracts.

Space-occupying and rapidly growing tumours cause the lymph tracts to be compressed or constricted (Schingale 2011). Any necessary surgery, radiation or infusions and the resulting scars and wounds will exacerbate the situation. In parallel, there may often be causes for **dynamic** or **high-volume insufficiency,** e. g. severe vascularisation of the tumours, immobility and most commonly cardiac failure, leading to interstitial venous congestion. Often, very pronounced levels of oedema (stage 3 or 4) may involve multifactorial, mixed forms.

Further causes for the development of oedema may be:
- hepatic disease (reduced bodily protein production);
- intestinal disease (bodily proteins excreted in the faeces);
- renal disease (bodily proteins excreted in the urine);
- diminished strength and immobility (reduced muscle pump, muscular atrophy);
- pulmonary failure and dyspnoea (cardiac failure);
- albumin deficiency;
- malnutritional oedema (nutrients can no longer be broken down).

Lymphoedema staging (AWMF 2011)

- **Stage I (latent oedema):** impaired, but compensated lymph drainage conditions which become manifest as a result of exogenous factors (insect bites, bruising, contusion of a joint, e. g. the ankle); complete resolution when positioned appropriately.
- **Stage II (reversible oedema):** swelling in the evening and sensation of heaviness in the affected extremity; reduction overnight.
- **Stage III (chronic, irreversible oedema):** non-pitting, firm on palpation; can no longer be reversed by positioning (➤ Figure 2.17).
- **Stage IV (lymphostatic elephantiasis):** swelling is advanced and unresponsive causing gross deformation of limbs with significant impact on function. Skin changes including fibrosis and lymphorrhoea (where interstitial fluid may seep through skin pores or breaks in the skin). In the most severe cases, untreated lymphoedema can develop into a rare form of lymphatic cancer called lymphangiosarcoma which can prove fatal if left untreated.

Impact of lymphoedema in palliative care patients

If lymphatic drainage is impaired, oedema develops and immobility increases due to the **heaviness of the**

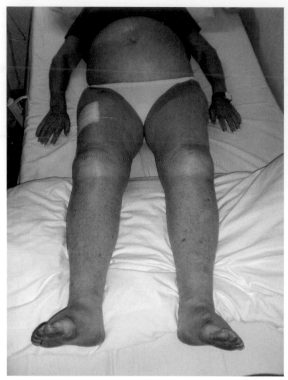

Figure 2.17 Lymphoedema stage III: chronic irreversible oedema [0597]

affected body parts. Proliferation of the affected tissue not only causes the oedematous extremities to feel heavy and cumbersome, but also renders them increasingly hard due to the accumulated protein and formation of connective tissue fibrosis. The patient will find it more and more difficult to change position or pursue activities that require mobility of the limbs (e. g. visiting the toilet, getting out of bed independently, etc.). Lymphoedema at end of life primarily presents as the accumulation of fluid in the arms or legs, but it can also affect the trunk, head and neck or genitalia. It may result in the following dysfunctions:
- impaired breathing (oedema in the abdomen and trunk);
- impaired sensory and physical perception (e. g. from eyelid oedema, neurological changes or reduced proprioception);
- impaired micturition and erectile dysfunction (oedema in the genital region).

Some further effects of tissue changes are painful skin tension as well as increasing problems with skin integrity. The result is parchment-like skin with reduced acid protection. Bacteria can infiltrate such very compromised and friable **skin** causing inflammatory and necrotic sores to develop. The wound healing processes that are triggered as a result lead to the affected

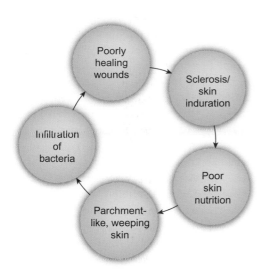

Figure 2.18 Vicious circle of untreated lymphoedema [M546/L157]

areas becoming highly vascularised; in turn, this increase in circulation intensifies the oedema (➤ Figure 2.18). If these processes are already well advanced, then according to the AWMF classification (AWMF 2010) a stage III chronic and irreversible oedema exists. This poses a further wound healing problem to patients at end of life and may impact on all the carers involved (Deng et al. 2012; Harris et al. 2012; Schingale 2011; Lawenda et al 2009).

Many palliative care patients generally refer to *'too much water in the body'* when talking about oedema, an aspect which is viewed as disfiguring, painful, immobilising and is also associated with physical and psychological distress. Relatives and visitors also become anxious or dismayed by the clearly visible physical changes.

A 64-year-old female palliative care patient with gastric and colon cancer gave a dramatic description of her secondary lymphoedema in the trunk and legs: *'My stomach and legs feel like a drum and two big sausages that are about to burst because the skin is too tight – I just don't want to live like this.'*

So it should be remembered that lymphoedema has other psycho-social effects aside from functional disorders, including:
- social isolation,
- changes in physical appearance, and
- anxiety

(Deng et al 2012).

2.5.3 Physiotherapy for lymphoedema in the palliative care setting

Examination and physical signs of lymphoedema

The most important **visual and physical examinations** and findings in the case of lymphoedema (as defined by the AWMF 2011) are:
- visual examination and palpation for oedema, sores, scars, skin changes and skin temperature;
- thumb pressure test: press for several seconds on the affected areas with the thumbs and then inspect visually or palpate for pathological indentation ('pitting');
- swelling of the extremities (first evident here due to the effect of gravity), spreading proximally to the trunk, and in lower limb oedema sometimes also to the genital region;
- oedema on the dorsum(a) of the feet/hands, with formation of deep folds at joint creases;
- Stemmer's sign: whereby the skin at the base of the second toe or finger joint cannot be lifted or pinched into a fold (Földi/Földi 2010; Cornely 2011);
- fibrosis (induration);
- lymphorrhoea: secretion of interstitial fluid through the skin, caused by a compromised venous and lymphatic system and porous cellular skin structures;
- evidence of fluid accumulation at the interface of tight clothing (e. g. socks welts);
- breathlessness, particularly if cardiac failure is an associated feature.

Suitable **methods of limb volume assessment** include:
- measurement of the limb circumference, using a tape measure (measure the length of the arm or leg, then define three points, e. g. at 10 cm, 30 cm, 60 cm), and comparison with the unaffected limb;
- use of a body scanner;
- displacement principle with water bath (e. g. hand) (Bringezu/Schreiner 2001).

Further assessments and standardised methods can be found in the relevant literature (e. g. AWMF 2011; Harris et al. 2012; Földi 2011).

Physiotherapy for lymphoedema

Complex physical decongestive therapy (PDT)

Treatment entails complex physical decongestive therapy (PDT) (Harris et al. 2012) and is applied both to primary and secondary lymphoedema. There are two phases to this lymphoedema treatment:

1. **reduction,** in which the oedema is primarily reduced by manual lymph drainage (MLD);
2. **maintenance,** in which reduction of the oedema is maintained first and foremost by compression therapy.

These components of PDT entail manual lymph drainage which increases the vasomotor activity of the lymphatic system by manual stimulation and filling of the lymphatic capillaries, and then compression, in conjunction with skin care and exercises to enhance muscle pump action.

Skin care in palliative care patients with lymphoedema

The acid mantle and epidermal differentiation of the skin cell structures are often impaired in palliative care patients with lymphoedema. As already mentioned, this can result in infections and sores. Because the body will attempt to heal such skin defects, the areas will become highly vascularised which in turn will intensify the propensity for oedema. Therapeutic compression will cause the skin to also lose oil and moisture, and the gentle, circular friction movements of MLD can be held responsible for abrasion of the corneocytes in the stratum corneum (Miller/Knetsch 2007). Cell debris and dead skin residues can be removed by cleansing the skin with a pH neutral, non-perfumed and surfactant-free soap, and the acid mantle supported by then applying a pH neutral cream. The elasticity of the skin is thus improved. According to Miller and Knetsch (2007), such an emollient cream should contain the following basic components: glycerol, urea, aluminium oxide and triclosan (beware of any allergies, however). A morning and evening skin care regime is an important part of therapy for palliative care patients with lymphoedema. The objective is to maintain and wherever possible restore the normal epidermal conditions and acid mantle for as long as possible.

Manual lymph drainage in palliative care patients

Excessive lymph can be drained into adjacent oedema-free quadrants by using lymphatic collateral circulation. Such therapy is applied very gently and slowly (for at least 30–45 minutes) to the skin, and is well tolerated by patients. When starting, the patient should be in a very relaxed, pain-free position and a comfortable environment; as a consequence, this will help to reduce the metabolism. The patient should be in lying if possible, with the head raised and supported by a pillow. If this starting position is not possible, however, the therapist will need to be flexible (as shown in the case study).

To begin with, minimal pressure is applied to influence the terminus and profundus region of the left and right angle of the jugular vein. These centrally applied manual techniques will stimulate the lymphangiomotor function at the junction of the superior vena cava and the influx of lymph from the oedematous quadrants. The affected lymphoedematous area is cleared by using circular strokes across the chest and back towards the corresponding truncal quadrant. After distal to proximal stimulation of the lymphangiomotor activity and collateral circulation, retrograde lymph drainage can take place. Any tissue induration in the drainage area should be carefully released by slow and intensive cross-fibre massage. The increase in lymphangiomotor function is sustained for up to 30 minutes after the stimulation has ended and then slowly recedes. Further localised massage followed by padding and compression bandaging as appropriate is then applied (Clemens et al. 2010; Schingale 2011).

> √ **GUIDANCE**
> **The added effect of touch**
>
> Due to long periods of enforced rest and lack of movement, the end of life patient increasingly loses important tactile stimuli that provide him with peace of mind, including impaired orientation and kinaesthetic sense. If such active and passive stimuli are lost on account of the patient's immobility, the hands-on techniques of manual lymph drainage and passive, assistive or active movement from compression in the larger quadrants of the body and extremities not only help to relieve the oedema but also have positive tactile and proprioceptive effects. At the same time, slow and gentle contact with the skin leads to the release of oxytocin, a pituitary hormone that reduces stress. (Gimpl/Fahrenholz 2001, Bartels 2004). Manual lymph drainage thus assumes an important, secondary palliative function. It engenders trust, reduces anxiety and elicits important tactile stimuli for the largest organ of the body, namely the skin.

Compression in palliative care patients with lymphoedema

Studies have demonstrated that lymphoedema can be reduced by appropriate compression therapy (McNeely et al. 2004). Effects achieved are as follows:
- reduction in capillary filtration;
- redistribution of fluid into non-compressed parts of the body;
- increased lymphatic reabsorption and stimulation of lymphatic transport;
- improved pumping of the veins;
- regeneration of tissue with fibrotic changes.

Compression is applied with non-elastic, short-stretch bandages. The advantage of short-stretch bandages is

Table 2.10 Compression classes in the palliative care setting (as defined by AWMF 2008)

Compression class	Pressure applied	Indications in palliative care patients
I	18–21 mm Hg	Thromboprophylaxis, alleviation of heaviness or fatigue in the legs, minor varicosis with a low risk of oedema. Often used in palliative care patients, as they can be managed by the patients themselves.
II	23–32 mm Hg	If the legs are swollen after smaller ulcers have healed and as relapse prophylaxis for healed ulcers. Second most common palliative compression class; help usually required with management.
III	34–46 mm Hg	For thrombosis, sequelae of post-thrombotic venous insufficiency, pronounced risk of oedema and dermatoliposclerosis as well as florid venous leg ulcer. Seldom used in palliative care as this compression class can only be applied by a relative or carer.
IV	>46 mmHg	Lymphoedema or elephantiasis. Very rarely used in palliative care. Management requires the help of an oedema therapist or experienced carer and is judged by most palliative care patients to be too rigid and tight.

Note: In different countries variations in compression classes may exist.

that they exert a high level of working pressure on movement, but less when lying down and at rest. The constant risk of vascular compromise from compression is thus reduced, and the compression produces intermittent peak pressures when walking and moving. Since the oedema suffered by palliative care patients is often very pronounced, daily compression therapy is preferable. Adaptation of the palliative care approach to the patient's needs should be the priority. This means for example that contrary to a school of thought that compression should be maintained during a 24 hour period, in palliative patients it may be waived during the night in order to improve the quality of sleep or, despite the possibility of an improved therapeutic outcome, it may be refused if it is subjectively perceived as too stressful. Palliative care patients who habitually remain in bed during the day may manage without compression therapy during such a time. Patients spending longer periods upright, either seated, standing or moving about, should receive supportive compression in order to prevent increased swelling and consequent skin damage. Made-to-measure compression garments are beneficial only in isolated cases of severe lymphoedema since the circumference of the extremity can change on a daily basis (Földi 2011; Brennan/Miller 1998).

Compression

Compression therapy involves wearing compression garments or bandages on the leg(s)/arm(s) which exert pressure and thus reduce the width of the veins (Panfil/Schröder 2010; Brennan/Miller 1998). A compression stocking or sleeve or appropriately applied bandage is designed such that the pressure exerted is graduated from distal to proximal (Sippel 2006).

Compression stockings, if used, are divided into different compression classes. These are outlined in ➤ Table 2.10.

Movement therapy and activity in palliative care patients with oedema

An ideal activity for the palliative care patient in order to get the muscles pumping is gentle, active, assisted and passive movement with a suitable supportive compression system. Such movement will at the same time improve the proprioception, coordination and strength of the patient. The lymphatic system will respond with increased lymphatic vasomotor function and intensified venous backflow, since the skin and bandage will act as a resistance, decreasing diffusion from the arterial branch of the capillaries and encouraging venous reabsorption and filling of the lymphatic capillaries (Földi/Stößenreuter 2011).

Depending on the patient's condition and well-being, the following therapeutic approaches and activities have proven successful:

- breathing exercises (lymphatic motor function is stimulated by the activity of the diaphragm);
- isometric muscle exercise;
- seated exercise programme;
- walking; if feasible with applied compression;
- nordic walking;
- cycling/exercise bike/cycloergometer;
- hydrotherapy at lukewarm temperatures (approx. 27 C), making use of the hydrostatic pressure (Földi/Stößenreuter 2011);
- any programmed training therapy may be combined with/without compression and/or sequential pump devices.

CASE STUDY
Patient autonomy in oedema therapy

Despite all the expertise and robust clinical reasoning skills applied by the oedema therapist, even including those of the highly specialist practitioner, a fully informed palliative care patient is at the centre of every treatment decision. Irrespective of whether the physiotherapist has provided a clear physiological explanation of the management plan, any interventions that may improve the patient's quality of life may be modified or even refused by the palliative care patient, and such a decision may not be viewed as detrimental to the patient. Quality of life is subjective, however serious the clinical picture may appear – as shown in the case study below:

Mr H. had bilateral secondary **lymphoedema in the legs with prostate carcinoma** and was undergoing PDT. Despite receiving logical and comprehensible explanation of the physiology and proposed management plan Mr H. refused to accept compression therapy with short-stretch bandages or stockings on both legs to 'maintain the therapeutic outcome between therapy sessions' His simple argument was: *'I enjoy your lymph drainage sessions and my legs always feel really light afterwards, but I've never been able to wear long stockings or bandages on my legs, … I've always hated them, even as a child. So why should I put myself through such torture now, when I'm about to die? The two hours are enough, when everything feels much lighter, to enable me to then bear the burden again.'*

Additional measures, support and precautions for lymphoedema in palliative care

Positioning

If patients' movements are not restricted, they are able to move around independently, reposition themselves in bed and alter position when up and around and when sleeping. However, a severely ill, immobile and oedematous end of life care patient often can only do this to a very limited extent, or not at all. A painless supported position will help to relieve the oedema during and between therapy interventions (Nieland 2009a). This entails not only elevating the extremities, but also regularly changing and modifying the patient's position as often as can be tolerated.

The following positioning principles should therefore be adopted when dealing with palliative care patients with oedema:

- To distribute the pressure, the supporting surface should be as large as possible.
- Alternate and combine hard and soft positions.
- Positioning intervals are determined individually by the patient and requests for a change in position should be observed.
- If the patient is not able to determine the positioning intervals, draw on previous experience and input from the family.

- The positions should promote and enable the patient's own activity (don't offer a helping hand too soon).
- Minimal traction when positioning helps to reduce pain and stress.
- Skin-damaging shear forces should be avoided as much as possible.

Alternative physiotherapeutic or complementary interventions

- Kinesiotape (only if the skin is intact);
- scar treatment;
- carbon dioxide bath (only if the skin is intact);
- curd poultices (including inflamed skin).

⚠ **CAUTION**
Instrumental intermittent compression (IIC): adjunctive therapy to PDT

The 'low tech, high touch' (Aulbert/Nauck/Radbruch 2011) principle applies in palliative care, namely that apparatus should only be used if really likely to be effective. Sequential gradient pumps can only be recommended to a certain extent, since they do not relieve proliferated tissue and cannot initiate collateral circulation. If used, there is a risk of circular protein fibrosis at the root of the extremities which can additionally cause the lymphatic drainage to worsen and thus exacerbate the oedema.

Nevertheless, studies have revealed that the effect of MLD can be supported by the use of IIC (Szuba/Achalu/Rockson 2002; AWMF Guidelines 2007; Brennan/Miller 1998).

Aids and appliances

- Stocking aids/sleeve applicators;
- positional wedges and pillows;
- walking sticks, crutches, walking frames, wheelchairs;
- ergonomically adjusted functional aids.

Precautions to observe for patients with oedema of the arms or legs

General warnings

- Avoid injuries, over-exertion, heat and cold. Also potential sources of risk: kitchen knives, animals, insect bites, hot water, ironing, cigarettes, caustic cleaning agents, heavy loads, thorns etc.
- Avoid prolonged or excessive flexed positions of the legs and arms.

Protection during activities of daily living

- Take care when sewing (use a thimble).
- Use oven gloves when cooking.
- Keep the arms covered and wear rubber gloves when doing housework.

Clothing

- Do not wear a watch/rings or other tight pieces of jewellery on the side of the body affected by the oedema.
- Bra straps should not cut into the body either on the shoulders or the chest (wear wide straps, light breast prostheses, avoid constricting support garments).
- Wear wide, comfortable shoes that fit properly (to minimise friction and risk of tripping).
- Do not wear underwear that cuts into the skin, tight belts or tight-fitting socks.

Personal care

- Personal hygiene should be meticulous.
- Nail care: do not cut or push the cuticles back; take care when filing.
- Avoid irritating cosmetics that may cause allergic reactions.
- Avoid saunas and sunbeds, infrared light and hot baths.
- Avoid pressure or friction in the area of the oedema.

Sport/outdoor activity

- Avoid excessively strenuous physical exercise.
- Protect from frost damage.
- Swimming, walking and cycling can be recommended.
- Avoid any activities or sports that involve sudden or precipitate movements of legs/arms, and all contact sports.
- Protect from contusions, bruising and accidental bleeding.

During the day

- Wear stocking(s)/sleeve(s) and bandages as prescribed.
- Perform specific (special) physical exercises in the compression garments.

During the night

- Elevate the oedematous arm(s) or leg(s).

Planning a holiday

- Avoid insect prone areas.

Visiting the doctor

- Do not allow blood pressure measurements to be taken on the side of the body that has undergone surgery or is oedematous.
- Do not allow any injections to be administered (either subcutaneous or intramuscular, venous or intra-articular) the taking of blood or acupuncture to oedematous areas (Harris et al 2012).

⚠️ **C A U T I O N**

Immediate medical attention

If the patient experiences any of the following conditions, signs or symptoms, a doctor should be contacted immediately:
- lymphatic fistula;
- inflammation in one of the affected extremities;
- fever/infections;
- onychomycosis; (fungal nail infection);
- dyspnoea;
- circulatory problems;
- vertigo/nausea;
- pain;
- cardiac decompensation.

Involvement of the family in palliative lymphoedema therapy

Aspects of family/carer involvement should be approached from various angles (➤ Chapter 2.1). The wishes of the patient, as well as the skills, willingness and preferences of the family must be taken into account. Once such issues have been adequately addressed, activities like positioning or gently massaging the arms and legs in the direction of the trunk are helpful components of oedema therapy that can be undertaken by members of the patient's family. In addition to its positive influence on lymphatic activity, there is also an important socio-emotional aspect to touch which can leave helpless family members feeling that they are making a difference. Information about cautionary measures and strategies (see 'Precautions') should also be conveyed to the patient's family. Take-home leaflets are helpful.

Complications and challenges of lymphoedema in palliative care patients

Erysipelas/cellulitis

Since the immune system is locally disabled by lymphoedema, patients are more likely to encounter an infection in areas that are oedematous. A common complication of lymphoedema is erysipelas or cellulitis, an inflammatory condition in the skin caused by bacteria. The protein-rich fluid that accumulates with lymphoedema is the perfect breeding ground for bacteria. As a rule, high-dose antibiotics (e. g. penicillin) are required, as life-threatening septicaemia can arise and erysipelas tends to recur (Földi 2011).

Lymphangiosarcoma

If painless, red, bruise-like patches appear on a lymphoedematous limb, this could be a malignant condition – namely lymphangiosarcoma. This rare complication is seen only if lymphoedema goes untreated, or is treated incorrectly. Patients receiving optimal care rarely develop such a malignant tumour since it most commonly arises as a result of chronic lymphoedema (Sordillo et al. 1981; Faul et al. 2000). If signs of a malignant tumour develop a biopsy is indicated. In rare cases of diagnosed lymphangiosarcoma the affected extremity may be amputated to prevent early and rapid spread of metastases which can be life-threatening (Földi 2011).

Fungating (Ulcerating) tumours

Fungating tumours in an oedematous region are a very challenging aspect of therapy in the palliative care patient. These often malodorous and disfiguring growths demand a balance between a pragmatic and professional approach on the part of the therapist. In the author's experience, any obvious and offensive odour should not be ignored or played down. Honesty and integrity are an essential part of the palliative care approach in such cases – such as: *'Yes, Mr X, the tumour really doesn't smell very nice. I'm sure it can be quite unpleasant. But I'm still going to treat the oedema surrounding the tumour.'* Collaboration with complementary therapists with regard to the use of essential oils can be helpful. In a clinical setting, the author has found that therapist-to-patient positioning can mitigate effects of the odour by approaching the oedema from a proximal direction towards the ulcerating tumour. This makes use of the suction effect of the stimulated lymphangiomotor system.

Wound healing disorders, necrosis, ulcers and pressure sores

The same rules apply here as for fungating tumours. It is important to extend the oedema therapy as far as the wound margins. Fresh, wound-healing, interstitial fluid, and the nutrients and immune defences found therein, can only be effective if the toxins have been removed from the venous and lymphatic system. Though the metabolic status of palliative care patients steadily deteriorates, therapeutic measures are important for decelerating such a process and improving quality of life.

Scars

Scars are artificial drainage barriers. Even if increased vascularisation in oedematous areas is otherwise avoided, local scar treatment is undertaken in the case of scars that are hindering drainage. Old and hardened scars may also be treated by firm transverse massage techniques as tolerated as well as lifting the scar. Intensified vascularisation can cause lymphatic vessels, blood vessels and peripheral nerves to proliferate again locally (Widgerow 2010).

Genital oedema

Genital oedema presents a particular challenge to the physiotherapist in end of life care, and the associated anxiety, distress and resultant debility demands a creative approach. More common in males due to anatomical differences and gravitational effects, oedema can be very dramatic, but compression must be treated with caution, as the scrotum has a very poor blood supply. Management tends to be conservative in approach; primarily through modified supra-pubic and lower trunk quadrant lymphatic drainage combined with the application of appropriate support. Diaphragmatic breathing, abdominal and pelvic floor exercise regimes together with scrupulous skin care, mobilising support and encouragement; these all have a role to play. Supportive and padded briefs can address vulval and labial oedema, while penile and scrotal oedema may be managed by modified bandaging, padded cycling shorts, or a range of specialist support slings (Whitaker 2009).

Lymphorrhoea

Transcutaneous secretion of interstitial fluid is a common problem with extensive, high-volume oedema because the diseased body is no longer able to maintain its total serum protein concentration within the normal range, making the metabolic conditions more difficult in terms of venous diffusion and reabsorption. First-line care entails systematic complex physical decongestive therapy (PDT). Applying bandages and thereby facilitating an increase in interstitial pressure, effects a drop in venous diffusion and rise in reabsorption of interstitial fluid and thus is at the forefront of therapy.

Questions on absolute and relative contraindications

Right ventricular failure and PDT in palliative care patients?

Herpertz (2010) views any disease of the right ventricle to always be associated with left ventricular failure. If oedematous fluid is mobilised by MLD, dyspnoea and pulmonary oedema can develop as a result of the increased quantity of blood and in the worst case scenario may lead to death. This absolute contraindication must be noted.

In the experience of the author, palliative care patients are usually under constant medical supervision and receiving pharmacological therapy. Such patients cope well with the small quantity of lymph released and transported by MLD. The oedema in palliative care patients with right ventricular failure can be attenuated slightly if they are under daily medical supervision, effective pharmacological therapy and 24-hour monitoring in a palliative care setting. This relative contraindication must always be clarified individually with the attending doctor, and also applies to gentle compression therapy (Lawenda et al 2009).

Thrombophlebitis/phlebothrombosis and occlusive arterial disease (OAD)

In end of life care, a number of absolute contraindications are being modified into relative contraindications with a view to improving quality of life. Commencement or continuation of palliative lymphoedema therapy is possible with thrombophlebitis, phlebothrombosis and occlusive arterial disease once the symptoms are managed with pharmacological therapy (Földi 2011).

Increased metastatic infiltration from palliative lymph drainage?

Herpertz (2010) also writes: *'Malignant lymphoedema is a relative contraindication to PDT.'* This implies that a doctor experienced in oncology, palliative care and lymphoedema therapy is entitled, in agreement with the attending physiotherapist or oedema therapist, to lift the contraindication and allow MLD to be performed. There is no evidence to support that lymph drainage influences the development of metastases. For a long time, clinicians believed it was theoretically conceivable to mechanically influence a tumour using lymph drainage, massage or other so-called physical methods, but in individual cases this tends to be unlikely.

One type of tumour could possibly be an exception: in the case of tumours of the head and neck, experts cannot entirely rule out the possibility – based on individual observations – that lymph drainage may increase the risk of metastases (May/Herberhold 1997). Lymph drainage possibly forces residual cancer cells into healthy tissue, where they may then take hold. Patients with tumours of the head and neck in particular often suffer (depending on their therapy) from severe lymphoedema in the face which will not reduce in size without drainage. Hence,

each patient must consider the benefits and risks together with their doctor (AWMF 2011); as a rule lymph drainage is absolutely essential if the symptoms are to be alleviated (Schingale 2011; Pinell et al 2007). The following currently applies to all tumour types: a correlation between massage, lymph drainage and metastasis has not been proven (Flor et al. 2009; Godette et al. 2006).

Diuretics

Diuretics are effective only in the case of low-protein lymphoedema and are not indicated for high-protein oedema; they do in fact increase urine production, but due to the oncotic pressure of the proteins remaining in the tissue, oedema will again begin to immediately develop (Herpertz 2010).

Late sequelae: why treatment is important

If lymphoedema goes untreated for a long time, there is an increased likelihood of late sequelae:

- **Impaired mobility and asymmetry:** because of the swelling, joint mobility is often diminished or exertional changes occur in the musculoskeletal system. As a consequence, contractures, pain and restricted activities of daily living are observed.
- **Changes in the lymphatic vessels:** the lymphatic vessels widen (vesiculation) in some patients with marked, chronic lymphoedema. These can also be referred to as lymphatic cysts. If these lymphatic cysts burst, lymphatic fistulae can develop. Since they link the inner to outer surfaces of the body, they can present an opening to bacteria. Such developments are rare if treatment is systematic.
- **Tumour risk:** in very rare cases pronounced chronic lymphoedema, which is difficult to treat, can itself become a tumour (Brown/Fletcher 2000; Jakob 2010). The tissue changes increase the risk above all of lymphangiosarcoma (refer to "Complications and challenges" above). Other types of tumours have also been associated, in individual cases, with severe lymphoedema.

The critical, most important question: is therapy for lymphoedema at end of life still worthwhile?

Rehabilitation means restoration and the alleviation of suffering (and can also have psychosocial perspectives) (Pschyrembel 2008).

In palliative care patients, lymphoedema is a very common symptom that is stressful and disfiguring. Often, even the most expertly administered PDT can only offer temporary relief. In the author's opinion, the severe and progressive nature of the disease seldom produces a measurable therapeutic outcome. Classic goals cannot be as easily defined or may be unachievable. Having read this chapter, would you feel confident to recommend and tackle effective management therapy if your patient has lymphoedema?

Note In the UK, the delivery of PDT or equivalent lymphoedema management approaches requires a specialist qualification recognised by the British Lymphology Society (BLS)

2.5.4 Reflective questions

- When would you advise your palliative care patient to undergo compression – and when not?
- How could you realistically manage and optimise the elements of PDT in your inpatient or outpatient setting?
- What experience do you have in the use of PDT for oedema of the head, and what form could compression take here?
- What forms of lymphoedematous proliferation have you dealt with particularly well?
- Which diseases have presented you with the most difficulty in terms of oedema therapy, and how were you able to improve the situation?
- What is your opinion of the thumb pressure test?
- What was the particularly challenging clinical picture that provoked the development of oedema in your patient?
- When considering oedema therapy, how do you manage your clinical time, and how do you de-stress after undertaking a strenuous session?

REFERENCES

Aulbert E, Nauck F, Radbruch L (eds). Lehrbuch der Palliativmedizin. 3rd ed. Stuttgart: Schattauer, 2011.

Association of the Scientific Medical Societies of Germany (AWMF). Instrumental intermittent compression according to the guidelines of the German Society of Phlebology. AWMF Register No. 037/007, 2007.

Association of the Scientific Medical Societies of Germany (AWMF). Compression classes according to the guidelines of the German Society of Phlebology. AWMF Register No. 037/009, 2008.

Association of the Scientific Medical Societies of Germany (AWMF). Diagnostics and therapy of lymphoedema. Guidelines of the Gesellschaft Deutschsprachiger Lymphologen. AWMF Register No. 058/001, 2011.

Bartels A. Zeki S. The neural correlates of maternal and romantic love. Neuroimage 2004;21(3):1,155–1,166.

Brennan MJ, Miller LT. Overview of treatment options and review of the current role and use of compression garments, intermittent pumps, and exercise in the management of lymphedema. Cancer 1998;83(12 Supplement American):2,821–2,827.

Bringezu G, Schreiner O. Lehrbuch der Entstauungstherapie. Vol. 1&2. Stuttgart: Springer, 2001.

Clemens KE, Jaspers B, Klaschik E, Nieland P. Evaluation on the clinical effectiveness of physiotherapeutic management of lymphoedema in palliative care patients. Jpn J Clin Oncol 2010;40(11):1,068–1,072.

Cornely M. Operative Lymphologie. Part 3: Die Vorbereitung des Paradigmenwechsels beim sekundären Lymphödem. Phlebologie 2011(5):268–273.

Deng J, Ridner SH, Dietrich MS, et al. Prevalence of secondary lymphedema in patients with head and neck cancer. J Pain Symptom Manage 2012;43(2):244–252.

Faul J, Berry GJ, Colby TV, et al. Thoracic lymphangiomas, lymphangiectasis, lymphangiomatosis, and lymphatic dysplasia syndrome. Am J Respir Crit Care Med 2000;161(3):1,037–1,046.

Flor EsM, Flor EnM, Flor AM. Manual lymph drainage in patients with tumoral activity. J Phlebol Lymphol 2009;2:13–15

Földi E. Das postoperative Lymphödem. Das klinische Problem: Diagnostik und aktuelle Behandlungskonzepte. Phlebologie 2011(3):123–126.

Földi M, Földi E. Das Lymphödem und verwandte Krankheiten. 9th ed. Munich: Elsevier, 2009.

Földi M, Földi E. Lehrbuch Lymphologie. 7th ed. Munich: Elsevier, 2010.

Földi M, Földi E. Lymphostatische Krankheitsbilder. In: Földi M, Földi E (Hrsg.). Lehrbuch der Lymphologie für Ärzte, Physiotherapeuten und Masseure/med. Bademeister. 7th ed. Munich: Elsevier, 2010: S. 175–263.

Földi M, Stößenreuter R. Grundlagen der Manuellen Lymphdrainage. 5th ed. Munich: Elsevier, 2011.

Gimpl G, Fahrenholz F. The oxytocin receptor system: structure, function, and regulation. Physiol Rev 2001;81(2):629–683.

Godette K, Mondry TE, Johnstone PA. Can manual treatment of lymphedema promote metastasis? J Soc Integr Oncol 2006;4(1):8–12.

Harris SR, Schmitz KH, Champbell KL, McNeely ML. Clinical practice guidelines for breast cancer rehabilitation. Syntheses of guideline recommendations and qualitative appraisals. Cancer 2012;118(8 Suppl):2,312–2,324.

Herpertz U. Ödeme und Lymphdrainage. Diagnose und Therapie von Ödemkrankheiten. 4th ed. Stuttgart: Schattauer, 2010.

Jakob L. Klinik und Prognose kutaner Angiosarkome und Kaposi-Sarkome. Doctoral dissertation, Dermatological University Hospital Tübingen, Dept. Dermatological Oncology, 2010.

Brown F, Fletcher C: Problems in Grading Soft Tissue Sarcomas. Am J Clin Pathol 2000;114(Suppl):S82–S89.

Lawenda BD, Mondry TE, Johnstone PA. Lymphedema: a primer on the identification and management of a chronic condition in oncologic treatment. CA Cancer J Clin 2009;59:8–24.

Martin ML, Herández MA, Avendaño C, Rodriguez F, Martinez H. Manual lymphatic drainage therapy in patients with breast cancer related lymphoedema. BMC Cancer 2011;11:94.

May R, Herberhold C. Möglichkeiten und Grenzen der Lymphdrainage in der HNO-Heilkunde. 2. Jenaer Fort- und Weiterbildungskurs „Onkologie in der HNO-Heilkunde", 7.–8.11.1997.

McNeely ML, Magee DJ, Lees AW, Bagnall KM, Haykowsky M, Hanson J. The addition of manual lymph drainage to compression therapy for breast cancer related lymph-edema: a randomized controlled trial. Breast Cancer Res Treat 2004;86(2):95–106.

Miller A, Knetsch K. Hautpflege bei lymphatischen Ödemen. Lymphologie in Forschung und Praxis 2007;11(1):29.

Nieland P. Einsatz der Physiotherapie in der Schmerzbehandlung. In: Aulbert E, Zech D (eds). Lehrbuch der Palliativmedizin. 1st ed. Schattauer, 1997.

Nieland P. Physiotherapie in der Palliativmedizin. Z Palliativmed 2009a(2):87–99.

Nieland P. Schmerz – Schmerzfreie Lagerung. pflegen: palliativ 2009b(1):28–32.

Panfil EM, Schröder G. Pflege von Menschen mit chronischen Wunden. Bern: Hans Huber, 2010: 229.

Pinell XA, Kirkpatrick SH, Hawkins K, Mondry TE, Johnstone PA. Manipulative therapy of secondary lymphedema in the presence of locoregional tumors. Cancer 2008;112(4):950–954.

Pschyrembel Klinisches Wörterbuch. 261th ed. Berlin: Walter de Gruyter, 2008.

Schingale FJ. Gesichtslymphödeme. Eine schwerwiegende Folge von Lymphgefäßstörungen im Kopfbereich. Phlebologie 2011(3):139–144.

Sippel K, Jünger M. Kompressionstherapie bei Varikose und chronisch venöser Insuffizienz. Gefäßchirurgie 2006;11:203–216.

Sordillo P, Chapman R, Hajdu SI, Magill GB, Golbey RB. Lymphangiosarcoma. Cancer 1981;48(7):1,674–1,679.

Szuba A, Achalu R, Rockson SG. Decongestive lymphatic therapy for patients with breast carcinoma-associated lymphedema. A randomized, prospective study of a role for adjunctive intermittent pneumatic compression. Cancer 2002;95:2,260–2,267.

Whitaker J. Genital oedema. Journal of Lymphoedema 2009 Vol. 4; No 1, 67–71.

Widgerow A. Scar management – marrying the practical with the science. Wound Healing Southern Africa 2010;3(1).

2.6 Fatigue and weakness
Sinead Cobbe

2.6.1 What is fatigue?

Fatigue is the most common symptom in palliative medicine (Radbruch et al. 2008; Sweeney/Neuenschwander/ Bruera 2005). It is strongly associated with advanced diseases such as cancer, AIDS, renal, cardiac and respiratory conditions (Solano/Gomes/Higginson 2006). Fatigue has traditionally received little attention from physicians (Stone et al. 2000), and treatment has lagged behind that of other symptoms such as pain (Collins et al. 2008).

The mechanisms of fatigue are poorly understood and are usually multifactorial. Attempts to link the severity of fatigue to disease progression have proved inconclusive and treatments themselves can be a contributing factor. The ubiquitous nature of fatigue in palliative care demands that knowledge of the condition be used when designing physiotherapy programmes. As pharmacological treatments for fatigue are still in their infancy, there is an opportunity for physiotherapists to step to the forefront of this developing field. The following case study illustrates some key aspects of fatigue management.

2.6.2 Case study

Mr J. N. was a 50-year-old farmer, married with one child. He had been referred by the palliative nurse and was assessed by a physiotherapist as an outpatient in the gymnasium of his local health centre. Initially he attended accompanied by his wife.

Diagnosis   Kidney cancer, with brain metastases.

Medical History   Nephrectomy and chemotherapy 2 years previously. Recent grand mal seizures.

Medications   Steroids to reduce brain swelling, anticonvulsant for seizures, analgesia for pain, sedative for agitation at night.

Subjective history   Mr J. N. reported the following significant physical factors:
- generalized fatigue, with gradual onset for 2 months; severity 4/10 at best, 10/10 after seizures; sometimes relieved by rest; worse after pain and seizure medications;
- difficulty sleeping from taking steroids, resulting in frequent daytime naps;
- de-conditioning: sedentary for prolonged periods during the day;
- left foot drop for previous 2 weeks;
- unsteady walking when tired.

Psychosocial factors further affecting his fatigue levels were:
- anxiety about the future;
- inability to work or drive, impacting on mood.

His goals were to:
- exercise for leisure;
- decrease fatigue levels;
- participate in family outings.

Objective examination   Gait independent. Slight foot drop; used a high-stepping gait. Oedema around ankles; proprioception poor in left foot. Strength in all 4 limbs normal, except that left dorsiflexors were 3/5 on Oxford scale. Exercise tolerance: walked 347 m in 3 minutes. Cycled 10 minutes at rate of 5 on the perceived exertion scale (see ➤ Figure 2.22 below).

Treatment Treatment options were fully discussed with Mr J. N., and sessions were planned for twice a week for 6 weeks initially before further review. Mr J. N. was provided with a walking stick and a foot drop splint to reduce the work of walking. He was also supplied with a wheelchair for outings with his family. His physiotherapeutic regime included:

- aerobic training: cycling: 10 minutes legs, 5 minutes arms;
- balance exercises for proprioception;
- resistance exercises: rubber bands for endurance: 30 repetitions × 2 sets for quadriceps, shoulder flexors, biceps;
- additionally, the patient was educated in energy conservation, sleep hygiene and relaxation techniques for night-time restlessness.

Multiprofessional team input Further liaison with other members of the team ensured a holistic approach to Mr J. N.'s fatigue. A doctor reduced the steroids to improve sleep patterns, prescribed diuretics to reduce ankle oedema, and rotated his pain medication to reduce impact on his fatigue. Social work input provided counselling for him and his family, an occupational therapist supplied equipment for energy conservation and finally music/art therapy sessions helped relaxation, self-expression and well-being.

Outcome at 6 weeks Mr J. N. continued to attend his twice-weekly physiotherapy sessions regularly, and a review showed:

- improved sleep; fewer daytime naps;
- improved exercise tolerance: 3 minute walk distance increased by 95 m;
- strength and fitness gains: 40 repetitions × 3 sets attained, 20 minutes lower limb cycle and 10 minutes upper limb cycle;
- general fatigue improved to 2/10 in severity;

- anxiety reduced as the patient gained more subjective control over his fatigue.

The patient's condition then began to gradually deteriorate, and he died about 2 months later with occasional physiotherapy intervention only for his mobility needs until the last week of his life.

Prevalence and effects of fatigue

The prevalence of fatigue in disease states is generally high and may be considerably more with advanced disease. It is therefore reasonable to assume that a high proportion of palliative patients experience some degree of fatigue. It not only has a detrimental effect on quality of life (QOL) and physical function, but has strong links with depression and anxiety (see ➤ Table 2.11). **Fatigue severity however does not always correlate with disease progression,** as patients with advanced disease may not be fatigued while those with less disease can be severely affected. Moreover fatigue tends to be under-prioritized by palliative patients themselves and only becomes more pressing when other symptoms have been controlled (Strömgren et al. 2006). This suggests that screening for fatigue by physiotherapists should be routinely carried out.

Aspects of fatigue

The terms used to describe fatigue include drowsiness, lethargy, asthenia, weakness, exhaustion, lack of energy, tiredness and desire for rest. Radbruch et al. (2008) defined fatigue in palliative care patients as *'a subjective feeling of tiredness, weakness or lack of energy'*. Fatigue is inherently different from sleepiness (Shen/Barbera/Shapiro 2006) even though they may be described in similar ways. It presents in three different dimensions:

Table 2.11 Prevalence and effects of disease-related fatigue

Disease	Prevalence	Detrimental effect on QOL	Link with anxiety or depression	Link with disease progression	Link with poor function
Advanced cancer	78 %–100 %	✓	✓	only towards end of life	✓
Motor neuron disease (MND)	44 %	✓	✓	X	no studies found
Multiple sclerosis (MS)	76 %–92 %	✓	✓	may be linked	✓
Chronic heart failure	90 %–100 %	✓	✓	✓	✓
Parkinson's disease	37 %–56 %	✓	✓	X	✓
HIV/AIDS	50 %–88 %	✓	✓	X	✓
Advanced renal disease	over 80 %	✓	✓	X	✓
Chronic lung disease	36 %–95 %	✓	✓	no studies found	✓

- physical: difficulty with practical tasks and maintaining performance;
- cognitive: detrimental effect on memory, concentration and psychological function;
- affective/emotional: reduced motivation, onset of depression, feeling of tiredness.

Before devising treatment plans, care must be taken to clinically reason which of these aspects are predominant. Also, fatigue may be hugely influenced by motivational and emotional factors.

Disease fatigue and normal fatigue

Fatigue is appropriate in acute illnesses and is part of the syndrome of 'illness behaviour' (Andrews et al. 2004), which also includes depression, nausea and anorexia. The role of fatigue in ongoing diseases is less well understood. For many years in cancer patients it was considered unavoidable (Stone et al. 2000) but this view has changed. Consensus opinion is that disease fatigue does not differ in *quality* from normal fatigue, except in its *intensity* (Chandhuri/Behan 2004; Olson et al. 2008; Radbruch et al. 2008).

'Physiological fatigue' is the kind of fatigue related to tiredness after activity, and this occurs in the general population. When physiological fatigue occurs, there is gradual deterioration in the ability to do a task, resulting in 'task failure'. This occurs when:

- the cardiovascular system cannot deliver enough oxygenated blood to the muscles or fuel supply to the muscles becomes depleted (**peripheral fatigue**);
- the drive from the motor cortex is inhibited by increases in dopamine and serotonin, or when core temperature rises to about 40 C (**central fatigue**) (Muhamed 2008).

In disease states, the sensorimotor system can become faulty, affecting movement and directly causing fatigue (Chandhuri/Behan 2004). Impairments above the level of the spinal cord lead to a greater propensity to central fatigue, while impairments below this level are more likely to lead to greater peripheral fatigue. In healthy persons, central fatigue has a minor role in task failure (Davis/Walsh 2010), but in patients with terminal disease it is believed to play a particularly strong role. **Patients can experience both disease fatigue and physiological fatigue.**

Pathophysiology of fatigue in disease states

A key feature of disease-related fatigue is that it does not respond to rest in the same way as normal fatigue. Disease fatigue is defined as both primary, that is due to disease itself, and secondary, when it is caused by treatments, concurrent syndromes or co-morbidities. ➤ Figure 2.19 outlines the main pathways of disease-related fatigue.

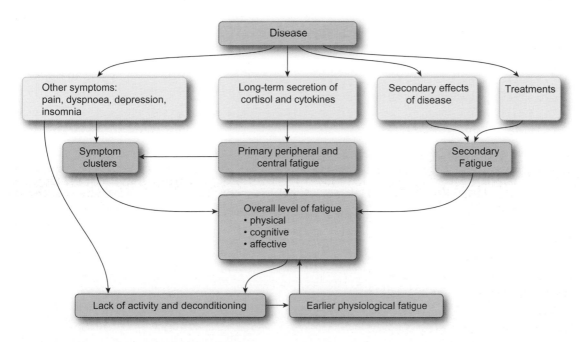

Figure 2.19 Pathways of disease fatigue [M545/L157]

Primary fatigue

In reaction to disease, cells release pro-inflammatory cytokines, which are designed to attack foreign bodies. The hypothalamus in the brain releases 'stress hormones', such as cortisol, to prepare the body for attack (Andrews et al. 2004). Prolonged exposure to cytokines and cortisol has detrimental effects on the sensorimotor system (➤ Table 2.12).

Secondary fatigue

In palliative care patients, a very large number of secondary factors tend to contribute to fatigue. Careful clinical reasoning is needed to take these into consideration when treating the fatigued patient at end of life. These multifactorial aspects are outlined in ➤ Table 2.13.

Table 2.12 Peripheral and central factors in primary fatigue and their implications

Mechanism impacting on fatigue	Implications
Loss of muscle mass occurs, due to cachexia or de-conditioning.	Increased muscle breakdown and less muscle bulk results in reduced strength and earlier physiological fatigue.
Changes in muscle function take place; fewer contractile elements in renal disease; loss of type I fibres in cardiac disease and cancer.	Fewer contractile elements means lower capacity to utilize oxygen. Loss of type I fibres leads to early onset of anaerobic metabolism and excess lactate levels.
Poor blood supply affects oxygenation of muscle.	There is early onset of anaerobic metabolism, and therefore early physiological fatigue.
Slower muscle recovery from exercise is found in renal disease and cancer.	There is early onset of anaerobic metabolism.
There may be altered perception of fatigue in the muscle ergoceptors. These perceive muscle work rate and are linked to the ventilatory system.	Ergoceptors are very active in cachexic patients, and cardiac patients, possibly leading to greater perception of fatigue.
Neurological disease leads to changes in muscle tone and strength.	There is often dissociation between electrical and mechanical properties in muscles, making movement more inefficient.
Central neural/hormonal control is disturbed, leading to lower muscle tone and a subjective feeling of being tired.	These are possibly the main pathways for fatigue in neurological diseases, and there is growing evidence of a role in cancer fatigue.

Sources: Andrews et al. 2004; Davis/Walsh 2010; Davis et al. 2011; Lou/Weiss/Carter 2010; Piepoli et al. 2006; Sweeney/Neuenschwander/Bruera 2005; Witte/Clarke 2007

Table 2.13 Secondary causes of fatigue and implications for physiotherapists

Secondary cause	Implications	Advice
Severe anaemia (Hb < 8 g/dl)	Anaemia, present in 70 % of palliative care patients, reduces exercise tolerance.	Careful pacing is necessary, as is liaison with medical team.
Infection	There is acute reduction in energy.	Careful pacing is necessary, as is liaison with medical team.
Fever	There is acute reduction in energy.	Careful pacing is necessary, as is liaison with medical team.
Nutritional deficits, including dehydration	Poor nutrition is suspected to have a role in fatigue, but improvements do not always mitigate.	Ensure sufficient hydration, nutrition, and control of gastro-intestinal symptoms when receiving physiotherapy. Liaise with dietitian.
Electrolyte imbalance (sodium, potassium, calcium, magnesium)	Low sodium or potassium can result from diuretic use; hypomagnesaemia from chemotherapy; hypercalcaemia is found in bony cancers. All can cause increased lethargy.	Liaise closely with medical team.
Cachexia/anorexia	Present in cancer, AIDS, and most end-stage diseases. These are associated with fatigue but it can exist independently of them; energy for vigorous activity may be greatly reduced.	Discuss nutrition with dietitian. Ensure that realistic goals are discussed with the patient.

Table 2.13 Secondary causes of fatigue and implications for physiotherapists (cont.)

Secondary cause	Implications	Advice
Endocrine disorders (diabetes, adrenal insufficiency, hypothyroidism, hypogonadism due to hormone treatments)	These can cause slow onset fatigue. Steroid withdrawal causes acute adrenal insufficiency and sudden reductions in energy.	Pace activities accordingly.
Side effects of treatments such as surgery, chemotherapy, radiotherapy	Chemotherapy fatigue peaks 4–5 days after treatment. Radiotherapy fatigue increases gradually and peaks at the end of treatment.	Plan timing and duration of treatments to avoid fatigue 'lows'.
Medications	Many medications cause fatigue as a side effect. Opioid toxicity is a common cause of acute drowsiness.	Be alert for sudden onset of fatigue associated with medication changes.
Neurological dysfunction	Peripheral neuropathies are a common side effect of chemotherapy and AIDS treatments. Paraneoplastic syndromes can result in localized neurological signs. Neurological changes contribute to fatigue through functional impairment.	Use corrective and adaptive support/strategies. Use balance and coordination techniques.
Autonomic dysfunction	This is present in over 50 % of cases with advanced cancer and may increase falls risk.	Use balance training and falls prevention.
Respiratory dysfunction: hypoxia, impaired respiratory muscles	There is increased daytime fatigue, reduced respiratory reserve and reduced recovery times on exertion	Night-time non-invasive positive pressure ventilation can improve daytime fatigue in MND and in end-stage respiratory diseases.
Deconditioning	Palliative patients can spend up to 5 hours per day sitting. This causes early onset physiological fatigue during daily activities.	Give guidance about pacing of activities of daily living and exercise
Cardiac dysfunction	Cardiomyopathy can be present in MND, cachexic patients and after chemotherapy.	Liaise with medical team and monitor exercise closely.
Ascites (fluid in abdominal cavity)	This makes movement tiring and cumbersome. Patients benefit from paracentesis but they may be weak for a day or two afterwards.	Careful timing and pacing of treatment sessions is needed.
Uncontrolled symptoms	Pain, depression, nausea, breathlessness, sleep disturbance and anxiety all contribute to fatigue.	Liaise with medical team. Use appropriate physiotherapy techniques.

Sources: Argilés et al. 2005; Lou/Weiss/Carter 2010; NCCN 2011; Oechsle et al. 2011; Radbruch et al. 2008; Rudnicki/Dalmau 2000; Stone et al. 2011a; Sweeney/Neuenschwander/Bruera 2005

Symptom control impact on fatigue and symptom clusters

Certain symptoms – depression, anxiety, and sleep disturbance – although contributing to fatigue, are not considered just as secondary causes. Indeed, many aspects of fatigue are also symptoms of clinical depression (Reuter/Härter 2004). Aspects of pain, nausea and breathlessness, if poorly controlled can also influence fatigue. Furthermore, symptoms co-exist and interact with fatigue and with each other. This is described as a **'symptom cluster'**, and is defined as *'three or more concurrent symptoms that are related to each other'* (Dodd/Miaskowski/Paul 2001). Established clusters associated with fatigue in cancer are outlined in ➤ Figure 2.20. This concept suggests that by impacting primarily on other symptoms, physiotherapists can influence and improve patients' fatigue.

2.6.3 Physiotherapy and fatigue

Physiotherapy assessment of fatigue

When assessing fatigued patients, physiotherapists must be mindful of the burden placed on patients. Comprehensive assessments rarely happen in one session, and time must be allowed for the patient and physiotherapist to explore symptoms together. An assessment and treatment regime is outlined; however, adaptations will be necessary for each patient.

Radbruch et al. (2008) recommend a single question for screening: *'Do you feel unusually tired or weak?'* Severity is assessed using the following question: *'How would you rate your fatigue on a scale from 0–10 over the*

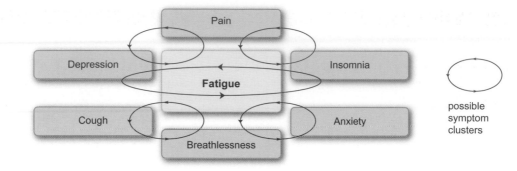

Figure 2.20 Symptom clusters associated with cancer fatigue [M545/L157]

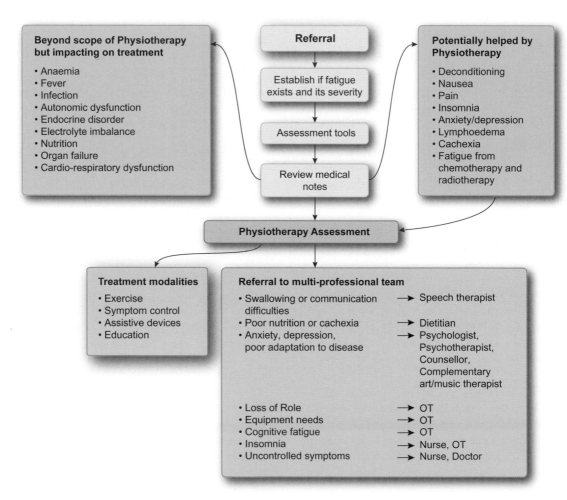

Figure 2.21 Assessment pathway for physiotherapists [M545/L157]

past 7 days?' (NCCN 2011). The medical history alerts the physiotherapist to the following:

- conditions outside the remit of physiotherapy but that can impact on fatigue;
- factors that might be improved by physiotherapy or require multiprofessional input (➤ Figure 2.21).

Assessment tools

There are a number of relatively short self-assessment tools suitable for assessing fatigue in palliative care patients. In the author's opinion, simple visual analogue scales (VAS) or the fatigue severity scale (Krupp et al.

Table 2.14 Subjective assessment

Aspects	Questions and reasoning
Onset and duration	Sudden onset is usually due to medical causes. Slower onsets may be amenable to physiotherapy. Does the history suggest de-conditioning?
Change over time	Does the pattern vary at times of the day, or with certain treatments?
Aggravating/alleviating factors	Is fatigue made worse by activity? If so, then some degree of physiological fatigue may be present.
Nature	Is the patient describing sleepiness, muscle weakness, generalized fatigue or cognitive fatigue? Are there memory problems or difficulties in concentrating? Muscle weakness and generalized fatigue can be treated with physiotherapy.
Other co-existent symptoms	Have the presence of pain, dyspnoea, nausea, cough and their severity been established?
Sleep disturbance	Is the problem getting to sleep, staying asleep or waking early? Waking early is associated with depression. Is pain, anxiety or something else preventing sleep? Does the patient nap during the day?
Interference with function	What can the patient *not* do because of fatigue? How much time each day is spent in bed or sitting? What is the effect on leisure/social activities? Consider the contribution of de-conditioning.
Food intake	Is there loss of appetite or difficulty eating/swallowing? Is the patient reducing fluid intake to prevent frequent toileting? Is fuel intake sufficient for his or her activity level?
Emotional effects	Is the patient anxious or depressed? Does fatigue make this worse? How does fatigue affect him or her emotionally? Does it impact on his or her family/carers?
Beliefs	What does the patient know about fatigue? What does it signify to him or her? Does he or she have any means of controlling it?
History of falls	Are there any falls, near falls or is there a feeling of unsteadiness? Are these linked to times when the patient is extra tired? Falls in palliative patients have been linked to a fear of falling, delirium, neuroleptic drugs and not wanting to ask for help (Pautex/Herrmann/Zulian 2008; Schonwetter et al. 2010).
Goals	What does the patient want to be able to do? Are the goals realistic?

1989), a 7 point Likert scale, can be easily used, and they work well. In addition, a multidimensional assessment tool, such as the *Multidimensional Fatigue Inventory* (MFI-20) (Smets et al 1995) although longer, appears to be widely used across the disease spectrum. These tools assess severity, impact on function or dimensions of fatigue. Disease-specific tools may also be used if available. The *Edmonton Functional Assessment Tool* is another tool, not specific to fatigue, that measures function and many other aspects affecting fatigue (Kaasa/Wessel 2000). Satisfaction or qualitative measures may be appropriate in very fatigued patients, for example: rating satisfaction or usefulness of treatment on a simple scale of 1–10. **It is vital to always use scales that are validated in the patient's own language,** as the literature shows that translation of descriptors can be ambiguous, and interpretation is then at risk.

Subjective assessment

Due to the multidimensional facets of fatigue, a thorough physiotherapy assessment will involve many broad-ranging questions and advanced level clinical reasoning. ➤ Table 2.14 outlines the main aspects of

assessment of the presentation that are relevant to the physiotherapist.

Objective assessment

Quick and pragmatic methods are used to assess the contributing factors to fatigue and the impact on function (➤ Table 2.15).

Treatment

Pharmacological treatments are used to treat fatigue in palliative patients with varying degrees of success (Yennurajalingam/Bruera 2007). It is beyond the scope of this chapter to evaluate these, but physiotherapists should be acquainted with such treatments as medications may improve fatigue irrespective of physiotherapy input. For example, steroids can cause dramatic improvements in fatigue and function.

The role of physiotherapy management of fatigue hinges on the following:
- recognition of factors outside the remit of physiotherapy;

Table 2.15 Objective assessment

Aspects to assess	Factors to consider
Observation: ascites, lymphoedema, cachexia	Is ascites making transfers/gait more tiring? Is lymphoedema making limbs heavy or difficult to move? Is cachexia present?
Physical function	Can the patient walk, transfer and do leisure activities? Could function be made easier with equipment?
Gait	Can the patient walk independently? Is walking limited by fatigue or something else? Would walking aids reduce the work of walking?
Strength	Measure strength of muscles involved in functional tasks. Proximal weakness may be due to steroid-induced myopathy. Localized weaknesses are noted. Strength can be measured clinically using (1) the Oxford scale, (2) a hand held dynamometer or (3) formulae that predict the one repetition maximum (1RM) (LeSeur et al. 1997).
Endurance	Ask the patient to perform a task that he or she finds easy. If the patient cannot repeat it more than 15 times, endurance is a problem. Lifting weights or doing functional tasks such as sit-to-stand can be used for the assessment.
Exercise tolerance	Is exercise limited by fatigue or another factor? The 6-minute walk test (ATS 2002) can be used, or alternatively measure the time spent on a stationary cycle before fatigue occurs. Physiological fatigue can be measured using the perceived exertion scale (see ➤ Figure 2.22 below) or changes in heart rate.
Balance	Falls are twice as common in palliative patients as in the elderly (Stone et al. 2011b). Falls may be linked to autonomic disturbance, so test initial standing balance. Cognitive balance tests, such as the dual task 'timed up and go' test (TUG), are important in patients with cognitive fatigue. Compare balance tests done when the patient is fatigued, with tests done when the patient is *not* fatigued.
Neurological testing	This is important if localized muscle weakness or primary brain disease exists. Weakness may be due to paraneoplastic syndromes or chemotherapy. What tasks are made more tiring by the deficits?

- ability to combat symptoms, including those involved in symptom clusters with fatigue, namely breathlessness, pain, insomnia, anxiety and depression;
- ability to directly impact on fatigue with exercise; exercise is also used to combat de-conditioning, and may benefit sleep, mood and symptoms such as pain and nausea;
- reduction of the functional work load with assistive devices;
- education of patients and carers to improve their understanding of fatigue and improve coping mechanisms.

Recognizing factors outside the remit of physiotherapy

Many possible causes of fatigue are medical or treatment related, and cannot be alleviated with physiotherapy. Physiotherapists need to recognize these and know which team members to refer to (➤ Figure 2.21). As fatigue is multifactorial, the most beneficial strategies typically involve joint approaches with other members of the multidisciplinary team (MDT). Multidisciplinary input is central to palliative care, and a coordinated team effort is most likely to be of benefit. **It is crucially important to coordinate treatments so that multiple treatments do not occur in a particular day or week, thereby adding to patient fatigue.**

Combating other symptoms

Combating other symptoms is possibly the most important consideration when dealing with fatigue in palliative patients. Treating other symptoms has a potentially powerful impact on reducing fatigue. Anxiety/depression, breathlessness, pain and insomnia are all involved in symptom clusters with fatigue and can all be alleviated with physiotherapy techniques. (➤ Chapter 2.2, ➤ Chapter 2.3, ➤ Chapter 2.4 and ➤ Chapter 2.7). Lymphoedema increases the workload of functional activities and can potentially be alleviated by physiotherapy (➤ Chapter 2.5). In addition, mood, sleep disturbance and nausea can all be alleviated by exercise or working in groups.

Relaxation

Relaxation techniques are used to alleviate anxiety, which can directly improve sleep patterns and therefore improve fatigue. They potentially dampen the effect of sympathetic 'stress' hormones, promoting release of parasympathetic hormones (Payne 2005). Since stress hormones, such as cortisol, are believed to add to central fatigue, these techniques may also directly impact on fatigue. **Inappropriate techniques may add to patient burden** (Kondo/Koitabashi/Kaneto 2009) so they must be tailored to the stress experienced:

- **Physical stress:** Tight muscles can be relieved by progressive relaxation techniques, breathing and massage. Breathing exercises alone can be effective (Bell/Saltikov 2000).
- **Cognitive stress:** Distressing thoughts can be relieved with cognitive behavioural techniques, meditation, distraction and imagery (Payne 2005, p. 11).

Relaxation techniques, including deep breathing, can also be used for severely fatigued patients, when other more vigorous activities are not appropriate.

Sleep management

By using physiotherapy to alleviate pain, anxiety or breathlessness, sleep patterns can be improved, resulting in less daytime fatigue. Sleep management techniques are also proven to benefit cancer fatigue (Mitchell/Berger 2006). These include:

- **sleep restriction:** restricting time in bed to time spent sleeping, and adhering to a 'sleep schedule';
- **sleep hygiene:** avoiding daytime naps; avoiding nicotine, alcohol and caffeine close to bedtime; having a quiet restful environment in bedroom;
- **relaxation techniques:** using relaxation techniques before bedtime and for sleepless episodes during the night (O' Donnell 2004).

Exercise in palliative care

Exercise is the most effective non-pharmacological treatment for reducing cancer fatigue, including during chemotherapy or radiotherapy (NCCN 2011). In patients who are non-symptomatic and functioning well, exercise is possibly the most important tool physiotherapists can use to impact on fatigue. Exercise trials in palliative cancer patients are outlined in recent systematic reviews (Beaton et al. 2009; Lowe/Watanabe/Courneya 2009) and one hospice trial (Buss et al. 2010). Fatigue improved, was unchanged, or the rate of advancing fatigue was reduced. The latter is probably a more appropriate measure of efficacy, as fatigue is realistically expected to increase in palliative patients over time. Quality of life improved in nearly all trials and few adverse events were recorded.

Patients often believe that exercise worsens fatigue (Borneman et al. 2011); exercise counselling is therefore advised. The benefits of exercise should be discussed with carers as many try to protect the patient by discouraging activity (Donnelly et al. 2010). Discuss their fears or dislikes about exercise, and also the precautions required to allow them to exercise safely. Make exercise

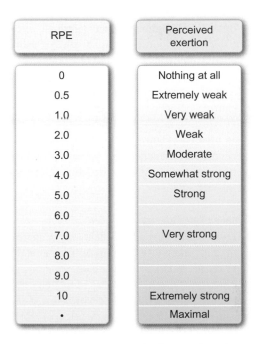

Figure 2.22 Borg category ratio scale of perceived exertion. Borg's category ratio scale includes a numerical rate of perceived exertion (RPE) scale as well as descriptive categories (CR-10) to aid with allocating a numerical perceived exertion score (Noble et al. 1983). [F324/L157]

enjoyable or meaningful by choosing one that enhances QOL, such as walking the dog; functional tasks such as daily chores; or fun and innovative interventions such as using interactive-technology exercise devices.

Aerobic exercise in palliative care

For cancer survivors, the *American College of Sports Medicine* (ACSM 2010) advises similar guidelines as for healthy adults: 3 times/week vigorous exercise for 20–60 minutes *or* 5 times/week moderate exercise, 30–60 minutes per day. For cancer patients, exercise is recommended to start at 30 %–45 % of heart rate reserve (HRR) for sedentary individuals with poor health (Schneider/Dennehy/Carter 2003). This should be at level 1–3 on the perceived exertion scale (➤ Figure 2.22). Those with moderate health and average fitness can start training at 50 %–60 % of HRR, or level 4–5 exertion.

Target heart rate

Calculate target heart rate as follows (Schneider/Dennehy/Carter 2003, p. 39):

- maximum heart rate (HR_{max}) = 220 minus the person's age
- HRR = HR_{max} minus resting HR
- target heart rate = resting HR + (% of HRR, as recommended)

Physiotherapists often start programmes with 5-minute slots throughout the day, gradually increasing the duration (Donnelly et al. 2010). For palliative care patients, moderate or low intensity exercise is appropriate, but in some trials this was progressed to high levels of intensity (Beaton et al. 2009; Lowe/Watanabe/Courneya 2009). Exercise can have a positive or negative effect on fatigue, depending on the degree of exertion used. ➤ Figure 2.23 is a guide to the degree of exertion that is beneficial for patients with fatigue, based on research into MS patients. This can be adapted for palliative patients.

Resistance exercise in palliative care

Resistance exercises are an excellent way of increasing strength and endurance in muscle groups. Loss of strength relates to loss of muscle bulk, whereas endurance is linked with oxygen delivery to the muscles. **Fatigue from radiotherapy is linked with reduced endurance rather than reduced strength** (Alt et al. 2011). In patients with chronic obstructive pulmonary disease (COPD), muscle endurance, not strength, was linked with decreased physical activity (Serres et al. 1998). This suggests that lack of endurance is a more important determinant of fatigue than lack of strength. Conversely, gains in endurance may reduce fatigue.

Resistance exercises are also believed to benefit cachexic patients by increasing protein synthesis, when combined with dietary supplements (Dudgeon et al. 2006). Cachexia is defined as loss of more than 5 % of pre-morbid weight in the preceding 6 months, and is due to decreased protein synthesis and increased muscle breakdown (Argilés et al. 2005).

When commencing resistance exercises it is advisable to start as advised for older/sedentary adults. This is a 40 %–50 % of 1RM, 10–15 repetitions for strength (ACSM 2011), using lower weights and 15–20 repetitions for endurance. Resistance bands, core exercises and functional tasks such as step-ups, can also be used to train strength and endurance: if the patient tires after 10–15 repetitions of an exercise, then the exercise can be used to train strength. If they tire after 15–20 repetitions or more, it can be used to train endurance. Start with one set of repetitions and progress to multiple sets. Recovery time of muscle is delayed in many diseases; therefore the rest period, normally 2–3 minutes between sets, should be extended. Courneya et al. recommend progressing to three sets before increasing resistance (Courneya/Mackey/McKenzie 2002). Forty-eight hours rest is advised between sessions; therefore **leaving a day's rest for muscle groups, or rotating exercised muscles on successive days helps to aid recovery.** In some trials, up to 80 % of 1RM was used on well functioning palliative patients (Beaton et al. 2009); therefore progression to higher weights can be done safely using clinical judgement. If treatment has to be postponed, the resistance or repetitions are reduced when resuming the programme (Schneider/Dennehy/Carter 2004).

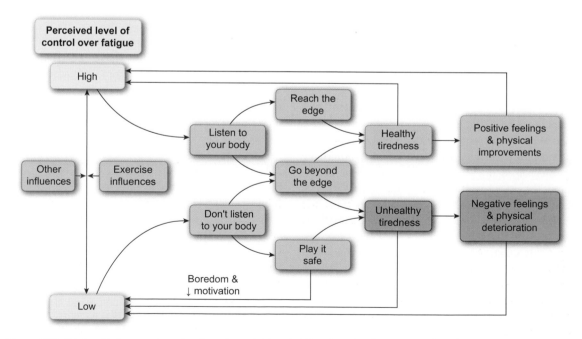

Figure 2.23 Relationship between intensity of exercise and fatigue in MS patients (Smith et al. 2009) [F323]

Stretching exercises in palliative care

Stretching exercises are appropriate for all palliative care patients. They are particularly useful for severely fatigued patients, when other forms of exercise cannot be done. They may reduce pain from static limbs, stretch scars from surgery/radiotherapy, as well as being relaxing. Stretching may help patients regain body awareness and a degree of control over their bodies. Deep breathing combined with stretches has an added possible effect on the visceral organs. T'ai chi, yoga and pilates all incorporate stretches and are regularly used for fatigued cancer patients (Donnelly et al. 2010).

Reduce the work of functional activities

Many functional tasks can be made easier by using adaptive equipment or compensatory techniques. This aspect should be assessed in conjunction with an occupational therapist who can discuss with the patient ways to reduce the energy expenditure of daily tasks. for example:

- Rolling walkers assist gait and require no lifting.
- High chairs are easier to rise from.
- Hoists assist transfers.
- Bed rails help bed mobility.
- Moving the bed downstairs avoids using the stairs.
- Using a commode reduces the energy used to walk to the bathroom.

Decisions to use assistive equipment can be distressing for the patient and family, but if they are explained in positive terms of **reducing energy expenditure,** patients may choose to use them rather than feeling that it signifies the loss of independence. Initially, they may need to use them only when very fatigued, which makes it easier to accept the changes occurring.

Patient and family education

Education of family/carers is an important aspect of fatigue management. Co-habiting patients report more fatigue (Collins et al. 2008; Stephen 2008), possibly because they worry about the impact on their loved ones. Benefits of exercise should be discussed, as **carers may try to protect the patient by discouraging activity** (Donnelly et al. 2010).

In general, patients and families find fatigue quite distressing and do not easily understand its causes or presentation. Explaining the fluctuating nature of fatigue is key in helping patients manage this complex symptom; patients can have 'good fatigue days' and 'bad fatigue days', and their levels of function need to be self-assessed and adjusted accordingly each day.

Multiprofessional fatigue groups are the ideal forum for providing education about coping with fatigue, cognitive behavioural techniques and advice on pacing and activities of daily living. **It is useful to use the analogy of money: energy is likened to a deposit in an'energy bank'.Patients may choose to spend it all on an important task and then feel fatigue. Or they can spend it in small amounts throughout the day, making it last the whole day.** Fatigue and/or sleep diaries can be helpful self-management tools, and patients should also be encouraged to discuss fatigue with their doctors. Sudden changes in fatigue levels may well be due to a reversible cause, such as infection, so patients should be urged to report any changes to their palliative nurse or physician. Explaining fatigue may not change its intensity, but it may improve coping mechanisms, thereby reducing distress. **Involving carers to help with exercise programmes or relaxation techniques may be of tremendous benefit to both carer and patient, if this is the wish of the patient.**

✓ **G U I D A N C E**

Strategies for patients living with fatigue:
- Accept fatigue, and don't fight it.
- Prioritize important tasks, and avoid unnecessary ones.
- Spread tasks throughout the day/week.
- Plan activities, including rest time.
- Sit for daily chores if possible.
- Delegate.
- Use assistive equipment to reduce workload.

⚠ **C A U T I O N**

End of life fatigue

In the last weeks of life:
- fatigue is inevitable and may be protective (Radbruch et al. 2008);
- fatigue may no longer cause distress to patients (Hagelin/Wengström/Fürst 2009), so physiotherapy intervention may no longer be indicated.

2.6.4 Conclusion

It is clear that fatigue is a highly complex symptom with numerous possible causes, and as a symptom it is hugely affected by the background medical condition. When physiotherapists work primarily to address fatigue, then it is important to understand in depth the most obvious factors that contribute. Skill lies in being then able not only to discuss these factors openly with the patient, but also to refer on to appropriate team members for other supportive strategies. The cognitive, physical and emotional consequences – which are often under-reported –

greatly affect patients' abilities and confidence at the end of life. Physiotherapists have the knowledge and tools to impact on fatigue at many stages of the disease trajectory, and good management involves both symptomatic and psychosocial interventions. Patients are very distressed by fatigue, and if we can alleviate their stress and help them understand it more, then we can reduce its impact on their lives, even if we cannot always change the intensity. **Above all, it is the patients' perception of control that will contribute most to quality of life.** Other benefits to the patient include improvements in function, strength, and independence.

Physiotherapy should play a leading role in fatigue management in palliative care. Collaboration with members of the MDT is both necessary and beneficial. By working together to address this major end of life symptom, physiotherapists are seen to play a key role not only for the patient and family but also by commissioners of service delivery in all end of life settings.

2.6.5 Reflective questions – fatigue

- How would you devise a multidisciplinary fatigue management programme in your workplace?
- How would you measure its effectiveness?
- What aspects should be incorporated into a fatigue information leaflet?

2.6.6 Group work in palliative care
Lorna Malcolm, Kate Norman

Historical context of groups in palliative care

Therapeutic groups are well established in palliative care. Particularly in day care, art therapy, music therapy and bereavement, groups are used to assist patients and their families come to terms with their disease and provide mutual support. Groups are also established modes of service delivery by physiotherapists for various conditions. Cardiac and pulmonary rehabilitation and back-care groups are well researched as effective programmes for improving function and exercise tolerance and are widely used in primary care throughout the UK.

Historically, in the UK, palliative care patients have mostly received one-to-one physiotherapy treatment. Principally this not only preserved some degree of discretion, but was a way of protecting vulnerable individuals from observing deterioration in others and being exposed

to reinforcement of their own morbidity and mortality. This one-to-one model also served to ensure that individuals' needs were singularly met, both physically and psychologically. However, interestingly, research has shown that **group work in palliative care can in fact reduce anxiety** (Lui et al. 2008). There are a number of benefits discussed below that suggest that group work may be not only an equally appropriate model but a preferred choice for many among this patient population.

The challenge facing physiotherapists working in end of life care today is the provision of therapy to patients who are surviving longer and with more co-morbidities. Patients may be unaware of the value of being active. Previous exercisers are often unsure if and when they should start exercising again, how much they should do, and how much they should push themselves. These perceptions are discussed further in ➤ Chapter 1.5. **One of the key issues facing physiotherapists in this field therefore is how to empower patients to choose activity** and to set realistic goals within the parameters of their symptoms and disease (Dahlin et al. 2009).

Advantages of group work

The NICE guidelines (2004) refer to the research of Braden and co-workers who suggest that structured, patient-centred interventions with elements of counselling and support, provided to groups, have beneficial outcomes for patients (Braden/Mishel/Longman 1998). It is an appropriate context to deliver support and information to cancer patients. **Group physiotherapy provides a mutually supportive setting where patients can increase or maintain their fitness and activity in a safe environment with professional supervision.** *'I think it's a really good class because it's hard to get motivated on your own, especially when you are in pain. Working with other people, seeing how you should do it is good'* (Mrs L.).

In the authors' experience, whilst exercising patients often share their stories and experiences, and banter and joke with each other. *'You are more inclined to do the exercises and enjoy it more when in a group. You can have a laugh, and it takes the seriousness away'* (Mrs A.) **This group support naturally evolves from a shared experience and, while encouraged, is initiated and sustained primarily by the patients, not the therapists.**

Group therapy is easily targeted to different physical abilities; using seated groups for less able patients, and gym equipment or more active standing exercises for the more able. Individual assessment and tailored programmes ensure that both the level of exercise and the type of activity is appropriate for the patient.

Educational element

A group structure provides an excellent opportunity for patient education by presenting a controlled situation allowing patients to learn from each other. Short presentations given within exercise sessions can empower patients and give them confidence to gradually increase their activity outside the group setting. The presentation style depends on aims and objectives, type and number of people within the group, group setting and available resources. An example of one style follows:

- setting: weekly one hour group exercise session with educational component;
- presentation: a 10-minute presentation at the start of each session;
- style: 5–6 presentation slides containing simple points on one of these key topics:
  - breathing and pacing;
  - falls prevention;
  - the components of health/fitness;
  - mental attitude to exercise/activity;
  - exercising at home.
- conclusion: time for interaction and questions.

Sometimes education may be the main focus of a group. Management of specific symptoms such as breathlessness, anxiety, fatigue and difficulty coping can be discussed in a group setting facilitated by various members of the MDT.

In this **next example, which addresses fatigue and breathlessness,** a range of topics is covered. Reasoning behind combining these symptoms is primarily because they are often experienced in combination. However, this also proves to be a useful strategy to mitigate the anxiety that could undermine a group focused on each symptom in isolation. Carers are also welcome to attend, and insight can be gained to supportive strategies:

- setting: weekly one hour fatigue and breathlessness group;
- presentation: focused on educational elements;
- style: slides, discussion, interspersed with exercises. Multiprofessionally led. Includes one of the following topics each week:
  - pacing, prioritization and planning (occupational therapist);
  - exercise and activity (physiotherapist);
  - breathlessness management (physiotherapist);
  - sleep hygiene (complementary therapist);
  - nutritional build-up (dietitian);
  - cognitive strategies for coping with symptoms (cognitive behavioural therapist).

√ **GUIDANCE**

Key considerations for successful group work

- Space: area available, health and safety regulations, lighting, temperature regulation;
- staffing: ensuring adequate physiotherapist-to-patient ratio;
- transport: provided by the facility, or patient's own; implications for attendance;
- equipment: use according to budget, space and availability;
- promotion: how and by whom will the programme be promoted? Who can refer and how?
- timing: ensuring no clash with other activities, groups or services so that patients can still access what they want and need;
- length of programme: should this run on a continuous cycle or run for a specific number of weeks?
- evaluation of service: introduce periodic progress assessments and user feedback;
- multiprofessional interaction: consider availability and benefit of linking with other team members as education providers.

Challenges in group work

The deteriorating patient

Group work presents challenges in ensuring effective treatment of individual patients. By definition, palliative care patients will deteriorate over time, and the trajectory of deterioration will vary. Many patients will plateau or experience a period of functional improvement before deteriorating. **Observing others in the group physically deteriorating, leaving the group and learning of their death can be a sharp reminder of patients' own mortality.** This may have emotional and psychological consequences for the patient. While being helpful in allowing patients to be realistic about their disease, it may also lead to anxiety or depression and thus need further management by other members of the MDT. For the deteriorating individual, there is the potential to experience a sense of failure when no longer being able to participate at the same level. To manage this, **devising exercises targeted at differing abilities allows the deteriorating patient to remain involved and continue to experience the support of others in the group.**

The use of passive equipment such as computerized/ motorized movement therapy systems or gentle arm pulleys allows participation at some level when continued involvement is thought to benefit the patient psychologically and will optimize circulation and range of joint movement.

Managing group numbers

With increased survivorship, **there is the risk that individuals, by continuing to attend over long periods, become dependent on the group for their exercise and psychosocial needs, preventing the recruitment and inclusion of new members.** A way to address this is by running the group as a course over a defined number of weeks. The goal over 9 weeks (for example), is for the individual to develop a personalized exercise programme guided by the physiotherapist, receive education about exercise choices and direction towards community or home exercise plans. *'I wanted it to make me feel a bit better about myself and get a bit more movement in my arms. I have very much enjoyed the 9 week course and have far more mobility now than I had before.'* (Mrs E.) If, subsequent to this, functional ability deteriorates, patients can be re-assessed to see if attendance at a further course is indicated.

Meeting individual needs

A further challenge of group work is the risk that patients' individual physical needs could be lost in a general exercise session. To prevent this, an initial one-to-one assessment session sets individual goals, agrees a personalized programme and introduces the patient to the exercises. This 'trial' session also serves to increase a patient's confidence before joining an established group. After the course is completed a second individual session re-assesses the patient's status, reflects on the course and ensures that the patient has an appropriate home exercise programme to continue and/or can be referred on to community services.

Evaluating effectiveness

Evaluating the effectiveness of physiotherapy intervention in palliative care is as challenging for group work as it is for individual work because the effectiveness of treatment may be obscured by patients' medical deterioration. At the time of writing there are no 'physiotherapy in palliative care specific' outcome measures, although the St Christopher's Index of Patient Priorities (SKIPP) is a new tool developed for palliative care (Sykes/Addington-Hall 2010) that could have potential for use in end of life physiotherapy. Physiotherapists need to consider which of the established measures in existence are appropriate to their patient group. Validated physical measures, such as 'timed up and go' (TUG; Podsiadio/Richardson 1991), show any changes in patient performance; subjective measures such as the Hospital Anxiety and Depression Score (HADS; Zigmond/Snaith 1983) indicate changes in psychological status, and tailored questionnaires can be used to evaluate changes in coping and understanding or for providing feedback (➤ Table 2.16).

Conclusion

With ongoing financial restraints, innovative solutions to limited resources are crucial in maintaining a quality physiotherapy service. Groups are a way of achieving this with the added advantage of offering psychological and social support. In the authors' personal experience **physiotherapy group work in end of life care is extremely rewarding for both the therapists and**

Table 2.16 Advantages and challenges of different physiotherapy groups. Careful consideration must be given to matching patient to group, both with regards to class structure and patient ability.

Type of class	Suitable for patients who …	Advantages	Challenges
Seated exercise	• … are wheelchair bound; • … want to improve limb mobility, joint flexibility, core strength, and/or specific muscular strength; • … cannot stand for any length of time or are unable to stand due to anxiety; • … need a gentler introduction/initiation into exercise.	• Inclusive of wheelchair bound patients and patients who have difficulty standing • One staff member can teach a large group • Exercises easily transferable to the home environment	• Managing group with different skill levels • Group psychosocial dynamics • Sourcing appropriate community classes • Discharging patients who want to stay within the group • Evaluating the effectiveness of the service because patients may deteriorate • Effectiveness of input and progression when patients may only attend once a week

Table 2.16 Advantages and challenges of different physiotherapy groups. Careful consideration must be given to matching patient to group, both with regards to class structure and patient ability (cont.).

Type of class	Suitable for patients who …	Advantages	Challenges
Standing exercise	• … are able to stand with no support or minimal support; • … need to work on their general fitness, strength, stamina and balance following specific treatment or remission of illness.	• Equipment-free, so can be delivered in many environments • Incorporates educational element to encourage independence on discharge from service • Allows patients to explore increased activity in supervised environment and gain symptom feedback from therapists • Exercises easily transferable to home environment	• Ensuring that staffing, number and disability level of patients correlates to guarantee patient safety • Preventing patients becoming dependent on the service for their exercise needs • Evaluating the effectiveness of the service as patients deteriorate
Circuits	• … are safe to move independently between equipment; • … can independently follow a written exercise programme; • … need to work on their general fitness, strength, stamina and balance following specific treatment or remission of illness; • … are anxious about increasing their activity alone, but would like to do more.	• Able to adjust written programme to suit individual patients' needs • Incorporates education element to encourage independence on discharge from service • Allows patients to explore increasing activity in a supervised environment and to gain feedback on symptoms from therapists	• Ensuring that staffing, number and disability level of patients correlates to guarantee patient safety • Preventing patients from becoming dependent on the service for their exercise needs • Managing the patient who places his or her hope of recovery in the gym environment and is reluctant to move on • Evaluating the effectiveness of the service as patients deteriorate • Accessibility to equipment in alternative settings
Education	• … experience symptoms or circumstances specific to the education session; for example: breathlessness, anxiety, fatigue or carer moving and handling; • … are able to hear, listen, understand and tolerate sitting for the duration of the session.	• Educates patients/carers to empower them to self-manage symptoms • A time and resource efficient way to educate patients about their symptoms • Patients/carers give each other support and advice as they share their own experiences	• Managing discharge in a group that is often well-connected through shared experience • Coordinating and communicating changes, development and patient information with other members of the MDT • Evaluating a largely educational service involving many professionals and different topics

patients, and the benefits far outweigh any potential challenges. *'They are excellent. We've been going for several weeks. There is improvement in my breathing and my muscles are better. The physios are one of the prime things [reasons] for coming to the hospice. It will give you great benefit'* (Mr T.)

Physiotherapists working in palliative/end of life care need to be creative when setting up groups within the constraints of available resources, continually evaluating the effectiveness of individual groups and contributing to research in this evolving area of practice.

REFERENCES

Alt C, Gore E, Montagnini M, Ng A. Muscle endurance, cancer-related fatigue and radiotherapy in prostate cancer survivors. Muscle Nerve 2011;43:415–424.

American College of Sports Medicine (ACSM). American College of Sports Medicine roundtable on exercise guidelines for cancer survivors. Med Sci Sports Exerc 2010;42:1,409–1,426.

Andrews P, Morrow G, Hickok J, Roscoe J, Stone P. Mechanisms and models of fatigue associated with cancer and its treatment: evidence from preclinical and clinical studies. In: Armes J, Krishnasamy M, Higginson I (eds). Fatigue in Cancer. New York: Oxford University Press, 2004: pp. 51–87.

Argilés J, Busquets S, Felipe A, López-Soriano F. Molecular mechanisms involved in muscle wasting on cancer and ageing: cachexia versus sarcopenia. Int J Biochem Cell Biol 2005;37:1,084–1,104.

Beaton R, Pagdin-Friesen W, Robertson C, Vigar C, Watson H, Harris S. Effects of exercise intervention on persons with metastatic cancer: a systematic review. Physiother Can 2009;61:141–153.

Bell J, Saltikov J. Mitchell's relaxation technique: is it effective? Physiotherapy 2000;86:473–479.

Borneman T, Koczywas M, Sun V, et al. Effectiveness of a clinical intervention to eliminate barriers to pain and fatigue management in oncology. J Palliat Med 2011;14:197–205.

Braden CJ, Mishel MH, Longman AJ. Self help intervention project: women receiving breast cancer treatment. Cancer Pract 1998;6:87–98.

Buss T, de Walden-Galuszko K, Modlinksa A, Osowicka M, Lichodziejewsken-Niemierko M, Janiszewska J. Kinesitherapy alleviates fatigue in terminal hospice patients: an experimental controlled study. Support Cancer Care 2010;18:743–749.

Chandhuri A, Behan P. Fatigue in neurological disorders. Lancet 2004;363:978–988.

Collins S, de Vogel-Voogt E, Visser A, van der Heide A. Presence, communication and treatment of fatigue and pain complaints in incurable cancer patients. Patient Educ Couns 2008;72:102–108.

Courneya K, Mackey J, McKenzie D. Exercise for breast cancer survivors: research and clinical guidelines. Phys Sportsmed 2002;30:33–42.

Dahlin Y, Heiwe S. Patients' experiences of physical therapy within palliative cancer care. J Palliat Care 2009;25:12–20.

Davis M, Walsh D. Mechanisms of fatigue. J Support Oncol 2010;8:164–174.

Davis M, Kisiel-Sajewicz J, Yue G, Seyidova-Khoshknabi D, Walsh D. Muscle fatigue changes biceps brachii muscle twitch force properties in healthy controls but not in cancer-related fatigue. In: 12th Congress of the European Association of Palliative Care: Palliative care reaching out. Newmarket: Hayward Medical Communications, 2011: p. 156.

Dodd M, Miaskowski C, Paul S. Symptom clusters and their effect on the functional status of patients with cancer. Oncol Nurs Forum 2001;28:465–470.

Donnelly C, Lowe-Strong A, Rankin J, Campbell A, Allen J, Gracey J. Physiotherapy management of cancer-related fatigue: a survey of UK current practice. Support Care Cancer 2010;18:817–825.

Dudgeon W, Phillips K, Carson J, Brewer R, Durstine J, Hand G. Counteracting muscle wasting in HIV-infected individuals. HIV Med 2006;7:299–310.

Hagelin C, Wengström Y, Fürst C. Patterns of fatigue related to advanced disease and radiotherapy in patients with cancer: a comparative cross-sectional study of fatigue intensity and characteristics. Support Care Cancer 2009;17:519–526.

Kaasa T, Wessel J. The Edmonton functional assessment tool: further development and validation for use in palliative care. J Palliat Care 2000;17:5–11.

Kondo Y, Koitabashi K, Kaneto Y. Experiences of difficulty that patients faced in the learning process of progressive muscular relaxation. Jpn J Nurs Sci 2009;6:123–132.

Krupp LB, LaRocca NG, Muir-Nash J, Steinberg AD. The fatigue severity scale: application to patients with multiple sclerosis and systematic lupus erythematosis. Arch Neurol 1989;46(10):1,121–1,123.

LeSuer D, McCormick J, Mayhew J, Wasserstein R, Arnold M. The accuracy of prediction equations for estimating 1RM performance in the bench press, squat and deadlift. J Strength Cond Res 1997;11:211–213.

Lou J, Weiss M, Carter G. Assessment and management of fatigue in neuromuscular disease. Am J Hosp Palliat Med 2010;27:145–157.

Lowe S, Watanabe S, Courneya K. Physical activity as a supportive care intervention in palliative care patients. J Support Oncol 2009;7:27–35.

Lui C, Hsiung P, Chang K, et al. A study on the efficacy of body-mind-spirit group therapy for patients with breast cancer. J Clin Nurs 2008;17:2,539–2,549.

Mitchell S, Berger M. Cancer-related fatigue: the evidence base for assessment and management. J Palliat Support Care 2006;12:374–387.

Muhamed A. Physiological models of fatigue during exercise. ISN Bulletin 2008;1:11–18.

National Comprehensive Cancer Network (NCCN). NCCN Clinical Practice Guidelines in Oncology: Cancer-Related Fatigue. Version 1, 2011. Available at: http://pfizerpro.com/resources/minisites/oncology/docs/NCCNFatigueGuidelines.pdf (last accessed August 2012).

National Institute for Clinical Excellence (NICE). Guidance on Cancer Services. Improving supportive and palliative care for adults with cancer: research evidence. 2004. Available at: http://www.nice.org.uk/nicemedia/live/10893/28818/28818.pdf (last accessed August 2012).

Noble B, Borg G, Jacobs I, Ceci R, Kaiser P (1983) A category-ratio perceived exertion scale: relationship to blood and muscle lactates and heart rate. Med Sci Sports Exerc 1983;15(6):523–528.

O'Donnell J. Insomnia in cancer patients. Clin Cornerstone 2004;6:S6–S15.

Oechsle K, Jensen W, Schmidt T, et al. Physical activity, quality of life, and the interest in physical exercise programs in patients undergoing palliative chemotherapy. Support Care Cancer 2011;19:613–619.

Olson K, Turner R, Courneya K, et al. Possible links between behavioural and physiological indices of tiredness, fatigue and exhaustion in advanced cancer. Support Care Cancer 2008;16:241–249.

Pautex S, Herrmann F, Zulian G. Factors associated with falls in patients with cancer hospitalized for palliative care. J Palliat Med 2008;11:878–884.

Payne R. Relaxation Techniques. A Practical Handbook for the Allied Health Professional. 3rd ed. Edinburgh: Elsevier Churchill Livingstone, 2005.

Piepoli M, Kaczmarek A, Francis D, et al. Reduced peripheral skeletal muscle mass and abnormal reflex physiology in chronic heart failure. Circulation 2006;114:126–134.

Podsiadlo D, Richardson S. The timed 'up and go': a test of basic functional mobility for frail elderly persons. J Am Geriatr Soc 1991;39:142–148.

Radbruch L, Strasser F, Elsner F, et al. for the Research Steering Committee of the European Association of Palliative Care. Fatigue in palliative care patients: an EAPC approach. Palliat Med 2008;22:13–32.

Regnard C, Hockley J. Fatigue, Drowsiness, Lethargy and Weakness. In: Regnard C, Hockley J (eds). A Guide to Symptom Relief in Palliative Care. 5th ed. Oxon: Radcliffe Medical Press, 2004: pp. 97–104.

Reuter K, Härter M. The concepts of fatigue and depression in cancer. Eur J Cancer Care 2004;13:127–134.

Rudnicki S, Dalmau J. Paraneoplastic syndromes of the spinal cord, nerve and muscle. Muscle Nerve 2000;23:1,800–1,818.

Schneider C, Dennehy C, Carter S. Exercise and cancer recovery. Champaigne: Human Kinetics, 2003.

Schonwetter RS, Kim S, Kirby J, Martin B, Henderson I. Etiology of falls among cognitively intact hospice patients. J Palliat Med 2010;13:1,353–1,363.

Serres I, Gautier V, Varray A, Prefaut C. Impaired skeletal muscle endurance related to physical inactivity and altered lung function in COPD patients. Chest 1998;113:900–905.

Shen J, Barbera J, Shapiro C. Distinguishing sleepiness and fatigue: focus on definition and measurement. Sleep Med Rev 2006;10:63–76.

Smets E, Garssen B, Bonke B, De Haes J. The Multidimensional Fatigue Inventory (MFI) psychometric qualities of an instrument to assess fatigue. J Psychosom Res 1995;39(3):315–325.

Smith C, Hale L, Olson K, Schneiders A. How does exercise influence fatigue in people with multiple sclerosis? Disabil Rehabil 2009;21:685–692.

Solano JP, Gomes B, Higginson I. A comparison of symptom prevalence in far advanced cancer, AIDS, heart disease, chronic obstructive pulmonary disease and renal disease. J Pain Symptom Manage 2006;31:58–69.

Stephen S. Fatigue in older adults with stable heart failure. Heart Lung 2008;37:122–131.

Stone C, Nolan B, Kenny R, Lawlor P. Prospective study of the prevalence and prognostic utility of autonomic dysfunction in ambulant patients with advanced cancer. In: 12th Congress of the European Association of Palliative Care: Palliative care reaching out. Newmarket: Hayward Medical Communications, 2011a: p. 88.

Stone C, Lawlor P, Nolan B, Kenny K. Falls: Is this geriatric giant an even bigger issue in palliative care? In: 12th Congress of the European Association of Palliative Care: Palliative care reaching out. Newmarket: Hayward Medical Communications, 2011b: pp. 56–57.

Stone P, Richardson A, Ream E, Smith AG, Kerr DJ, Kearney N. Cancer related fatigue: inevitable, unimportant and untreatable? Results of a multi-centre patient survey. Ann Oncol 2000;11:971–975.

Strömgren AS, Sjogren P, Goldschmidt D, Petersen MA, Pedersen L, Groenvold M. Symptom priority and course of symptomatology in specialized palliative care. J Pain Symptom Manage 2006;31:100–206.

Sweeney C, Neuenschwander H, Bruera E. Fatigue and asthenia. In: Doyle D, Hank G, Cherny N, Calman K (eds). Oxford Textbook of Palliative Medicine. 3rd ed. Oxford: Oxford University Press, 2005: pp. 560–568.

Sykes N, Addington-Hall J. New outcome measures for palliative care. National Council for Palliative Care: Inside Palliative Care, 2010;14:14–16.

Witte K, Clarke A. Why does chronic heart failure cause breathlessness and fatigue? Prog Cardiovasc Dis 2007;49:366–384.

Yennurajalingam S, Bruera E. Palliative management of fatigue at the close of life. JAMA 2007;297:295–304.

Zigmond AS, Snaith RP. The hospital anxiety and depression scale. Acta Psychiatr Scand 1983;67:361–370.

BIBLIOGRAPHY

Armes J, Krishnasamy M, Higginson I (eds). Fatigue in Cancer. New York: Oxford University Press, 2004.

Dittner A, Wessely S, Brown R. The assessment of fatigue: a practical guide for clinicians and researchers. J Psychosom Res 2004;56:157–170.

Whitehead L. The measurement of fatigue in chronic illness: a systematic review of unidimensional and multidimensional fatigue measures. J Pain Symptom Manage 2009;37:107–129.

2.7 Anxiety in the context of palliative physiotherapy

Rainer Simader

This chapter mainly discusses the fears that have a direct or indirect effect on the mobility and function of critically ill individuals. Aside from the causes and effects, it also addresses the positive side of physical therapies in situations overlaid with anxiety.

2.7.1 Case study

The patient   Mrs K., 77 years old, is referred to a mobile palliative care team by her oncologist for symptom control (severe dyspnoea) and assessment with a view to assistance in activities of daily living. Mrs K. lives with her 35-year-old son in a two-storey house. She was diagnosed eight weeks ago as having metastatic and incurable small-cell lung cancer. At their first meeting, the home care nurse advises admission to a hospice since the patient is clearly in need of a much more intense programme of support. Mrs K. is described by her family and friends as having been highly independent, active, lively and immaculate until the day of her diagnosis.

Initial assessment   Mrs K. is brought to a ward of the hospice on a Thursday lunchtime by the ambulance service. The physiotherapist sees her that same afternoon because of her serious breathing difficulties. He observes a somewhat unkempt, old-looking lady sitting in an armchair in her room, but not leaning against the back of the chair. The only movement visible or even audible from her otherwise completely rigid body is very rapid breathing with marked inspiratory effort (she is on 2 L oxygen via nasal cannula). Her eyes are wide open and fixed on the blank wall. Mrs K. hardly responds at all when first addressed. The therapist asks nonetheless whether he can stay with her and explain the purpose of the hospice and in particular what his role will be. Occasional, brief eye contact is established, especially when the therapist explains that physiotherapy will play an important part in treating the breathing difficulties and facilitate as much independence as possible. Little physical contact is achieved, however, with the patient's rigidity being very powerful and 'overwhelming'. The therapist's interpretation is that fear could be a major factor. After about 10 minutes, he volunteers an opinion: '*Mrs K., if I look at your body I have the feeling that fear is a serious consideration here.*' (Note: it is important to describe one's own interpretation as it really is. Also, the therapist has applied the technique of externalisation (➤ Chapter 3.1)). He hardly finishes the sentence before eye contact is sustained and the patient starts to cry (with her breathing becoming calmer as a result).

The physiotherapeutic strategy Mrs K. then describes how she felt *'struck down'* by her diagnosis and that she is very frightened, both of dying and of the hospice, which she sees as a *'house of death'*. She also reports that her family has relieved her of all her activities since the day she was diagnosed and they, along with her friends, constantly demand that she take it easy and *'look after herself'*. But because of the shock, she doesn't feel at all able to make decisions for herself and sees this as her fate. She reports anxiety caused by the distressing breathing difficulties and her loss of self-confidence as regards being able to walk. She reports that at home she can only reach the toilet from her living room (where she is now sleeping as well), just four metres away, by stopping a number of times on the way.

Her breathing has now become a little deeper, and posture slightly relaxed. With a view to the pending weekend, the therapist devises the following **plan:**
• information on breathlessness;
• simple exercises for coping independently with the dyspnoea;
• initiation of an active exercise programme for improving mobility and subjective security (an important objective is to assign the patient an active role).

The following **actions** are to be pursued in the first couple of days:
• information about the pathophysiology of breathlessness, basic anatomy of the lungs, importance of expiration (the patient was initially afraid of breathing out due to the experience of not getting enough air), proposal and information concerning walking aids (initially rejected by the patient); a brochure on managing dyspnoea is left behind, in a prominent position, both as a reminder and also for informing visitors;
• self-management programme: exercises for expiration, active depression of the pectoral girdle, positioning of the arms and supporting the lumbar spine when sitting, permission to request active support from team members at any time; use of a fan;
• exercise programme: extension of the knees when seated, getting up from and sitting down on an armchair, thoracic rotations.

The plan and activities are also documented in order to keep the weekend staff informed of the strategy.

Ongoing physiotherapeutic strategy Mrs K. performs the exercises over the weekend, and the subjective experience of the dyspnoea clearly improves. At the interdisciplinary team meeting, consideration is given to discharging Mrs K. with the appropriate support and symptom control, since this would respect the patient's wishes and is also believed by the team to be feasible. In light of the scheduled discharge, the physiotherapy goal is 'mobility at home'. To achieve this, the following **treatment plan** is drawn up with the patient after evaluating Mrs K. and her functionality:
• continued dyspnoea management, also on exertion;
• increased walking distance and trial with a walking aid;
• general activity for regaining self-confidence and security.

The following strategies are undertaken:
• participation in dyspnoea group therapy accompanied by her son (➤ Chapter 2.4, ➤ Chapter 2.6);
• incorporation of the adopted activities in daily one-on-one therapy (breathing in stressful situations, finding a comfortable walking speed, managing pauses correctly);
• commence walking with a walking frame and mobile oxygen system (referred to by the patient after the first attempt: *'This could be love at first sight.'*);
• after one week: participation in an exercise group (one hour/three times a week);
• home visits from occupational therapist (analysis of aids and appliances).

Ongoing management The patient spent a total of 17 days at the hospice; her mood improving exponentially. Mrs K. was able to walk about 300 metres with the frame and also managed to tackle a flight of stairs. Nevertheless, when at home she decided from then on to live on the ground floor. During the day the shortness of breath no longer proved a problem except when there were a lot of visitors and much talking. Mrs K. was discharged home and attended a once-weekly exercise group for a further eight weeks. She was readmitted after 10 weeks and died shortly thereafter.

2.7.2 Anxiety in palliative care patients

General anxiety

Working in the palliative care setting and living in an environment – whether in an elderly care home or one's own house – where the subject of death is 'omnipresent' can be full of emotions. In light of this and the

Table 2.17 Prevalence of anxiety and depression (Mitchell et al. 2011)

Diagnosis	Palliative care setting	Oncological/ haematological setting
Major depression or episode of major depression	14.3–16.5 %	14.9–16.3 %
Minor depression	9.6 %	19.2 %
Adjustment disorder	15.4 %	19.4 %
Anxiety	9.8 %	10.3 %

fact that a person's life is about to come to an end, it is not abnormal for anxiety to spread – in fact it can simply become a matter of course. A specific assessment will help determine whether and, if applicable, which members of a multiprofessional team should deal with the said anxiety.

Figures vary concerning the frequency with which patients at end of life are diagnosed with a psychiatric condition requiring treatment. The figures in ➤ Table 2.17 were collected by Mitchell et al. (2011) in a meta-analysis of the frequency of depression, anxiety and adjustment disorders in cancer patients in the palliative and non-palliative care setting.

Wilson et al. (2007) also report that anxiety and depression often co-exist and that those affected experience much greater suffering than patients who suffer only one of the two conditions. It should also be noted that, significantly, the existence of one or both of these conditions is accompanied by an increased sense of general malaise, pain, numbness, nausea, weakness and also shortness of breath. Mitchell et al. (2011) note that such conditions are often inadequately identified, diagnosed and treated, and hence there is a considerable discrepancy between the needs and the willingness of those affected to undergo treatment. The diagnosis of psychiatric and psychological disorders, together with any appropriate psychotherapeutic treatments, is important. The experience shows that physiotherapeutic interventions and training are an effective form of treatment.

Anxiety concerning the body, movement and activity

Jolliffe and Bury (2002) and Oldervoll et al. (2006) report that physical condition and function are one of the most important determinants for quality of life in palliative care patients. Physical function includes respiration or excretion on the one hand, but also walking, visiting the toilet independently, etc., on the other. The fear of being physically dependent on somebody else and having uncontrollable symptoms (pain, dyspnoea, etc.) contributes considerably towards diminishing quality of life (Heyland et al. 2006, Lloyd-Williams et al. 2007, Mystakidou et al. 2005). Kolva et al. (2011) describe how patients suffering from anxiety more often have a diminished level of physical functionality. Physical function and mobility also enhance self-confidence in palliative care patients (Jolliffe/Bury 2002, Kieslinger 2001). Conversely, self-confidence is reduced when such functions are lost and in turn this can lead to anxiety.

Lloyd-Williams et al. (2007) report similar findings in the elderly. A number of older people talk of a 'good death' if physical autonomy is preserved for as long as possible. There is also a tremendous desire to remain in the home environment, particularly if disease progresses.

Mobility, activity and also the associated ability to manage certain – not just physical – interactions are very important marks of identity to humans. They are often self-evident in the daily routine of a healthy individual and an automatic part of human life. If during a phase of severe illness *'the body suddenly begins to lecture the patient'*, as Dreßke (2005) writes, anxiety can be anticipated as a result of this loss of control.

Physical loss of control engenders fear

In palliative care patients, aspects related to the body that engender fear include the loss of functional ability, awareness of physical changes (e. g. sores, odours, etc.) and also the associated change in one's own identity. As a result the patient is confronted physically with an external loss, and mentally with a frightening, inner **loss of control.**

From defining the physiotherapeutic goals to devising a plan of action and implementing the appropriate interventions, it is very important to support the patient in gaining self-control and realising his own capabilities. Cicely Saunders formulated it thus: *'to enable the dying person to live until he dies, at his own maximal potential performing to the limit of his physical and mental capacity with control and independence whenever possible'* (Saunders 1998). This is also commensurate with the basic human need for autonomy and control – even, and above all, at the end of life.

Anxiety is also a palpable and visible physical sensation that interacts very intensely with emotional fears. Thoughts and physical sensations play a major role in the intensity of the anxiety experienced (➤ Figure 2.24).

2

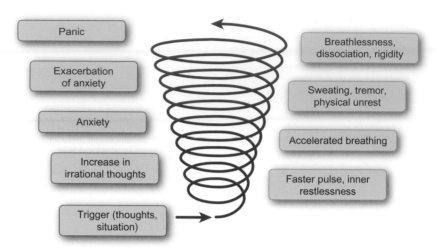

Figure 2.24 Spiral of fear [M547/L157]

Fear avoidance – reasoning and behaviour

In palliative physiotherapy, fear must always be considered before commencing activity itself. In the author's experience, there are two factors that are often significant to such a process.

On the one hand there may have been a **bad experience with movement** during the course of the disease. Patients over-exert themselves and therefore find that their symptoms worsen (e.g. fear of increased movement due to shortness of breath, pain or a fall caused by over-exertion or carelessness). *For the patient* the logical reasoning may be that this type of movement is dangerous or even harmful. Such a mind-set is known in chronic pain emergence as 'fear avoidance reasoning'. This change in attitude, which to the patient is logical, will include avoidance of the potentially 'dangerous' activities. This is referred to as 'fear avoidance behaviour'. The pattern of emergence has been closely researched and described in patients with chronic pain conditions and it can be assumed that the mechanisms will be similar in patients with severe, life-limiting diseases.

The second factor may be **transferral of fear** to the patient by another individual through remarks that are often incidental and appear to lack consideration. Even patients not presenting with specific symptoms are repeatedly urged by their family, social surroundings and even members of the medical professions from whom they are receiving care to 'take it easy' (= you're sick and weak), and so are relieved of activities by being told to 'Leave that, I'll do it' (= I no longer trust you with that, or: I can do it quicker), etc. Hence the patient is quickly 'pigeonholed' by society as being seriously or chronically ill, an attitude that actively engenders fear. Danger can be construed from many of the messages a sick person

receives – even danger to life or survival in the case of a life-limiting illness. Fear emerges above all if a message is articulated by members of the medical professions whom the patient would never question or 'has to' believe, or on whom he or she feels dependent. Avoidance behaviour can also be 'programmed' in such a way, though evidence suggests that the *promotion* of activity in palliative care patients is important (➤ Chapter 1.4, ➤ Chapter 2.6).

Such patterns are globally recognised in physiotherapy. One possible pattern can emerge in patients with incurable diseases, as illustrated in ➤ Figure 2.25:

Sometimes, behaviour to the contrary can be seen. Existential fear can also be engendered by patients attempting with all their available energy to train intensively or be excessively active in order to prevent the impending threat, namely their physical demise.

Fear as an important means of protection

Another possible reason why patients avoid activity and movement at the end of life may be that they are protecting themselves. Fear not only has a destructive aspect that worsens quality of life, but **fear can also prevent negative encounters.** It is neither physically nor mentally agreeable to have to repeat activities that also involve truly negative sensations such as pain, dyspnoea, nausea, etc. Tremendous care needs to be taken with fear, therefore, and the **fear protective function should not be broken by a hyper-motivated 'we can do it' mentality.** An extensive, interdisciplinary approach to symptom control, for the purposes of ameliorating the fear, is essential in such a case.

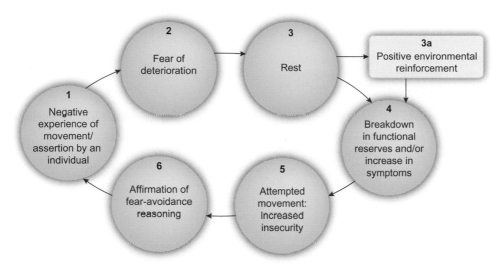

Figure 2.25 Emergence of the fear of movement [M547/L157]

✓ **G U I D A N C E**

Helpful therapeutic approaches to fear

- Even palliative care patients wish to achieve certain goals.
- It is important to consider your attitudes: Do you feel that patients at end of life are capable and have the right to achieve things?
- Patients have every right to be fearful.
- Fear can protect patients from negative experiences.
- Fear can be contagious, requiring the therapist to be strong and self-confident.
- It is not possible to take a patient's fear away; what is important is to offer the patient help in order that he can learn how to better manage his fear
- Fear is also a physical sensation; so there is a possibility to intervene with physically orientated therapy.

2.7.3 Specific and practical assessment methods related to anxiety

The assessment of anxiety is important for different diagnostic reasons (Mitchell et al. 2011). The question of whether a physical symptom such as palpitations, dyspnoea, sweating or indigestion has arisen from anxiety or from the underlying disease is significant to further therapy (Pessin/Rosenfeld/Breitbart 2002).

Specific assessments

- **Hospital Depression and Anxiety Scale (HADS)** (Zigmond/Snaith 1983): measures the level and course of anxiety, without looking in more detail at physical effects and symptoms.

- **State Trait Anxiety Inventory (STAI)** (Spielberger/Gorsuch/Lushene 1970): a much more lengthy assessment, as well as being more differentiated.
- **Anxiety Rating Scale (HAM-A)** (Hamilton 1959): examines a range of physical symptoms (muscular, cardiovascular, respiratory, etc.).
- **Beck Anxiety Inventory (BAI)** (Beck/Steer 1993): assesses a number of physical changes related to anxiety.

Other specific questionnaires that examine anxiety, physical symptoms (mostly pain), physical behaviour and activity are generally derived from musculoskeletal physiotherapy and have not been evaluated in palliative care patients. Examples are the *Fear Avoidance Beliefs Questionnaire* (Waddell et al. 1993), the *Pain Anxiety Symptoms Scale* (McCracken/Zayfert/Gross 1992) or *Tampa Scale for Kinesiophobia* (Miller/Kori/Todd 1991). In terms of the fear of falling, the *Fall Efficacy Scale* (Tinetti/Richman/Powell 1990) can be used.

Individual questions from these assessments can also be used with palliative care patients, though the physiotherapist should be more flexible in his choice of words. In the opinion of the author, the term 'pain' can be replaced by the terms breathlessness, weakness or other symptoms, where applicable.

The following **questions** with a view to discerning anxiety and evaluating the physical behaviour and attitudes of the patient are useful for the future therapeutic plan.

- Are you afraid that your condition (specify: breathlessness, pain, fatigue, etc.) will deteriorate (specify: walking, standing up, climbing the stairs, leaving the house, etc.) when you move?

- Do you believe that training, exercises, etc. are useful in your situation?
- Do you feel that you now (specify: since diagnosis, because of metastasis, due to shortness of breath, etc.) have to be especially cautious or avoid certain activities? If so, which?
- What do you do (how do you behave) if your symptom (specify) becomes obvious? Responses that could indicate anxiety are: immediately lying down, immediately taking a break, can't think of anything else, etc.

Aside from all the assessments and specified questions, the therapist should not forget the most important question: "Are you afraid?" or "What are you afraid of?" Anxiety is a feeling that is seldom welcomed in society, and a topic that is often neglected or taboo even in the medical environment.

From the author's experience, basic skills in resource-orientated conversational techniques are helpful when working with palliative care patients and their families (➤ Chapter 3.1 and ➤ Chapter 3.2).

> ✓ **GUIDANCE**
>
> **Is it dangerous to address the matter of fear?**
>
> All the questions listed above will enable the patient to express his anxiety in words, and help him to differentiate as well as allay such fears. It is not unusual for a therapist to be anxious about specifically addressing the subject and asking questions – mostly for fear of then triggering or potentiating any anxiety or other intense reactions.
>
> **Such apprehension is misplaced, since** …
> - … nothing will develop or emerge from the patient that hasn't already existed;
> - … the verbal expression of an inner feeling brings great relief to the patient, but is ultimately also beneficial to the therapeutic process;
> - … having the opportunity to articulate important worries and fears during therapy is a crucial aspect of care that fosters a good relationship between the patient and therapist;
> - … even if a patient starts to cry or otherwise reacts very emotionally, he will also stop doing so at some point.

Other methods for assessing anxiety

Most of the assessment tools mentioned are based on **patient self-evaluation.** As many as possible of the patient's cognitive functions must still be intact in order for him to be able to make valid statements regarding his experiences.

There are no specific assessment tools for evaluating anxiety in individuals with cognitive disorders (e. g. dementia). In this case the PACSLAC Scale (Fuchs-Lacelle/Hadjistavropoulos 2004) could be used (➤ Chapter 2.8), whilst consultation with the team and family is essential.

It is important to always take note of the physical signs of anxiety, since it should not be presumed that patients are always able or willing to formulate their fears verbally.

When observing very anxious individuals the most noticeable **non-verbal features,** according to Pessin et al. (2002), are:
- high muscle tone;
- gripping/clinging;
- shallow and possibly rapid breathing;
- reduction in general mobility;
- refusal to move;
- vegetative symptoms (increased sweating, tremor);
- nausea;
- dizziness or vertigo.

2.7.4 Physiotherapeutic interventions related to anxiety

Active interventions should be prioritised where possible, since there is a risk of losing self-control (➤ Figure 2.25). Support can and should be offered on both a verbal and physical level. Verbal interventions are designed to differentiate the anxiety, develop coping strategies and solutions, define realistic goals and – very important with anxiety – provide information. The objective of physical intervention is to work through situations in which anxiety develops, experience movement, recognise one's own limits, improve the use of resources (such as pacing), gain self-confidence, increase physical strength and endurance, and relax by integrating relaxation techniques.

> ⚠ **CAUTION**
>
> Anxiety can have a 'paralysing' effect and some palliative care patients are fearful of making their own decisions. Over the course of their disease, patients constantly have to make decisions that involve a great deal of uncertainty and ultimately may also bring disappointment (e. g. deciding for or against treatment). The challenge of making a decision or doing something can trigger anxiety, even if it 'only' involves physical training or further (physio)therapeutic interventions. To provide the patient with some relief from this, the therapist can make recommendations and assure him that he will 'take good care of him'.

Basic approach

The physiotherapist's task is to mark out a protected space and, using his knowledge, abilities and skills, suggest ways in which the patient can learn to deal with his anxiety and judge his own mobility as well as make the best possible improvements. The patient dictates the pace. Any external pressure will cause the patient anxiety and generate resistance, even if the therapist is convinced that the patient does actually possess the necessary ability. And even if the patient decides against expanding that space or if goals cannot be reached because of a progression in the disease, it is very important that the patient takes advantage of all his own available resources in this secure space.

Differentiation of anxiety

Under certain circumstances the patient will find it difficult, in the beginning, to describe his anxiety precisely. There may be a feeling of impotence ('having no strength'). Differentiation is possible by asking what the patient is really afraid of. If a patient has suffered a fall, for instance, he may simply be anxious about falling again, or he may be frightened that he can no longer get up from the floor on his own. Through differentiation, the planned therapy and interventions will also change.

Definition of realistic goals

If unrealistic goals are pursued, disappointment and anxiety result. It is helpful to pursue part-objectives and distinguish important goals from those that are less important (➤ Chapter 2.1).

Clarification and modification of less helpful beliefs

"Make the patient an expert in his problem and its solution". Knowledge can reduce anxiety; many fears emerge if the information allows too much room for interpretation or if conflicting and incorrect information, or no information at all, is provided. It is very helpful if patients and their families receive the correct basic information about the disease, physiology, anatomy, therapeutic possibilities, exercise intensities, the importance of activity, 'normal' reactions after training, etc., from a physiotherapist.

A practical example elucidates how important this is: Due to its prevalence in almost every participant, the subject of breathlessness was addressed in a therapy group of eight palliative care patients. The therapist asked how large the patients believed their lungs to be. Almost all of those asked spontaneously made a fist with one hand to demonstrate the size. When asked where the lungs are actually positioned in the body, again almost all of them placed their fists against the upper third of the sternum (representing as it does the part of the body where breathlessness is often perceived or described as most intense).

It seems logical that this incorrect assumption will lead to anxiety or, perhaps, an unwillingness to move. It

is essential when planning therapy to specifically ask about the type of advice or recommendations that patients and their families have received regarding activity and movement, their previous experience of physiotherapy, the extent of information the patient has found on the Internet or how patients believe their problems can be solved. Inappropriate or unhelpful information must be corrected by the therapist. Only very few patients have a medical background, hence it can be assumed that such a consideration will be of tremendous importance.

Dealing with deterioration

If there is a deterioration in activity or function, the patient should know how to recognise a reversible deterioration and determine the cause. He should also be able to identify signs of serious decline, however. In either case, he should have enough knowledge in order to be able to cope.

Strategies for handling acute anxiety

In the event of true anxiety/panic, the patient needs to implement coping strategies (➤ Chapter 3.2 and ➤ Chapter 2.4).

Accurately assessing one's own abilities and limitations

Patients find it helpful to know their own limits and above all their own abilities. Such awareness will help to differentiate and, if necessary, allay any anxiety. In patients with very little self-confidence it is wise to enable a self-assessment prior to any activity (e.g. How far do you think you can walk? How many repetitions do you think you can manage? How much help do you think you might need?) and compare the achievements afterwards with the actual predictions.

Physical activity and training

Various studies have demonstrated that physical activity – that is, practising everyday activities, weights and endurance work (adapted to the ability of critically ill individuals) – both individually and in group therapy, improves quality of life and self-confidence and thus also reduces anxiety (Oldervoll et al. 2006, Lowe et al. 2009b). The available data, which are very promising, assume that physical activity is linked to improved quality of life in the critically ill (Lowe et al. 2009a). To date there are no binding guidelines as to how intensive such activities or training need to be for achieving positive effects. An initial attempt is made by Lowe et al. (2009a) who report that quality of life is improved and symptoms (including anxiety) lessened, the more time that is dedicated to being active. A major contributing factor is likely to be the change in the perception of an activity, i. e. one which was previously associated with fear does not or no longer engenders fear to the same extent.

In order to again pursue activities of daily living without anxiety, it is beneficial for patients to **learn how to balance their energies** correctly (➤ Chapter 2.4). This includes rationalisation of breathing and movement just as much as pacing activity effectively and using aids and appliances.

Where patients have discovered that movement can be hazardous (e. g. after falling, over-exertion and the development of major symptoms), it is helpful if the therapist can **practise the activity that ultimately caused the anxiety in a secure setting.** In such a way, a patient who has fallen will learn that the floor can again be a 'safe foundation' by practising getting down onto the floor and up again (Knuchel/Schädler 2004).

To reduce anxiety, the patient may need an **appropriate aid.** This can on the one hand help to minimise certain symptoms that cause anxiety (e. g. walking frames for dyspnoea, slings for pain), while on the other hand, if selected appropriately, can empower patients to increase their movement somewhat more (diverse walking aids, rails, devices for getting in and out of bed independently, shoe horns, appropriate footwear, etc.). An appropriate multidisciplinary approach will lead to a clear improvement in anxiety, as Pituskin et al. (2010) have demonstrated. Aids and appliances can also have a considerable influence on the likelihood of a sick individual being able to remain at home.

Group physiotherapy can also be a very helpful (adjuvant) approach to managing anxiety (➤ Chapter 2.6).

Massage techniques

Proximity and touch – if desired by the patient – are often found to be agreeable and helpful in the case of anxiety. Unlike other professional groups, physiotherapists have the advantage of being able to maintain lengthy and intensive physical contact. Certain studies have revealed that treatments such as traditional massages or foot reflexology (Cassileth/Vickers 2004), or massages combined with aromatherapy (essential oils) (Kyle 2006, Wilkinson et al. 1999), can reduce anxiety in palliative care patients. The results of such studies have mostly demonstrated that although anxiety is reduced very rapidly, the effect is only limited. Massage can be used if it suits the objectives or also if appropriate for patients whose ability to move is greatly impaired. In addition, a

massage is a highly structured approach in a setting that otherwise involves little contact (➤ Chapter 2.5)

Relaxation techniques

Anxiety is associated with a high degree of muscular tension. Physical relaxation techniques are therefore highly appropriate, particularly so when working with people who are seriously or terminally ill. A study in oncology revealed that Jacobson's technique of progressive muscle relaxation is effective (Cheung/Molassiotis/Chang 2003), offering advantages over many other theoretical approaches: it is simple to learn, easy to apply on account of the purely physical intervention, and ensures concentration on the body when thoughts are otherwise dominated by anxiety.

2.7.5 Conclusion

Fear of movement is common in severely ill patients and has a huge impact on autonomy, participation and quality of life. Because of the associated physical symptoms, anxiety is a very specific and immediate issue. It is precisely because of this physical dimension that physiotherapy is helpful and can promote activity.

Since the fear of losing self-control is seen as a major feature in palliative care patients, priority should be given to as active an approach to therapy as possible. Because the symptoms that frequently occur in palliative care patients (e. g. pain, dyspnoea, oedema or constipation) can also cause anxiety, physiotherapy is a very effective 'anxiolytic' for alleviating or controlling the symptoms with few related side effects.

Courage is the opposite of fear. Anxious palliative care patients can also be very courageous in response to their situation. A similarly brave approach and courageous attitude should also form part of a physiotherapist's armoury.

2.7.6 Reflective questions

- Are you afraid of losing your own physical abilities and independence, and what would you want from your treatment team?
- If you think about your very anxious patients, what are the typical physical postures and tensions you encounter and how could they benefit physically from your work?
- What in your opinion are the 'positives' when it comes to anxiety?

REFERENCES

Beck AT, Steer RA. Beck Anxiety Inventory Manual. San Antonio: Harcourt Brace and Company; 1993.

Cassileth B, Vickers A. Massage therapy for symptom control: outcome study at a major cancer center. J Pain Symptom Manage 2004;28:244–249.

Cheung Y, Molassiotis A, Chang A. The effect of progressive muscle relaxation training on anxiety and quality of life after stoma surgery in colorectal cancer patients. Psychooncology 2003;12:254–266.

Dreßke S. Sterben im Hospiz. Der Alltag in einer alternativen Pflegeeinrichtung. Frankfurt: Campus Verlag, 2005.

Fuchs-Lacelle S, Hadjistavropoulos T. Development and preliminary validation of the pain assessment checklist for seniors with limited ability to communicate (PACSLAC). Pain Manag Nurs 2004;5(1):37–49.

Hamilton M. The assessment of anxiety states by rating. Br J Medical Psychol 1959;32:50–55.

Heyland D, Dodek P, Rocker G, et al. What matters most in end-of-life care: Perceptions of seriously ill patients and their family members. CMAJ 2006;174(5):627–633 (online).

Jolliffe J, Bury T. The effectiveness of physiotherapy in the palliative car of older people. The Chartered Society of Physiotherapy, 2002.

Kieslinger M. Stellenbeschreibung für Physiotherapeuten im Hospiz bzw. auf der Palliativstation. Diploma thesis. Akademie für Physiotherapie am Kaiser-Franz-Josef Spital der Stadt Wien, 2001.

Kolva E, Rosenfeld B, Pessin H, Breitbart W, Brescia R. Anxiety in terminally ill cancer patients. J Pain Symptom Manage 2011;42(5):691–701.

Knuchel S, Schädler S. Auf Nummer sicher gehen. Sturzprävention beim alten Menschen. Physiopraxis 2004.

Kyle G. Evaluating the effectiveness of aromatherapy in reducing levels of anxiety in palliative care patients: results of a pilot study. Complement Ther Clin Pract 2006;12:148–155.

Lloyd-Williams M, Kennedy V, Sixsmith A, Sixsmith J. The end of life: a quality study of the perceptions of people over the age of 80 on issues surrounding death and dying. J Pain Symptom Manage 2007;34:60–66.

Lowe S, Watanabe S, Baracos V, Courneya K. Associations between physical activity and quality of life in cancer patients receiving palliative care: a pilot survey. J Pain Symptom Manage 2009a;38:785–796.

Lowe S, Watanabe S, Courneya K. Physical activity as a supportive care intervention in palliative cancer patients: a systematic review. J Support Oncol 2009b;7:27–34.

McCracken L, Zayfert C, Gross R. The pain anxiety symptoms scale: development and validation of a scale to measure fear of pain. Pain 1992;50(1):67–73.

Miller RP, Kori SH, Todd DH. The Tampa Scale: a measure of kinesiophobia. Clin J Pain 1991;7(1):51–52

Mitchel AJ, Chan M, Bhatti H, et al. Prevalence of depression, anxiety and adjustment disorder in oncological, haematological and palliative-care setting: a meta-analysis of 94 interview-based studies. Lancet Oncol 2011;12:160–174.

Mystakidou K, Rosenfeld B, Parpa E, et al. Desire for death near the end of life: the role of depression, anxiety and pain. Gen Hosp Psychiatry 2005;27(4):258–262.

Oldervoll LM, Loge JH, Paltiel H, et al. The effect of a physical exercise program in palliative care: a phase II study. J Pain Symptom Manage 2006;31(5):421–430.

Pessin H, Rosenfeld B, Breitbart W. Assessing psychological distress near the end of life. Am Behav Sci 2002;46(3):357–372.

Pituskin E, Fairchild A, Dutka J, et al. Multidisciplinary team contributions within a dedicated outpatient palliative radiotherapy clinic: a prospective descriptive study. Int J Radiat Oncol Biol Phys 2010;78:527–532.

Saunders C. Foreword. In: Doyle D, Hanks G, MacDonald N (eds.). Oxford Textbook of Palliative Medicine. New York: Oxford University Press, 1998: pp. v–ix.

Spielberger CD, Gorsuch RL, Lushene RE. Manual for the State-Trait Anxiety Inventory. Palo Alto, CA: Consulting Psychologists Press, 1970.

Tinetti M, Richman D, Powell L. Falls efficacy as a measure of fear of falling. J Gerontol 1990;45(6):P239–243.

Waddell G, Newton M, Henderson I, Somerville D, Main CJ. A fear-avoidance beliefs questionnaire (FABQ) and the role of fear-avoidance beliefs in chronic low back pain and disability. Pain 1993;52:157–168.

Wilkinson S, Aldridge J, Salmon I, Cain E, Wilson B. An evaluation of aromatherapy massage in palliative care. Palliat Med 1999;13:409–417.

Wilson KG, Chochinov HM, Skirko MG, et al. Depression and anxiety disorders in palliative cancer care. J Pain Sympt Manage 2007;33(2):118–129.

Zigmond AS, Snaith RP. The Hospital Anxiety and Depression Scale. Acta Psychiatr Scand 1983;67:361–370.

2.8 Dementia
Elisabeth Grünberger

The term dementia is Latin in origin and literally means 'without mind'.

In psychiatry, it is understood to be an organic impairment of the brain's general functionality associated with negative effects at the social level.

The continuous organic loss of mental capabilities leads to a chronic state of confusion with disorders affecting:

- memory and cognition;
- cogitation;
- attention;
- speech;
- visual and spatial awareness;
- executive function;
- orientation.   (Kieckebusch 2011).

√ **GUIDANCE**
Dementia and physical identity

To the physiotherapist, it is of utmost importance to note that impaired body experience and body awareness are very debilitating, rendering the affected individual incapable of identifying either the names or the functions of parts of the body. Unfortunately, he will no longer be in a position to adequately control his movements during the advanced stages of disease.

An increase in dementia-related diseases is foreseeable throughout Europe. Populations are ageing, and neither migration nor birth rates will help in making them any younger. This is a development that will also impact palliative care, and so requires careful planning. The topic of dementia is often discussed in different media. Nevertheless, the knowledge available in healthcare systems and society is still far too sparse. Primary prevention is certainly good to some extent, yet it will change little in terms of the evolution of the disease. There must be an increase and improvement in early diagnosis; if developments continue at the current pace, dementia will become *'one of the biggest, if not the biggest challenge in the care of what were once the baby boomers, but are now a booming geriatric generation'* (Psota 2011).

2.8.1 Development and types of dementia

Dementia is one of the most common psychological conditions of old age.

Changes of no pathological significance

In the differential diagnosis of dementia, i. e. differentiating a pathological condition from physiological changes in old age, the natural physiological processes that have **no pathological significance** are itemised.

Psychological changes:
- forgetfulness;
- associative disorders;
- benign old-age forgetfulness;
- age-related idiosyncrasies;
- age-related personality disorders.

Cognitive changes:
- diffuse decline in the ability to concentrate;
- reduced attention span;
- decreased tolerance;
- rapid exhaustion.

(Heuft/Kruse 2000).

Disorientation

Disorientation, as a mental disorder, is also very common in old age. It is mainly caused by physiological factors and has no specific boundaries. A distinction is made between acute and chronic, as well as reversible and irreversible disorientation, respectively. It very often takes the form of what is known as **'relocation stress syndrome'**. Changes in location which are highly emotional, such as entering a home or staying in hospital, but also frequent room changes or the quick turnover in neighbours, all contribute to such a disorder. It can mostly be remedied and reversed by rehabilitative exercises.

Further causes for disorientation are:
- dehydration (often the sensation of thirst is impaired in the elderly);
- metabolic disorders in diabetes;
- renal or hepatic damage;
- thyroid dysfunction;
- oxygen deficiency due to heart failure or cardiac arrhythmias;
- blood pressure changes, asthma, anaemia;
- noxae such as alcohol or incorrect medication doses and their side effects;
- external factors: loss of a partner or death of the person with whom they share a room, for example.

A variety of **symptoms** can result: most prominently factors related to orientation, mood, concentration, attention and short or long-term memory. Often, the affected individuals are unable to identify or recognise other people, certain situations, or even themselves.

Another typical manifestation is **impaired drive,** which can lead to impulsive activity and psycho-motor restlessness but in some cases also inactivity. Paranoid sensations and hallucinations are further symptoms of disorientation.

Types of dementia

There are various types of dementia which differ to some extent depending on their cause, development, symptoms and treatment. ➤ Table 2.18 provides an outline of the different types.

Criteria for dementia

In light of the various types of dementia as well as its distinction from disorientation and other neurological diseases, the ICD-10 and DSM-IV (American Psychiatric Association 1994) classifications describe exactly when and how dementia should be diagnosed. Dementia is chronic and progressive in its development, and to diagnose the condition the following disorders must primarily exist:

Table 2.18 Outline of the types and prevalence of dementia

Dementia	Prevalence
Dementia of the Alzheimer type	60 %
Vascular dementia	16 %
Alzheimer's and vascular dementia	8 %
Alzheimer's and Parkinson's disease	8 %
Parkinson's disease	1 %
Fronto-temporal dementia	1 %
Lewy body dementia	1 %
Creutzfeldt-Jakob disease	1 %
Other causes	4 %

Table 2.19 Severities of dementia (according to Gatterer 2003)

Mild dementia	Moderate dementia	Severe dementia
Patient can still live alone	Patient requires assistance on a daily basis, but can still be left alone	Patient is in need of care

Table 2.20 Seven stages of dementia (according to Reisberg 1982)

Stage	Cognitive condition	Development of dementia	Functionality
I	No cognitive decline	Normal	Functional disorder neither subjectively nor objectively identifiable
II	Very mild cognitive decline	Forgetfulness	Difficulty recovering items; subjective difficulties with work; everyday independence; good compensatory abilities
III	Mild cognitive decline	Early stages of confusion	Drop in professional performance; difficulties in orienting oneself; independent; endeavouring to maintain a façade
IV	Moderate cognitive decline	Late stages of confusion	Waning ability to manage complex activities; difficulties dealing with money; ADL maintained to the extent that living alone is possible
V	Moderately severe cognitive decline	Early-stage dementia	Help required with dressing and washing; requires daily support; can eat and drink independently; partially incontinent
VI	Severe cognitive decline	Moderately severe dementia	Difficulties dressing correctly; help needed with washing/WC; urinary and faecal incontinence
VII	Very severe cognitive decline	Late-stage dementia	Able to say 1–5 words; no verbal communication; stupor/coma

A. demonstrable impairment of short and long-term memory;

B. presentation of one feature:
   – abstract thought impaired;
   – ability to judge impaired;
   – changes in personality;
   – other impairments to higher cortical functions (aphasia, apraxia, agnosia, disorders to executive functions such as planning, organisation, following a sequence, abstraction).

C. disruptions to A and B are so severe that they clearly affect work, daily social activities or personal relationships with other people;

D. the disorder may not just exist during an episode of delirium (organic psychosyndrome, transition syndrome);

E. indications of an organic element based on history, physical findings or additional assessment;

F. work and social life disrupted;

G. consciousness not impaired;

H. evidence of a specific organic element or exclusion of depression.

Possible classifications of dementia

Dementia-related diseases can be classified in a number of ways: by phenomenological type, severity, or divided into seven different stages. In physiotherapy, cognitive performance as well as the ability to pursue activities of daily living are important. For this reason, the following two categories are addressed. ➤ Table 2.19 describes the severity classification, and ➤ Table 2.20 the seven stages of dementia.

Both methods of classification are useful for diagnosis, but also for planning therapy so that the goals of 'everyday competence' and 'autonomous care' can be pursued. A realistic estimation of the course of the disease and the applicable therapeutic possibilities must be considered by the physiotherapist if the person suffering from dementia is not to be under- or over-exerted.

Vascular dementia

In the case of vascular dementia (VD), circulatory disorders cause cerebral lesions to develop, resulting in transient or permanent neurological deficits. A subtype of vascular dementia is multi-infarct dementia (MID), which entails multiple small cerebral infarctions and gradually leads to corresponding cognitive deficits.

Causes, course, symptoms and therapy

The onset of this type of dementia is often sudden and intermittent. A characteristic of the condition is that the severity of the dementia symptoms may at some point improve, but also tend to fluctuate over time. Such episodes indicate a renewed phase of ischaemia.

The following **causes** are likely:

- multiple infarcts;
- anoxia/hypoxia (e. g. cardiac arrest);
- arteritis (immune disease);
- Binswanger's disease (diffuse vascular damage to the cerebellar medulla);
- arterio-venous malformations;
- consequence of subarachnoid haemorrhage.

(Wallesch/Förstl 2005)

Risk factors that can contribute to VD are hypertension, smoking, cardiac diseases (especially if associated with atrial fibrillation), diabetes and hyperlipidaemia.

Psychological examination will reveal the following disorders:

- impaired retentiveness;
- criteria (A–H) for dementia (ICD-10 and DSM IV);
- associative abilities and analytical reasoning markedly reduced;
- abstract thought, general knowledge, attention less affected;
- depressive moods;
- disorientation;
- emotional lability;
- delusions.

If **therapy** is initiated early enough, the cognitive impairments of MID will remain manageable. Progression can be prevented by eliminating the risk factors and causative conditions. Cognitive and mnestic exercises, as well as a structured plan to the day, help the affected individual to remain independent for as long as possible.

Dementia of the Alzheimer type

Dementia of the Alzheimer type (DAT) was first documented by Alois Alzheimer in 1970 and is the most widely known, as well as most common of all types of dementia.

It is characterised by neurodegenerative changes which become noticeable histopathologically as deposits of amyloid beta and other proteins between the nerve cells. The development of such amyloid plaques and a pathological change in the fibrils result in extensive cerebral atrophy.

The diagnosis can only be confirmed, however, if all other organic brain diseases – particularly vascular, inflammatory and space-occupying changes – can be ruled out. DAT cannot be diagnosed on the basis of cerebral atrophy alone (Lauterbacher/Gauggel 2010).

Dementia of the Alzheimer type (DAT) occurs at the age of 40 years or over. Above the age of 65, it is known as senile dementia of the Alzheimer type (SDAT).

Causes, course, symptoms and therapy (according to Kastner/Löbach 2010)

The exact evolution of DAT has not yet been explained, but the following parameters are likely indicators of the disease:

- diagnosis of dementia from neuropsychological testing using the *Mini Mental State Examination* (MMSE);
- deficits in two or more cognitive functions, such as local, temporal, situative, spatial orientation, impaired long and short-term memory, lack of personal orientation;
- progressive deterioration in memory;
- consciousness not impaired;
- onset between the ages of 40 and 90;
- absence of other diseases that cause dementia.

Diagnosis is supported by a progressive deterioration in cognitive functions such as speech and dexterity, and by altered behavioural patterns (e. g. daily routine). Genetic factors as well as a family history of DAT and lab results can likewise be of diagnostic help. Acute onset, accompanied by neurological symptoms (e. g. hemiparesis, scotoma, etc.), means that DAT is unlikely.

The **changes noticeable in everyday situations** are:

- apathy, lack of drive and passivity;
- stereotypical behaviour;
- aggression, change in impulse control;
- anxiety and panic attacks;
- running away, straying, constant searching, hoarding, concealing;
- repeated questioning, calling and shouting;
- eating disorders;
- confusing day and night.

➤ Table 2.21 provides a simple comparison of the two types of dementia.

Table 2.21 Differentiation between VD and DAT (according to Gershon/Herman 1982)

	VD	DAT
Onset	Often sudden	Gradual
Course	Incremental and variable	Gradual, progressive
Sex	More often men	Evenly distributed
Central nervous system pathology	Frequent	Usually absent
Pathology	Cerebral softening, infarctions, atherosclerosis	Neurofibrillary tangles, senile plaques

Mixed forms

VD and DAT

Basic neuropathological examinations in dementia sufferers will reveal signs of the Alzheimer type as well as pathological findings in the blood vessels. In very general terms, the older the individual with Alzheimer's disease, the more likely the brain will exhibit signs of vascular pathology (Lautenbacher/Gauggel 2010).

VD and Parkinson's disease

This mixed type is a subcortical form of dementia in which the primary pathology is suspected to be found in the deeper regions of the cerebral cortex. It is also known as Lewy body dementia (Lautenbacher/Gauggel 2010).

Other types of dementia

- Dementia with Creutzfeldt-Jakob disease;
- dementia with Huntington's chorea;
- progressive supranuclear palsy: atypical Parkinson's syndrome;
- fronto-temporal dementia.

2.8.2 Diagnosing dementia

In dementia, the diagnostic process involves examining mental performance and well-being as well as establishing the level of independence.

Early diagnosis

Early diagnosis is very important to the course of dementia, since it can be influenced considerably by prompt treatment and therapy whilst delaying the progression of the disease and thereby enhancing the quality of life of those concerned. Differential diagnosis is often problematic, however, due to issues of multimorbidity arising with advancing age. Also, speech problems (e.g. following insult) often make it impossible to test the cognitive functions.

Early diagnostic procedures can help to differentiate between the pathological and mental deficits typical of growing old. Determination of the severity and establishment of the degree of independence are the principles upon which further therapeutic measures are based. At an early stage, the cognitive functions will only be slightly impaired (mild cognitive impairment, MCI). Underlying deficits or minimal cognitive disorders are characteristic of MCI, especially if the disorders deviate from what is normal at that age, but are not sufficient either in their severity or attendant circumstances to make a clinical diagnosis (Markowitsch/Calabrese 2003).

Substantial differential diagnosis for dementia is therefore important for appropriately structuring a treatment plan to deal specifically with the behavioural and psychological disorders. Therapy includes medication, cognitive training and other targeted therapeutic methods, e.g. physiotherapy, occupational therapy, dance and movement therapy, relaxation techniques, psychosocial care and psychotherapy, music therapy, art therapy, animal-assisted therapy, etc.

Assessments

The following is a list of the basic assessments that are usually undertaken.

- GDS: *Global Deterioration Scale* by Reisberg (Reisberg et al. 1982);
- MMSE: *Mini Mental State Examination* (Folstein/Folstein/McHugh 1975): suspected dementia – introduction of screening methods;
- SLUMS test: *Saint Louis University Mental Status Examination* (Tariq et al. 2006);
- CLOCK Completion Test (Shulman et al. 1993);
- CERAD: test battery of the *Consortium to Establish a Registry for Alzheimer's Disease* (Aebi 2002);
- AKT: Alters-Konzentrations-Test (age concentration test) (Gatterer 1990), as a non-verbal strike-through test.

Aside from general assessments for dementia, the physiotherapist will find it quite a challenge to record the individual medical symptoms, not least because pain is a major symptom.

⚠ **C A U T I O N**
Dementia and pain

As dementia progresses, the way in which pain is managed and perceived will also change. Pain may be perceived either as more or less intense. In care homes, roughly 80 % of residents suffer from chronic pain. Sensitivity to pain does not generally recede, but the assessment of the pain changes as it is sometimes perceived as a greater threat (Kunz 2009, Kunz et al. 2009).

The degree of verbal communication can be limited in dementia sufferers and thus result in the underestimation and inadequate perception of the said symptoms during their therapy and care. To this end, non-verbal assessments are available specifically for documenting pain in dementia patients. The test described in the 'pain measurement' box can be used both for examining as well as for determining the course of the pain, which is by no means less important.

√ GUIDANCE
Pain measurement in dementia

In practice it is noticeable that dementia sufferers need more time to react and respond to questions such as 'can you feel pressure, pulling, piercing?'. Voluntary information is impossible to obtain in the advanced stages of dementia.

The **PACSLAC test** is a standardised test for assessing pain in dementia sufferers (Fuchs-Lacelle/Hadjistavropoulos 2004). Standardised geriatric pain assessments for people with impaired cognitive skills include:
• PAINAD: *Pain Assessment in Advanced Dementia* (Warden/ Hurley/Volicer 2003);
• ECPA: *Echelle comportementale de la douleur pour personnes âgées non communicantes* (French and German) (Morello et al. 2002);
• DOLOPLUS (Wary/Serbouti 2001).

To conclude it should be mentioned that a geriatric assessment – whether for general diagnosis or for examining the specific symptoms of dementia – is the basic premise for further medical treatment and therapy. Geriatric assessments entail a multidimensional, interdisciplinary and diagnostic procedure aiming to document the medical, psychosocial and functional problems and resources of the elderly.

2.8.3 Dementia and the body

Ageing itself is perceived, described and communicated primarily on a physical level. As a result, the anti-ageing attitude of society focuses on the *negative* changes in our bodies. Working with resources in physiotherapy requires all the more attention to 'what can be done' rather than 'what can no longer be done' if the ageing patient is to be treated with dignity and respect.

At the point where communication comes to a halt, physiotherapy requires new, creative approaches to treatment for achieving therapeutic goals such as maintaining and promoting mobility, body awareness and, in turn, independence.

Physical impact of dementia

Cognitive deficits of any nature – local, temporal, spatial, situative and related to oneself – considerably affect one's physical experience and perception of one's own body.

In general, psychomotor sequences and, in particular, awareness of one's own body have not been adequately addressed by the literature in relation to dementia sufferers. The author has gained the following experience in this respect:
• Parts of the body can be named or recognised only to a limited extent or not at all.
• Parts of the body cannot be identified by their function.
• Sensory perception (severe/mild, strong/gentle, etc.) and feeling are restricted, distorted or lost entirely.
• Temperature perception is often vague or lacking; if present, cold is mostly the complaint.
• The spatial recognition of movements is restricted or lost, movements or distances cannot be estimated.
• Instructions to move cannot be translated or understood.
• Pain sensitivity can be greatly increased or may even be decreased.

Symbolic language

Dementia sufferers make use of symbolic language. Physiotherapists can work at the level of the body's symbolic language, though knowledge of the patient's biography is essential if such language is to be understood correctly. When the dementia begins, therefore, sequences of movement, gestures and actions arising from the life or personal biography of the patient can be easily adopted and implemented. Mostly they involve events that are intensely emotional.

An example is a female patient with moderate dementia who, having covered a distance of several kilometres by walking around the ward and surrounding departments during the course of the day, explained her compulsion to wander thus: *'It's terrible being tied down. Your body forgets to move and is good for nothing.'*

The more advanced the dementia, the more varied and, to us, distorted the symbolic messages displayed by the affected individual. However, this is often the only way in which those with severe dementia can express themselves. The symbols used by those with dementia relate to things or people that have actually existed in the past. A hand may become a baby to a disoriented woman, for example, or the wheelchair table may become an old gentleman's desk.

√ GUIDANCE
Symbolic language

The more disoriented the person, the more physically resemblant the symbolism becomes. It is important in physiotherapy to 'enter into' this world, 'adopt' the elderly and their symbols and possibly even communicate in his or her symbolic language.

The swaying movement of the upper body, as an example, can express the need for comfort, for one's mother, for pleasure, or a need for security. **The emotional memory continues to function despite all other losses.** Owing to these memories dementia sufferers fortunately remain very responsive (Feil 2005).

2.8.4 Principles of supportive physiotherapy in dementia

According to Mitchell et al. (2009) advanced dementia should be viewed as a terminal illness requiring palliative care.

Family members and advocates or authorised proxies, if necessary, should be included in the planning of the treatment and care.

Treatment plan and therapeutic objective

A physiotherapist needs to be very flexible when dealing with dementia patients and administering their therapy.

⚠ CAUTION
Flexibility in the therapeutic process

Experience has shown that the more fragile the physical and mental state, the more flexible, but also the more stable the structure must be for physiotherapeutic management. This applies to both physical and emotional aspects.

Being flexible in this context means that the treatment plan should be part of a therapeutic process in which each intervention by the interdisciplinary team is tailored and reflects the individuality of the patient.

Stability in physiotherapy can be achieved by consistency and dependability on the part of the therapist, who should administer the measures in a setting that offers security. Security entails that which is familiar and customary – actions that the patient can cope with during therapy. Often they may be simple, basic daily activities such as picking up a glass, combing the hair, eating, etc.

It is wise to broaden the therapeutic approach to physiotherapy by applying the existing principles of developmental and depth psychology, thereby lending a new dimension to physiotherapeutic techniques and even basic interventions.

Movement and kinaesthetic perception are often used in order to initiate and structure the therapeutic process. This is then reflected and processed verbally. Verbal commentary, e. g. "you're now moving your leg" or "you can feel my hands on your lower leg", is used to encourage the realisation and integration of experiences of the body and movement, and is an effective element of therapy.

Even at the advanced stages 6 and 7 and/or if additional neurological disorders are hindering communication, verbal commentary is useful. The therapeutic process will be successful if it is based on empathy, creativity, presence and a regard for 'otherness'.

The family often has unrealistic, but also understandable expectations of physiotherapists in terms of mobilisation, ability to walk and other activities. Physiotherapy is frequently seen as the last resort for halting the decline in strength as well as mental agility. On the other hand, physiotherapists can engender a great deal of trust by focusing on the resources than can best preserve a patient's functionality and enhance the quality of life.

For physiotherapy to be most effective, the physiotherapist must also look after himself (➤ Chapter 5).

The body as a means of structuring relationships

A basic knowledge of psycho-physical therapy is advantageous when it comes to physiotherapy in dementia, as well as other psychological and cognitive disorders in old age. In such a way, physiotherapeutic techniques, methods and theories are enriched by human encounters, thereby opening up new pathways.

√ GUIDANCE
Healing properties of the body and movement

A key feature, also in physiotherapy, is the fact that the body and mind are constantly interacting with one another and that the processes of the body and movement have healing properties. To the dementia sufferer, the reinvention of movement and body experience represents an extension of his or her limited feeling of 'being in the world'.

The aim is to perceive and, if possible, reduce structural deficits by means of body awareness and develop a realistic image of the body, as well as to acquire new ways of structuring movement and relationships.

The physiotherapeutic approach

Approach in this context refers to the 'upright attitude' of respectful contact in the physiotherapeutic sense. Aside from selecting the appropriate physiotherapeutic techniques, the inward and outward approach to the treatment of dementia sufferers determines how sustainable and successful the relationship and therapy will be. A relationship between the physiotherapist and patient that is based on security and trust helps considerably in coping with the limitations.

D. W. Winnicott's reference to *'good enough holding'* (Winnicott 1965) is a good therapeutic foundation. By this, Winnicott means creating a 'good enough holding environment' that embraces physical, spiritual, psychological and social components.

Dementia sufferers are neither babies nor children, but it is remarkable that many of their movements, postures and attitudes suggest the opposite. The physical cycle of life appears to want to come full circle at this point.

The effects of the disease can trigger feelings of impotence and helplessness in the physiotherapist, but should not encourage a need to 'cosset' the elderly and demented patient.

Making contact with the body

In the majority of cases the way in which contact is made can be crucial to further therapy, which should only ensue if therapeutic contact has truly been established.

It is important in particular to afford this process plenty of time and patience so that the individual boundaries of such an experience can be respected and safeguarded.

Here the principle of 'less is more' applies. Not every act of contact will become immediately apparent – or at least, not in the same way as with those who do not have dementia. Thus we may only perceive the response of the dementia patient to our establishing contact as modified breathing or facial expressions.

The thoughts and emotions that actually move a dementia patient cannot be verified, of course. The reality can only ever be approximated. The following account by a patient could provide the professional carer with valuable insight.

'I'm lying in bed and reminiscing about my wonderful husband who had passed away; shame that he had to go before me, … my eyes are closed so that I can see him more clearly, and what he looked like: Hans, my husband. Did someone just speak to me? My hearing's not good as it is. I can sense a warmth nearby. Maybe someone's entered the room, I'm not really sure. Yet somehow it's different, so I'm a little curious and try to slowly open my eyes. Again it's as if someone is talking to me … the warmth next to me is so nice; though I see only shadows, I think I recognise the voice; a soft, young voice has come to my bedside. Then I feel a touch on my hand. Thin fingers gently wrap themselves around mine. How warm these hands are, and now I gradually make out a face. The young man that visits every day. It must be about lunchtime, as he always comes around then, and he looks a little like my grandson. It's nice that he has so much time for me. He holds my hand in his, keeping it safe and steady. So nice when he holds my hand like that. It soothes me and now I feel a little more at peace …'

From the therapist's perspective, these ten minutes could have transpired thus: *'I'm standing by Mrs K.'s room and I bring up her biography in my head. I know that her husband, who looked after her at home, died a year ago and she moved to the home shortly afterwards. I knock gently on the door, as per 'our routine', then stand at the end of the bed for a while and say hello. I can see her breathing. Quick and shallow. She seems a little flustered. Slowly I start to reflect the rhythm of her breathing from a distance. Her eyes are closed, but I can see that her breathing and eye movements beneath her eyelids are beginning to slow down. I move a chair into position on her left, to where her head is turned, and where her hand is lying on the blanket. Her hand looks soft and tender. All the things this hand has seen and done? Slowly I touch her hand. With a confident move, I then take her frail fingers in my hand. They're much warmer than I expected. She briefly opens her eyes, and I mine, and she looks at me. Maybe …'*

Tips for dealing with disorientation and dementia

It is a challenge not to over- or under-exert individuals who are disoriented and have dementia. The following **behaviour** should be considered as guidance in physiotherapeutic interventions (Feil 2005, Feil 2007):
- Therapeutic actions should convey emotional sensitivity (cognitive demands should be reduced).
- Review internal attitude, posture and empathy.
- Maintain presence and attention, and constant therapeutic contact with the patient.
- Consider a familiar environment, gently deflect conflict.

- Use straightforward, intelligible and clear verbal and non-verbal communication.
- Adopt synchronous and consistent speech, touch, vision and movement.
- Avoid contradictions.
- Consider biographical history.

A **useful concept** to keep in mind is that dementia patients can sense the inward attitudes and emotions with which they are approached.

For physiotherapy to be effective, it is useful to modify the approach to the therapeutic process by considering the following:

- Focus on a topic of discussion or potential movement.
- The therapist is active, guiding the patient towards the present task/issue.
- Work slowly: formulate clearly, repeat key statements, devise manageable units.
- Multimodal process: speak, show, do, work with pictures and symbols that can be converted into movement.
- Memory aids: leave notes and other reminders.
- Strategies for sustained attention: shorter sessions, taking breaks.
- Review opinions and negative expectations concerning 'body and movement'.
- Use the surrounding resources, e.g. garden, bed, familiar environment.

The focus of the physiotherapist must be continually sharpened, readjusting and reacting with tremendous flexibility to the surroundings and the perception of individuals with dementia. Physiotherapy should be characterised primarily by interventions that deliver assurance, support and trust. Physiotherapists are not helpless when it comes to dealing with dementia patients, but rather they can create an understanding environment based on each patient's individual biography.

2.8.5 Patient cases and physiotherapeutic interventions
Louis Hollander

Patients with dementia tend to become increasingly passive, especially during the last stage of the dementia process. Physiotherapy as a specialized profession concerned with movement commonly tends to be one of the first disciplines to be discontinued, although it has been shown that movement has a positive effect on cognition (Eggermont et al. 2009; Scherder et al. 2007). If movement therapy takes place in the context of patient groups the effect is even more explicit. Re-activation, re-socialization and effective functioning are stimulated (Droës

1997). In general, 'active exercise therapy' – such as that employed in 'fitness' classes – empowers the patient during the declining process of dementia.

The following patient cases show that physiotherapy can be indispensable right up to the last phase of care. The cases are not entirely representative of all dementia patients. They have been chosen to illustrate that in the last phase of care therapeutic strategies are based more on intervention using mainly non-verbal approaches, such as eye contact, body language and touch. The physiotherapist is a specialist in manual contact, i. e. in therapeutic touch. Touch can, for example, turn anguished wailing into a contented humming.

Case study 1: Patient resistance during the care process (> Figure 2.26)

Presentation Mrs S., a patient in the last phase of dementia, had contractures and suffered pain during all care procedures. Muscle tone had increased recently. The care process was burdensome not only for her but also for the nurses involved in her daily care. Sensation could not be formally assessed due to cognitive impairment. Mrs S. cried out and moaned loudly during all personal care. Occupational therapy had a role in addressing positioning issues.

Physiotherapy referral The aims of the physiotherapy referral were:
- non-pharmacological intervention for hypertonia and pain during the care process;
- education and training for nursing staff with regard to strategies for approaching and managing Mrs S. during the care process.

Observation and evaluation Paratonia or gegenhalten, which is defined as an active but involuntary

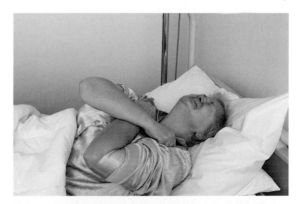

Figure 2.26 Patient with typical 'resistance posture' [0596]

resistance to passive movement, was present. Mrs S.'s cervical spine was held in extension and left rotation. Strong hypertonia of the sternocleidomastoid muscle led to increased extension of the cervical spine. This was exacerbated when her head and cervical spine were unsupported. Elbows and forearms were held strongly against the trunk. Extreme flexion of her fingers into the palms had led to skin breakdown. The fingers could be extended with slow passive stretch, but this seemed to provoke a lot of pain. Mrs S. had no palmar roll in situ. Because of the asymmetric paratonia and contractures (more severe on the left side than the right) her legs were deviated to the left and sometimes even displaced out of the bed. Gleno-humeral and acromio-clavicular joint ranges of movement were both severely limited and painful. Both humeri were displaced anteriorly and subluxed.

Observation of nursing care   Two nurses were required to wash and clothe Mrs S. due to her strongly defensive reactive behaviour. She demonstrated restlessness throughout the care process. Loud noises and bright light provoked motor disturbance in both trunk and legs. When giving general personal care, removing the bedclothes and any water contact led to both verbal and physical defensive behaviour including loud protestation (for example *'No, don't do that!'* and *'Leave me alone!'*) and also resistance. Turning her from side-to-side elicited shouting, grasping or pinching. When dressing Mrs S. the passive movements needed for the task provoked shouting and heightened tone in all four limbs. It appeared that pain increased during the care process.

Assessments   Following the observation of Mrs S.'s personal care, these additional physiotherapy assessments were conducted:
- **Pain:** Because Mrs S. was unable to verbalize her pain experience, a non-verbal pain assessment was implemented. The Pain Assessment Scale for Seniors with Severe Dementia (PACSLAC; Fuchs-Lacelle/Hadjistavropoulos 2007) was used, and PACSLAC scores were as follows:
  - facial expression: high;
  - activity/body movement (stiffness, rigidity): high;
  - other (physiological changes, eating, sleeping): high;
  - social/personality/mood (verbal aggression, not wanting to be touched): maximum.
- **Muscle tone and range of movement:** Further differential diagnostic tools were implemented:

- Paratonia Assessment Instrument (PAI; Hobbelen 2010): With the help of five criteria, this tool can assist the physiotherapist to distinguish paratonia from a Parkinson's-type rigidity or from spastic hemiparesis. Mrs S. demonstrated the presence of all five criteria.
- Modified Ashworth Scale (MAS): shoulder and elbow: 3; hand and fingers: 4; lower limbs: 3.
- Range of movement: severe restriction in extension, elevation and abduction of all joints.

Physiotherapeutic goals   The principle goal was to establish comfort during the care process. Comfort in the context of this demented patient is interpreted as follows:
- reduction of pain (PACSLAC total score <10);
- reduction of tone, impacting on restlessness (PACSLAC subscale activity/body movement);
- reduction of resistance (PACSLAC subscale social/personality/mood = 0);
- reduction of fear and anxiety.
Longer term goals included:
- prevention of further contractures: MAS and ROM stable;
- prevention of pressure sores.

Physiotherapeutic interventions   Of prime importance was the education of – and provision of information to – nursing staff to promote improved awareness of the positive influence of caring touch. This was combined with strategies to develop trust in the patient and carer relationship through slow moving and handling techniques.

√ **GUIDANCE**
- Provide reduced, low sensory stimuli; perhaps preferred music set at a low volume, which can lead to more restfulness (Guétin et al. 2009).
- Avoid cold stimuli; maintain warmth; use waterless washing methods.
- Weighted fleece blankets induce improved relaxation with reduction of hypertonia.
- Relaxed, open hands develop trust and engender relaxation (Bowlby 1979; Hall 1966).
- Slow rocking movements combined with gentle slow stretch reduce tone (Dijk 2006).
- Avoid rolling, or roll the patient slowly (for example in 5 or 10 second intervals).
- Delivering care to the patient via only one caregiver promotes more rest and relaxation.

Evaluation   With the practical care/advice and various support interventions, episodes of care were no longer a struggle. After two weeks the PACSLAC score during caring lowered significantly.

Outcome It was possible to observe a metaphor of the circle of life. At the end of her life, Mrs S. reverted to a foetal position. This anatomical position has negative implications for the adult, as it carries many complicated risks. These include restlessness, fear, contractures, hypertonia, pain and pressure lesions. Suffering from impaired kinaesthetic sense as a result of stimulus reduction; the patient tried to compensate for this by adopting a more flexed position in search of additional stimuli. The weight of bedclothes or placing of a hand roll can fulfil this need and help to reduce tone. **Suffering for Mrs S. is compounded by her inability to understand what is happening during the care process. At the end of her life she struggles with nurses whose intentions are good. This is frustrating not just for Mrs S. but also for the nurses as well.** In the Netherlands physiotherapists developed a care/treatment method especially for this target group. Called 'passivities of daily life' ('the PDL-method'; Dijk 2006), the key two pillars of the method are a safe, trusting, open body-oriented approach combined with a strict sequence of actions. It is possible to wash, clean and clothe the patient with just one rolling action into side lying. If practitioners work alone, instead of two caregivers, twice the time must be taken; but the benefit is that more rest is created for the patient during the caring process.

⚠ **CAUTION**
- Passive movement therapy is not effective in reducing paratonia in severely demented patients (Hobbelen 2010).
- Do not underestimate pain in the elderly, especially in the demented elderly (Epps 2001; Scherder 2003; Zwakhalen et al. 2006).

✓ **GUIDANCE**
- Good postural support diminishes paratonia.
- Collaborate with the occupational therapist to create good body support in lying.
- A horseshoe-pillow holds the cervical spine in supported flexion and protracts the shoulders. Cervical flexion with the pillow diminishes problems with swallowing. The full support can give a sense of embrace. The two side protrusions of the pillow can be positioned between the chest wall and the upper arms; they then prevent the upper arms from pressing against the chest and therefore prevent gleno-humeral adduction.
- The lateral aspects of the trunk should be supported to prevent flexed knees rotating to the side. A T-shaped foam pillow or support behind and between the knees will prevent both medial knee pressure and heel to glutei contact.
- A firm hand roll in the palm of the hand prevents claw hand deformity and associated skin breakdown. It will also help to reduce tone. By contrast, a soft hand roll can increase tone (Hobbelen 2010).

Case study 2: Walking again thanks to the vacuum cleaner (➤ Figure 2.27)

Presentation Ms H., aged 76, diagnosed with severe dementia (Alzheimer's disease), presented with very low awareness and understanding. Totally dependent, she needed feeding. Her oral behaviour displayed a tendency to put all kinds of things into her mouth. Ms H. had previously been able to walk, but two weeks prior to referral had fallen. The Ottawa Ankle Rules were negative (no pain) so there was a small chance for a fracture (Bachmann et al. 2003). Bruising of the ankle was present with slight localized oedema. After her fall Ms H. showed no initiative to walk and sat down the whole day. Nurses had tried to get her on her feet again but Ms H. exhibited both strong resistance and protest.

Referral to physiotherapy Although Ms H. was non-compliant with either exercise or mobility, mobilization post ankle contusion was requested.

Observation/evaluation On examination the patient presented the following picture:
- mild ankle oedema;
- inability to follow instructions for active movement tests;
- passive movements established moderate range of movement;
- inability to perform sit-to-stand-to-walk procedure;
- demonstration, guidance and inviting facilitation not effective;
- Ms H. remained passively sitting.

Intervention For the first three sessions the physiotherapist attempted sit-to-stand techniques, without success. By chance, before the following physiotherapy session, the domestic cleaner had left her vacuum cleaner

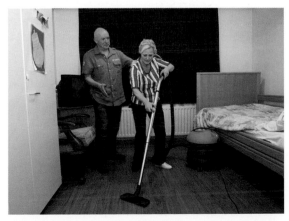

Figure 2.27 Vacuum cleaner as therapeutic instrument [O596]

in Ms H.'s apartment. The physiotherapist commenced role-playing action using the vacuum cleaner. When Ms H. saw, heard and then felt the cleaner in her hands it looked as if a button in her brain had been switched on. She suddenly became active, started to clean the floor, walked with the cleaner all around the apartment, even bending forward to pick up paper from the floor. After using the vacuum cleaner, she started to tidy and clean her wardrobe.

Evaluation   After this apparent 'small miracle', the physiotherapist advised the nurses to give Ms H. small house-keeping tasks. She simply needed to be guided. From that time onwards Ms H. cleaned the floor every day and helped the kitchen assistant with both shopping and cooking.

Outcome   The above mentioned 'reawakening' is probably based on sensory integration combined with motor memory. In earlier days Ms H. had been a housewife, responsible for caring, cleaning and cooking. Since the onset of dementia she needed to live in a nursing home, so was relatively institutionalised; she consequently became more and more passive. Lacking the stimulus to be active, the doors to her memory were locked, and Ms H. forgot the basic activities of daily living (ADL) skills.

√ **GUIDANCE**

With the help of sensory integration – in this case from a vacuum cleaner – the patient's mind subconsciously 'remembers' the skills again. Unaware of this, the patient rediscovers her ability to walk.

Case study 3: Repetitive movements calmed (➤ Figure 2.28, ➤ Figure 2.29)

Presentation   Ms L., aged 86, diagnosed with severe dementia (Alzheimer's disease), sat the entire day in a wheelchair with attached tray table. Although dysarthric, she had adequate communication skills. Ms L. was developing marked skin irritation due to constant finger rubbing.

Physiotherapy referral   Sedation medication was not medically indicated or appropriate; advice was therefore sought including the consideration of protective fixation or any other possible therapeutic strategies.

Observation   Ms L. did not appear to be nervous, sitting quietly in her well-adapted chair with an upright posture. However, her hands and fingers were continuously busy. Sometimes she closed her eyes and it looked as if she was focused on her hand activity. The hand and finger movements were quick and mostly well coordinated. Rubbing her fingers up and down, pinching and sometimes scratching her thumb and little (fourth) finger, this hyperactivity started on waking and continued throughout the entire day.

Sometimes the movements stopped, but only for a few seconds; then the activity started again.

The continuous movements of the hand, and fingers, almost endlessly repeated, seemed to have no purpose. It appeared obsessive.

Where the friction was worst, the skin turned slightly red. Occasionally the patient hurt herself because she hyperextended one of her fingers. It was possible to stop the movements by applying manual contact but this was only effective for a short period.

Reflection   These repetitive movements characterize the psycho-motor phase. Feil describes it as 'permanent motion' (Feil 2002). In the opinion of Reedijk **this motor behaviour is manifest as a result of the patient's need of a form of fear control.** He calls it *'the hypnotic function of stereotypical behaviour'* (Reedijk 2006). By these means the patient can lower sensory arousal and as a result fear will diminish.

Verdult emphasizes the importance of physical contact with the patient. His message is clear: *'Change stereotypical behaviour by offering human contact!'* (Verdult 2003). He also suggests that in accordance with retrogenesis theory (that is, that the progression of types of dementia occurs in reverse order from normal human development) we see motor behaviour from childhood (Verdult 2009).

The physiotherapeutic goal is not to suppress this motor behaviour but to manage it, channel it, reduce fear, and prevent the patient from self-harming.

Intervention   The physiotherapist tried to stimulate Ms L. to perform other motor behaviour with a ball and various equipment. Ms L. reacted best to a cuddly toy in her hand. Immediately her involuntary movements become slower and less intense. Also, the quality of motion changed: rubbing and pinching actions changed to petting and stroking. There was still movement but the sensory information was different.

Reflection   What is happening here? Is it fear control (as Reedijk propounds), is Ms L. lowering her arousal, or is it something different? The hands and fingers are our 'antennae' or 'scanners'; we use them to touch and sense

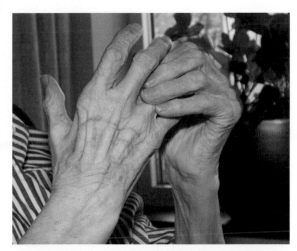

Figure 2.28 Repetitive movements with the hands [O596]

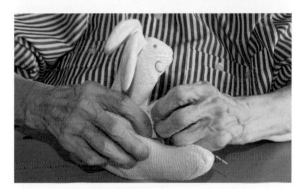

Figure 2.29 A soft toy calms repetitive movements [O596]

the environment. In the primary sensory and motor cortex in the evolutionary process a relatively large area has been dedicated to the control and coordination of the hand and fingers. In the author's opinion, it could be conjectured that when Ms L. performs certain hand movements – thereby positively activating these areas of the brain – rather than it acting only to lower arousal, the dementia effects are perhaps diminished. The reader can access interesting aspects of research concerning hand motor activity and cognition in Eggermont et al. (2009).

Outcome No further treatment was indicated. The family and nurses were informed and educated about the importance of human contact. In addition to this Ms L. was provided with 'feeling' materials.

✓ **GUIDANCE**
Do not always try to restrain repetitive movements, even when they may seem useless. They may have a function. More important is to structure or channel the movements and to prevent complications.

Case study 4: Constant wandering

Presentation Mr J., aged 84, diagnosed with severe vascular dementia, perpetually walked almost all day long round and round the care unit. He was constantly lost due to lack of orientation. In the morning he was balanced and safe, but after 4 pm he became progressively more tired with consequent unsteadiness.

Physiotherapy referral Mr J. was referred for falls prevention.

Observation/evaluation Mr J. walked obsessively. He only stopped for a short visit to the toilet. He was not amenable to group activities or individual activities. He was compelled to continually walk, resting for a maximum of two minutes. After several hours of wandering around the care unit, Mr J. leaned towards his left side and veered to the left. Mr J. was unable to follow instructions for the 6 minutes walking test or the Berg Balance Scale test. His heart rate during walking was 125 beats/minute.

Intervention and advice The physiotherapist attempted to control the patient's motor behaviour by means of fitness exercises, but Mr J. was non compliant. In consultation with the occupational therapist, nurses were advised to allow Mr J. to walk during the morning and then offer him a wheelchair after 2 pm. Mr J. was assessed as being capable of moving himself forward safely while sitting in his wheelchair and using his feet.

Subsequently a further problem emerged as transfers from his wheel chair from sitting to standing were unstable because Mr J. consistently forgot to use the braking mechanism. An innovation project was therefore implemented to create a wheelchair with automatic brakes; as soon as Mr J. lifted his pelvis from the seat the braking mechanism was activated.

Evaluation Mr J. was able to maintain independent walking if able and steady and also to move his wheelchair forward in a sitting position when tired or unsteady.

Outcome Although Mr J.'s urgency to walk was not resolved, he was however successfully protected against fall injury.

⚠ **CAUTION**
In falls prevention, fixation frequently leads to additional complications. Try to prevent falling by using alternative strategies without involving fixation. Be creative! (Tilly et al. 2006)

2

Case study 5: A wheel chair swing provides relaxation (➤ Figure 2.30)

Presentation   Ms G., aged 83, diagnosed with severe dementia, used to be a very active walker. Since becoming wheelchair dependent 6 months prior to referral, restlessness had increased. Sometimes she shouted out for her parents.

Physiotherapy referral   Observation and advice was requested in order to assess for non-pharmacological strategies to aid relaxation.

Observation/evaluation   Ms G. moved her trunk rhythmically forwards and backwards when sitting. Simultaneously she rubbed her hands along the armrests of her wheelchair. She did not appear to have pain but her facial expression showed despair. There were no possibilities for her to perform meaningful tasks, but she still yearned for physical activity.

Intervention   Input was multidisciplinary in discussion with the nurses and the occupational therapist. The physiotherapist advised trial of a rocking chair. The rationale was that Ms G.'s agitated trunk movements could initiate the rocking chair. Her restless movements would change into rhythmic rocking movements, and this could lull her into a relaxed state. The rhythmic frequency of this rocking chair was 30 times per minute: forward and backward per 2-second intervals. Although the patient was able to initiate the rocking chair movements she continued to look very restless; her face was still full of despair.

The physiotherapist then tried to hoist Ms G. into a wheelchair swing. This swing has a low frequency (6 times per minute). In this swing, Ms G. stopped her trunk movements, perhaps because she was now being moved by the swing.

The patient's physical restlessness diminished when in the swing. Her expression was peaceful, she closed her eyes, and it appeared that was surrendering herself to the rhythmic movements of the swing. After a few swings Ms G. started to hum an old cradle song. When listening carefully it was possible to understand the softly spoken words of an old lullaby.

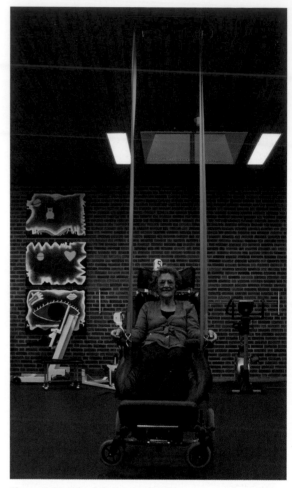

Figure 2.30 Wheel chair swing [O596]

✓ GUIDANCE

- Rocking rhythms relax. Explore how rhythm relaxes and what kinds of rhythms (and frequencies) are beneficial for the patient.
- Music influences mood up to the last stage of life. Because listening is passive, the patient experiences a sense of passive well-being (Guétin et al. 2009).

2.8.6 Conclusion

In all the preceding cases, referral to physiotherapy was to support or be a substitute for certain pharmacological treatment. Outcomes are sometimes astounding. The cases are presented in the hope that they will inspire physiotherapists to consider patients in a total and holistic way, and to be creative in finding treatment solutions, even if active movement and exercises are impracticable.

2.8.7 Reflective questions

Elisabeth Grünberger

- An Alzheimer patient cannot be motivated to undertake physiotherapy; he spends hours propelling himself up and down the corridor in his wheelchair, appearing completely absorbed and concentrated. What options do you think exist for establishing contact?
- How do you feel, as a physiotherapist, sitting by the bed of dementia patients and holding their hands? Is such an intervention already part of your therapeutic plan, or does it have no place in physiotherapy?
- The relative of a man with dementia asks you to do as much as you can so that his father regains his mobility and health. How would you explain your therapeutic plan to him?
- A woman with dementia does not recognise you as her physiotherapist. However, she always touches her right cheek when contact is established. How do you interpret this action and how could you use it in the physiotherapeutic process?
- You have set yourself the objective of always including new ideas in your therapy. Despite all your efforts, your therapy group of dementia sufferers appears to be increasingly restless and absent. Why is that, do you think?

REFERENCES

Aebi C. Validierung der neuropsychologischen Testbatterie CERAD-NP: eine Multi-Center-Studie. Doctoral thesis. University of Basel, 2002.

Bachmann LM, Kolb E, Koller MT, Steurer J, ter Riet G. Accuracy of Ottawa ankle rules to exclude fractures of the ankle and mid-foot: systematic review. BMJ 2003;326:417.

Bowlby J. The Making and Breaking of Affectional Bonds. London–New York: Routledge, 2000.

Droës RM. Psychomotor group therapy for demented patients in the nursing home. In: Miesen BML (ed). Caregiving in dementia: Research and applications, vol 2, 1997: pp. 95–118.

DSM-IV Diagnostic and Statistical Manual of Mental Disorders, 4th ed. American Psychiatric Association, 1994.

Eggermont LH, Knol DL, Hol EM, Swaab DF, Scherder EJ. A clustered randomized trial in nursing home residents with dementia: Hand motor activity, cognition, mood and the rest activity rhythm in dementia. Behav Brain Res 2009;196:271–278.

Epps CD. Recognizing pain in the institutionalized elder with dementia. Geriatr Nurs 2001; 22:71–77;quiz8–9.

Feil N. The validation breakthrough: simple techniques for communicating with people with Alzheimer's type dementia. 2nd ed. Health Professions Press, 2002.

Feil N. Validation. Ein Weg zum Verständnis verwirrter alter Menschen. München: Reinhardt Verlag 2005.

Feil N. Validation in Anwendung und Beispielen. München: Reinhardt Verlag 2007.

Fuchs-Lacelle S, Hadjistavropoulos T. Development and preliminary validation of the pain assessment checklist for seniors with limited ability to communicate (PACSLAC). Pain Manag Nurs 2004;5(1):37–49.

Fuchs-Lacelle S, Hadjistavropoulos T. Pain Assessment Checklist for Seniors with Limited Ability to Communicate (PACSLAC), 2007. Available at: http://ltctoolkit.rnao.ca/sites/ltc/files/resources/pain/PACSLAC.pdf (accessed June 2012).

Gatterer G. Alters-Konzentrations-Test (AKT). Göttingen: Hofgrefe 1990.

Gatterer G. Multiprofessionelle Altenbetreuung. Wien: Springer Verlag 2003.

Gershon S, Herman SP. The differential diagnosis of dementia. J Am Geriatr Soc 1982;30(11 Suppl):S58–S66.

Guétin S, Portet F, Picot MC, et al. Randomised, controlled study: Effect of music therapy on anxiety and depression in patients with Alzheimer's type dementia. Dement Geriatr Cogn Disord 2009;28:36–46.

Hall ET. The Hidden Dimension. New York: Doubleday, 1966.

Herrmann DJ, Searleman A. The new multimodal approach to memory improvement. In: Bower GH (ed). The Psychology of Learning and Motivation: Advances in research and theory. San Diego: Academic Press, 1990: pp. 175–205.

Heuft G, Kruse A. Lehrbuch der Gerontopsychosomatik und Alterspsychotherapie. München: Reinhardt Verlag, 2000.

Hobbelen HJM. Paratonia enlightened. Thesis. Enschede: Gildeprint Drukkerijen, 2010.

Kastner U, Löbach R. Handbuch der Demenz. München: Elsevier Urban&Fischer, 2010.

Kunz M. Veränderungen in der Schmerzverarbeitung bei Demenzpatienten: subjektive, mimische, motorische und vegetative Indikatoren. Doctoral thesis. Otto Friedrich University Bamberg, 2009.

Kunz M, Mylius V, Scharmann S, Schepelmann K, Lautenbacher S. Influence of dementia on multiple components of pain. Eur J Pain 2009;13(3):317–325.

Lautenbacher S, Gauggel S. Neuropsychologie psychischer Störungen. Berlin: Springer, 2010.

Markowitsch HJ, Calabrese P. Neuropsychologie des Gedächtnisses: In: Förstl H (eds). Lehrbuch der Gerontopsychiatrie und -psychotherapie. Stuttgart: Thieme. 2003.

Mitchell SL, Teno JM, Kiely DK, et al. The clinical course of advanced dementia. New Engl J Med 2009;361:1,529–1,538.

Morello R, Jean A, Alix M, Sellin-Peres D, Fermanian J. A scale to measure pain in non-verbally communicating older patients: the EPCA-2 study of its psychometric properties. Pain 2007;133:87–98.

Psota G. Oral presentation "Was brauchen Demente?" (What do demented people need?) at the Dementia Symposium, Eisenstadt 2011. Available at: http://www.volkshilfe-bgld.at/1068,,2.html

Shulman KI, Pushkar Gold D, Cohen CA, Zucchero CA. Clock-drawing and dementia in the community: A longitudinal study. Int J Geriatr Psychiatry 1993;8:487–496.

Reisberg B, Ferris SH, de Leon MJ, Crook T. The Global Deterioration Scale for assessment of primary degenerative dementia. Am J Psychiatry 1982;139:1,136–1,139.

Tariq SH, Tumosa N, Chibnall JT, Perry HM 3rd, Morley JE. Comparison of the Saint Louis University mental status examination and the mini-mental state examination for detecting dementia and mild neurocognitive disorder – a pilot study. Am J Geriatr Psychiatry 2006;14:900–910. Available at: http://medschool.slu.edu/agingsuccessfully/pdfsurveys/slumsexam_05.pdf (last accessed August 2012).

Tilly J, Reed P. Alzheimer's association: falls, wandering, and physical restraints. Interventions for residents with dementia in assisted living and nursing homes. Philadelphia, PA: Lippincott, Williams & Wilkins, 2006.

van Dijk G, Dijkstra A. Kraftlosigkeit anerkennen. Passivitäten des täglichen Lebens und palliative Pflege. Pflege Z 2006;59(6):362–365.

Scherder EJA, Sergeant JA, Swaab DF. Pain processing in dementia and its relation to neuropathology. Lancet Neurol 2003;2:677–686.

Scherder E, Eggermont L, Swaab D, et al. Gait in ageing and associated dementias: its relationship with cognition. Neurosci Biobehav Rev 2007;31:485–497.

van Dijk PT, Meulenberg OG, van de Sande HJ, Habbema JD. Falls in dementia patients. Gerontologist 1993;33:200–204.

von Kieckebusch, U. Psychologische Demenzdiagnostik. München: Reinhardt Verlag, 2011.

Verdult R. De pijn van Dement zijn [The pain of being demented]. Baarn: HB Uitgevers, 2003.

Verdult R. Prenatal aspects in Alzheimer's disease. J Prenat Perinat Psychol Health 2009;23:235–262.

Wallesch W, Förstl H. Neuropathologie der Demenzen. Stuttgart: Thieme, 2005.

Warden V, Hurley AC, Volicer L. Development and psychometric evaluation of the Pain Assessment in Advanced Dementia (PAINAD) scale. J Am Med Dir Assoc 2003;4(1):9–15.

Wary B, Serbouti S. Doloplus: validation d'une échelle d'évaluation comportementale de la douleur chez la personne âgée. Revue Douleurs 2001,2;1:35–38.

Winnicott DV. The maturational processes and the faciliating environment. Studies in the theory of emotional development. London: Hogarth Press, 1965.

Zwakhalen SM, Hamers JP, Abu-Saad HH, Berger MP. Pain in elderly people with severe dementia: a systematic review of behavioral pain assessment tools. BMC Geriatr 2006;6:3.

2.9 Physiotherapy in paediatric palliative care

Christina Plath, Sabine Schraut

⚠ **C A U T I O N**
"Children are not mini-adults."

2.9.1 Features of paediatric palliative care

According to the *Association for Children with Life-threatening or Terminal Conditions and Their Families* (ACT) paediatric palliative care is an active and far-reaching care concept that unites **physical, emotional, social and spiritual elements.** Its focus lies in achieving the best possible **qualify of life for the child** and provid-

ing all-round **support for the family.** The concept includes the treatment of distressing symptoms as well as providing respite, medical nursing and psychosocial support until death and also during the subsequent period of bereavement (Statement by the *Task Force Paediatric Palliative Care* of the *European Association for Palliative Care* during its *International Meeting for Palliative Care in Children* in Trento).

Four types of life-limiting disease are defined that may necessitate palliative care in children:

1. Life-threatening illnesses for which curative therapy (leading to recovery) is available but is often unsuccessful or in turn may lead to life-threatening complications, including cancer and organ failure (waiting for a transplant).
2. Illnesses in which premature death is unavoidable but appropriate symptomatic therapy will facilitate prolonged life commensurate with the child's age, e. g. mucoviscidosis or Duchenne muscular dystrophy.
3. Advanced illnesses with no chance of curative therapy, e. g. certain congenital muscular diseases or certain metabolic disorders.
4. Non-progressive diseases as a result of trauma that routinely involve complications and therefore end in premature death, e. g. severe brain injury before or during birth, certain severe, congenital deformities, serious traumatic brain injury.

More than half of those children requiring palliative care suffer from the consequences of congenital deformities, chromosomal damage, perinatal complications or trauma, combined with varying degrees of mental and motor disorders.

⚠ **C A U T I O N**
Distinguishing between children and adults in palliative care

Unlike adults, children often require many years of palliative care: they may have phases of relative well-being enabling them to participate in group activities with children of the same age that can alternate with phases in which they are seriously ill and death appears to be imminent.
The course is difficult to predict, and spontaneous changes repeatedly result in uncertainty on the part of the family and professional staff. **Not every episode represents the terminal phase, even if this may appear to be the case.**

Prevalent issues and their paediatric features

The 'classic' problems in the palliative care setting, especially at end of life, are mostly the same as those in adults but are manifested differently depending on age and therefore necessitate different therapeutic approaches.

Non-specific symptoms in childhood:

- listlessness;
- lack of appetite;
- disobedience/non-compliance;
- nausea.

In children who are not, or only partly, communicative, **vegetative symptoms** such as sweating, centralisation of the circulation, tachycardia or tachypnoea and changes (mostly increases) in tone are sometimes the only means by which severe pain or debilitating anxiety are manifested.

Drugs like opioids, sedatives, botulinum toxin and baclofen can also be used to good effect in the paediatric palliative care setting (➤ Chapter 2.2).

If the team of professionals works smoothly together, a maximum synergistic effect can be achieved through a combination of physiotherapy and drug treatment. Specific physiotherapeutic measures do not differ a great deal from those applied in adults, however children can be easily engaged by means of imaginative diversionary tactics, fantasy journeys, and also touch (e. g. massage).

Pain

Young children (at least until school age) are not able to relate their discomfort to a particular organ, even if their linguistic skills are already advanced. Stomach ache, for example, can be a sign of constipation but also of breathlessness. For therapy to be effective, careful consideration of the possible causes is very important: a full bladder or bowel will require different techniques to pain arising from a tumour or painful episodes of spasticity. The parents and carers who know the child well are best suited to identifying the relevant signs.

Assessments for establishing a child's pain

There are numerous **observational methods and measurements** that can be used to acurately assess a child's pain. The effects of therapy are easy to evaluate by using the same scale at the start, during and after treatment. Very detailed observational tools such as the *Puediatric Pain Profile* (Hunt et al. 2004) or *Non-Communication Children's Pain Checklist* (Breau et al. 2001) deliver a differentiated picture, but are too complex to be used regularly in physiotherapy.

In the experience of the authors, the two methods described below are effective and very simple to use: the German **KUSS Scale** (➤ Table 2.22) was originally designed for measuring postoperative pain in alert neonates and infants up to the age of four years.

Action must be taken if the total score exceeds 4. The scale can also be used in older children unable to communicate, and can be modified to assess other distressing symptoms.

An option that can be used in children above the age of about four who can communicate commensurate to their age is the **Faces Pain Scale** (➤ Figure 2.31)

The child should point to the face that best represents how he or she currently feels about the pain. The face on

Table 2.22 KUSS – Childhood discomfort and pain scale [Kindliche Unbehagens- und Schmerzskala] (Büttner 1998)

Observation	Assessment	Score
Crying	None	0
	Groaning, whining, crying	1
	Screaming	2
Facial expression	Relaxed, smiling	0
	Mouth distorted	1
	Mouth grimacing, eyes screwed up	2
Upper body posture	Neutral	0
	Unsteady	1
	Lurching, askew	2
Position of legs	Neutral	0
	Kicking, thrashing	1
	Drawn up tightly	2
Motor restlessness	Absent	0
	Moderate	1
	Restless	2
	Total	

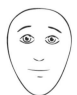 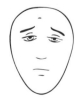 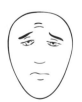 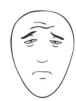 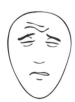 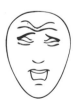

Figure 2.31 Faces Pain Scale – revised (Hicks et al 2001).
Reprinted with the kind permission of the *International Association for the Study of Pain*® (IASP®) [F148]

2

the left is scored as 0 (no pain) and those from left to right 2, 4, 6, 8 and 10 points, respectively. 10 points signify the most intense pain, represented by the face on the right. (**NB:** The patient must point to the picture; it is not the patient's facial expression that is being assessed.)

Anxiety

Fear of pain prevails during diagnostic and therapeutic procedures. The children generally have many years of experience in this area and just like healthy children have different ways with which to cope. Anxiety can cause a child who generally appears to be very mature to suddenly behave like an infant and no longer be responsive to well-intentioned propositions. The therapist first needs to gain the trust of the child so that he is assured that no harm will be done.

A doll or reference person can be used to demonstrate the various moves and exercises. This will also help the adults to better understand the child in the therapeutic setting. The **greater the trust,** the easier it will be to develop joint strategies for the pending medical and therapeutic interventions. Experience has shown that the more 'say' a child has in the therapeutic process, the greater the compliance.

Children with severe cognitive dysfunctions can also be plagued by fear – there need only be an unusual situation or strange sensation for anxiety and fear to be triggered. In a similar way to pain, non-specific **vegetative symptoms and changes in tone** can be observed. Assessment of the situation by the child's family combined with close observation of behaviour and facial expressions are most important.

A **parent's anxiety** will often be transferred to the child, especially if the fears cannot or should not be put into words.

Respiratory insufficiency and breathlessness

It is important to distinguish between respiratory insufficiency and the subjective sensation of breathlessness. The visible signs of respiratory insufficiency in childhood do not especially correlate with the subjective feeling of breathlessness. Hence, some children who clearly have objective symptoms can be quite active, whilst children with barely perceptible objective signs may appear to be seriously ill. The anxiety that accompanies breathlessness and causes it to worsen is relatively negligible in young children, and only becomes apparent in older children and adolescents.

Common causes for respiratory insufficiency are neurological diseases as well as severe scoliosis, recurrent

aspiration and insufficiency of the respiratory muscles, in addition to the causes already known in adults (➤ Chapter 2.3, ➤ Chapter 2.4).

Aside from the objective signs of reduced oxygen saturation displayed on a monitor, the typical symptoms are:
- accelerated breathing;
- nasal flaring;
- stridor;
- pale grey perioral skin pigmentation;
- cyanotic lips;
- use of accessory respiratory muscles (mainly the scalene and sternocleidomastoid muscles);
- use of abdominal muscles when exhaling;
- paradoxical respiration.

General measures and therapeutic interventions are described in ➤ Chapter 2.3 and ➤ Chapter 2.4.

✓ GUIDANCE

Measures appropriate for children with respiratory insufficiency/breathlessness

- The therapist or parent should sit with arms wrapped around the child from behind, controlling the breathing.
- Draw a face on the child's stomach, which will increase and decrease in size with the breathing pattern.
- Humming, singing of rhythmic nursery rhymes.
- Rhythmic reading of poems aloud.
- Breathing onto a mirror.
- Blowing a cotton wool ball.
- Blowing bubbles.

(Brocke 2003, Ehrenberg 2001)

Constipation

Children with severe and multiple disabilities are often very constipated. Other illnesses can also be associated with constipation, causes for which can be a lack of exercise, reduced intake of fluids and food, inability to defecate as a result of weakness and fear of pain during the process, disorders of the innervation of the rectum, adverse drug effects (particularly from opioids).

Children are not keen to dwell on such a subject; hence, even in communicative children it is important to look out for special signs in addition to the general discomforts listed above: a tender abdomen, lack of appetite and vomiting, malaise, bloating, flatulence or faecal overflow (which can often be erroneously interpreted as diarrhoea) can all be signs of constipation.

✓ GUIDANCE

Physiotherapeutic interventions for constipation

The potential physiotherapeutic interventions do not differ from those applied in adults. They can be used as an adjunct

to pharmacological therapy, are perceived as less unpleasant than laxatives, and can easily be undertaken by the carer. They mainly have a reflexive influence on intestinal motility:
• warm feet;
• respiratory therapy;
• colon massage;
• heat application to the abdomen;
• vibration plate beneath the feet when lying and standing;
• extensions of the adductor, piriformis and gluteus minimus muscles.

Nausea and vomiting

Vomiting is seldom perceived by young children as distressing and must be viewed in context.

Nausea, on the other hand, can be an insurmountable obstacle to therapy in children since total refusal may result. Diversionary tactics can therefore be of greater help than in adults. Nausea is very difficult to evaluate in children who are uncommunicative.

Fatigue

Fatigue is a topic that generally is still afforded too little attention in paediatrics. A few studies have been conducted into fatigue in children with chronic illness, and also in children with oncological diseases (Eddy/Cruz 2007). The measurement tools designed for children are not yet in widespread use and can only be applied to older children with cognitive skills appropriate to their age (➤ Chapter 2.6).

Development as a special feature

⚠ **CAUTION**
Development is the decisive resource on the basis of which children can be fundamentally differentiated from adults in any therapeutic situation, including palliative care.

Development is always restricted in a critically ill child and depending on the disease will generally be inconsistent. For example, a child with muscular dystrophy may be almost completely immobilised, but in intellectual terms be perfectly developed for his age; a child with a severe perinatal brain injury may have serious mental disorders in addition to marked spasticity; and a child with leukaemia may have fully developed intellectual and motor skills for his age and be far more advanced than his peers in terms of emotional maturity.

It is generally accepted and perfectly understandable that children who are constantly confronted by death and dying in a hospital will become aware of their own death much sooner than healthy children of the same age. Nevertheless, the nature and expression of such knowledge will reflect the corresponding stage of a child's development (Longaker 1997; Zernikow 2008).

Guidance on socio-emotional development in relation to disease, dying and death may divide children into the following age categories (Keller 1998, Largo 2001, Largo 2007, Niethammer 2008):
• **Children aged 0 to 1.5 years** see themselves as one unit with their person of reference, and have not yet developed any object permanence (or person permanence). Communication mostly takes place at the non-verbal level via physical contact and vocal sounds.
• **Children aged 1.5 to 3.5 years** realise that they exist independently of the person of reference, develop object and person permanence, but do not yet have any concept of time.
• **Children aged 3.5 to 7 years** live in a magical world full of fantasies, believing that death and disease are influenced by their own behaviour (e. g.: *'If something bad happens, it will be my fault because I wasn't good'*) and that death is another form of existence (life in heaven).
• **Children aged 7 to 10 years** recognise the finiteness of situations, understand that death is irreversible, can comprehend the internal organic causes of death and are often frightened about mutilation. Role playing, vivid descriptions or perhaps monologues are typical of this age group.
• **Children aged over 11 years** understand death as the termination of all human relationships. At this age, fear of death is most pronounced as children find themselves in a natural phase of disengagement and reorientation. Children at this age develop their own philosophical and spiritual views. Justice plays an important role (*'Is it fair that I am terminally ill when everyone around me is healthy?'*). Openness is replaced by reticence.
• **Adolescents** experience the loss of independence as an exclusion of realities of daily living such as vitality, fitness, beauty, the loss of which is seen as a loss of human dignity. Excessive parental protection and social isolation are problems to which adolescents feel they are subjected. Dying adolescents often give the impression of being detached and aloof. Most important at this age is to develop an understanding of the concepts and desires of an adolescent, and above all respect their right to choose or refuse treatments.

Autonomy has different meanings in the various age groups. On the one hand it means physical autonomy and independence, e. g. mobility, eating (or not eating), controlling one's bodily excretions, independent occupation or contact with the 'outside world'. The physiotherapist is important here for helping to maintain or develop such abilities. On the other hand autonomy in a child also means making one's own decisions. During the majority of their short lifetimes, decisions concerning seriously ill children have invariably been made by others. At the palliative stage, however, it is the last opportunity to let the child determine how to live – this also includes the right to refuse therapy.

The ability to make decisions not only advances as the psychosocial functions of a child develop, but is also dependent on the degree to which the cognitive skills are impaired (Wiesemann et al. 2003).

A particular challenge exists if the child is able to realistically judge his own condition, the therapist is aware but the parents refuse to accept it. Professionalism here means holding back without becoming insincere, and using team communication to ensure a common approach with defined roles

The crictally ill, dying child as part of the family system

Children are never sick on their own. They and their illness are part of the family system in which each individual (parents, siblings) has his or her own special place and role when it comes to dealing with the situation. Parents with a disabled or critically ill child organise their lives around their child's condition. They have fewer social contacts because there remains little time for such interaction or because former friends have withdrawn. The physiotherapist is often the only regular 'outsider' to appear in the household. This makes the role of the physiotherapist very demanding, and he or she is held in **high esteem by the parents as the specialist for their child.**

Parents who have not yet gained much experience in dealing with their newborn child require the support of a therapist in order to become experts.

Therapy becomes a dynamic exchange: between child and therapist, therapist and parents, parents and child (➤ Chapter 3.1).

⚠ **C A U T I O N**
The therapist in the family system

- Maintain an appropriate distance, professional yet warm, with the entire family.
- Parents sometimes have different ideas from the therapist.
- Parents sometimes have different ideas from the child.

Aside from the sick child, there may often be **siblings** who live a 'shadowy life'. They also need the attention of the physiotherapist, whether involving them in a short game at the start or end of the therapy session or by including them in the therapeutic process, etc. The time used for therapy can also become a special time for the parents to spend with their healthy child(ren).

2.9.2 Principles of physiotherapy with children and adolescents in the palliative care setting

Basics

The physiotherapeutic goal-setting process is fundamentally based on the following question: **Am I looking at skills that have never been developed that can now be initiated, or the loss of skills that had already been acquired for which we need to look for ways to compensate?**

✓ **G U I D A N C E**
Basic approaches

- Encourage, don't enforce.
- Partake in the here and now.
- Integrate into family life.

The child should join in with family life as much as his level of development and current situation permit, and be able to pursue his own activities (meals, trips, travel and visits together). It is challenging to design the therapeutic plan in such a way that the therapeutic goals can be adjusted at any time.

Physiotherapeutic assessments based on measurements are often difficult and not always necessary when administering palliative care to children; in children with no specific prognosis, however, they can be a reasonable basis for introducing aids and defining goals. In the palliative care setting it is sometimes difficult to put the improvement in quality of life as defined by the ICF (International Classification of Functioning, Disability and Health) into perspective. Nevertheless, physiotherapeutic interventions may be very helpful. Some forms of physiotherapy may still prove unpleasant to children in such a situation (e. g. clearance of mucus, laxative procedures or contracture prophylaxis), despite being effective and expedient in terms of palliative care.

Basic knowledge

The following basic knowledge is required if physiotherapy is to be successful in critically ill children:
- regulated motor development;
- regulated cognitive development;
- regulated socio-emotional development;
- deviations from such developmental steps specific to the illness.

If children are not (yet) able to recognise the benefit of a therapeutic intervention, their inner acceptance must still be obtained. This can be done by very closely observing and assessing any possible resistance on the part of the child (➤ Table 2.23). An evaluation by the parent(s) is important in case of any uncertainty.

Every child has at least one open channel of perception that the therapist can tap into. On identifying the widest channel, attention is drawn towards what the child can do and away from what he cannot do. Searching for such an opening is the way to build up a relationship with the child, as the basis for continued therapy – irrespective of how very sick the child is and the goals that are achievable.

The physical, mental and spiritual resources of a child can be divided, according to Söller (2007), into four levels. If it is possible to work at one of these levels, each of the other three will be positively influenced accordingly:
- physical/motor (posture and mobility, coordination, fine motor skills);
- emotional/social (intrinsic motivation, degree of interaction, emotions);
- cognitive (attention, curiosity, concentration, speech, exploration);
- sensory (sight, hearing, feel, taste, smell, perceptual processing).

Physiotherapeutic methods

Due to the often prolonged need for physiotherapeutic care, all the principles and procedures that generally apply to any child undergoing physiotherapy also have to be taken into account in palliative care children. The following treatment concepts can be considered in particular in paediatric palliative care:
- therapies for supporting and managing neuro-physiological development and therapy (e.g. Bobath, Castillo Morales);
- methods for supporting psychomotor development;
- animal-assisted therapy;
- basal stimulation.

Certain other methods, albeit not child-specific, are also worth mentioning e.g.:
- electrotherapy (TENS);
- vibration plate when lying and standing;
- taping, compression bandaging (e.g. for contractures and lymphoedema).

> ✓ **G U I D A N C E**
> - **Useful items in the therapeutic repertoire:** hand puppet, balloons, blowing bubbles, coloured fabric, torch, conkers, lentils, rice, acorns, sweetcorn, beans, small balls, cherrystone bags, shaving foam, feathers, cotton wool, oils, camera, etc.
> - **Useful items that can be used from the child's environment:** newspaper cuttings, polystyrene, rice for 'sprinkling', bubble bottle, warm water, ice cubes, makeup, clothes pegs, pillows, hand towels, bed linen, foam rolls, hairdryer, fan, spray humidifier, fancy-dress, hats, chalk, coloured pencils, black and white card for contrasts, instruments such as drums, rattles, bells, etc. Domestic pets can also be integrated into the therapy session.

Aids and appliances

One of the physiotherapist's important tasks, also in palliative care, is to ensure that adequate aids and appliances are to hand.

Aids should be used in line with the general criteria applicable to children. The baseline assessment should

Table 2.23 Comprehension in children with impaired verbal communication

Observation	Child feels well	Child feels unwell
Eye contact	Questioning, inviting, towards the therapist	Avoidance
Facial expression	Relaxed, smiling, changeable	Large eyes, knitted brows, wrinkled nose
Gesticulation	Pointing at objects, hands active	'Rigid'
Body language	Listens attentively, engaged, open, loose movements, relaxed	Generally restless, yawning, hands/fists in front of the eyes (suggesting tiredness), turns away, increased muscle tone, increased involuntary movements, hyperextended, frees himself from therapist's hands, brushes the therapist's hand away
Voice	Talking, making noises, whooping, laughing	Groaning, crying, whining In infants: single, prolonged exhalation (sigh)
Speech	As before (ask parents)	Louder, quieter, monotone, falling silent

establish the aids that have been used so far and the benefit they have brought, combined with suggestions of changes and additions. In the palliative care situation in particular, the laborious and time-consuming process of obtaining approval for such aids can be outpaced by rapid functional changes. The choices made must therefore be very flexible and forward-looking. This applies in particular if a child is discharged from hospital to return home, or is moved to a care facility or hospice. The physiotherapist's plan should take into account such a transition.

Positioning

Positioning is crucial if the child's condition deteriorates, specific symptoms develop or the terminal phase is reached. If contractures develop, the child's position

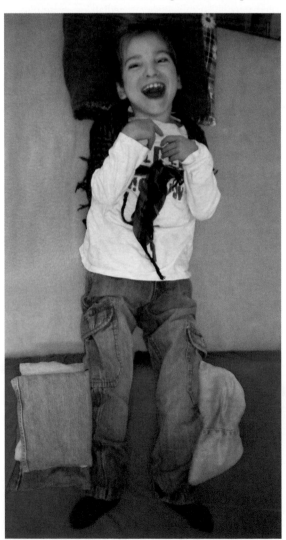

Figure 2.32 Position with shoulder support [O595]

should be adjusted accordingly. Creativity is demanded when it comes to making use of the materials available in the child's environment.

Depending on the objective, various supports – whether hard or soft – may be used, along with diverse materials and resources such as water, sand, cloths, pads, breastfeeding pillows, wedges, blankets, hand towels, cuddly toys, slings, etc.

Some examples:

- Half a roll of cardboard lined with pillows and positioned on a skateboard, permitting movement in all directions.
- The child can be carried and transported in blankets.
- An upper body wrap or shoulder support can be created from the mother's scarf (➤ Fig. 2.32).
- A semi-inflated ball or inner tube from a large car tyre facilitate maximum tactile awareness.
- The top and bottom ends of the bed can be used as alternative positions if the bed cannot be moved.

The **objectives of positioning** in paediatric palliative care:

- pain reduction;
- tactile awareness;
- alleviating the breathing/clearing mucus;
- improvement of circulation and ventilation;
- increased involvement in social life (➤ Fig. 2.33);
- improved mobility.

2.9.3 Special features of therapy in different situations

Children in hospital

When a critically ill child is in hospital or on the palliative care unit, this is generally a transitional phase involving myriad medical procedures undertaken for the purposes of diagnosis and optimisation of therapy. Close collaboration with the nursing staff will help integrate the physiotherapeutic programme into the everyday workings of the ward (➤ Chapter 1.3).

> **✓ GUIDANCE**
> Regular involvement of the physiotherapist in visits and case discussions will be beneficial when it comes to defining common therapeutic goals.

To have a paediatric palliative care unit with a team so well organised that the common therapeutic goal can be determined together with the family is certainly desirable, but seldom feasible. A **non-hierarchical structure** (collaborative and shared expertise from the various

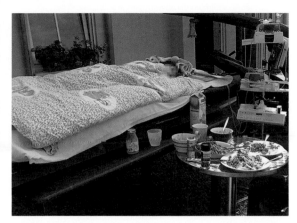

Figure 2.33 Position of a dying female patient on the terrace [0598]

professional teams) is highly beneficial to children, their families and all involved.

Children in a hospice/care facility

Like those in hospital, children in a hospice or care facility also spend a lot of time either sitting or lying down. A regular change in position and location, preferably according to a fixed schedule, is important for minimising pain from pressure sores, poor circulation, spasticity and contractures. It is also important for the nursing staff and other therapists to hold team meetings to devise and implement joint goals and allocate responsibilities.

✓ **GUIDANCE**

Group positioning

By placing children in a group and including art therapies or breathing components, they are both distracted and motivated while the various therapists are presented with the possibility to develop synergistic ideas.

Children at home

The child and family may feel more comfortable at home where they can live a 'normal' family life. They are not being controlled by outsiders and do not have to justify their every feeling and activity (e. g. outbreaks of sadness or anger, specific eating or sleeping habits). In addition, friends or also household pets are allowed unlimited access.

The attending physiotherapist arranges visits that necessarily suit the rules and rituals of family life.

2.9.4 Case study

History   Aaron, aged one year 8 months, receives therapy in the form of home visits (➤ Figure 2.34). *Past medical history:* Born at week 39 of pregnancy, 2,790 g, 46 cm, 35 cm. Suspected intrauterine finding of a heart defect. Admitted to the intensive care unit after spontaneous birth, diverse cardiac operations, tracheostomy fitted for laryngomalacia, insertion of a PEG tube for swallowing difficulties, closure of cleft lip/palate. *Medical diagnoses* on discharge after 6 weeks: CHARGE syndrome in the palliative setting, hypertrophic cardiomyopathy, severe psychomotor retardation, cleft lip/palate. *Medication:* Various drugs for stabilising cardiac function and circulation. *Aids:* Therapeutic chair, oxygen saturation monitor, suction equipment, resuscitation pack for controlling life-threatening situations. *Therapy and interventions:* Outpatient paediatric nursing service 4 times a week, physiotherapy once a week. *Prognosis:* Decompensated cardiac failure or deterioration in respiratory condition possible at any time. It is not possible to predict how long Aaron will live and what course the condition will take (a few months to a number of years).

Home and social environment   Aaron is living with his parents and four-year-old sister in a 30-square-metre apartment. The family has a migratory background. His

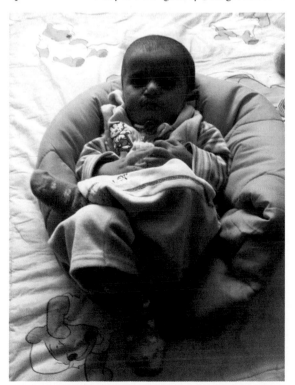

Figure 2.34 Aaron [M548]

mother is the main point of contact but has little speech comprehension so communication takes place primarily using hand signals. Aaron's sister is present during his therapy, and Aaron understands Arabic and German.

General impression   Good general, dystrophic nutritional state; receiving very good care. Levels of attention and vigilance depend on form on the day. The auditory canal is the main means of gaining Aaron's attention. He recognises the therapist and visually interacts with him very well.

Main issues at present   Inadequate control of the head due to reduced muscle tone in the trunk, no autonomous locomotion, not able to straighten independently and lacks perception in a number of the senses. This causes reduced coordination of voluntary movements, insufficient recognition and interpretation of sensory stimuli, and decreased communication skills with regard to his family and therapist.

Therapeutic goals   The following therapeutic goals are agreed with the parents:

Stage 1: Once adequate control of the head is achieved, Aaron can sit at the table and thus be part of the family's communal activities, especially at mealtimes (he can be fed at this time via his tube).

Stage 2: Autonomously holding himself upright when seated.

Stage 3: Introduction of independent locomotion.

Long-term: Creation of a resource-based management plan for the parents' planned return to their homeland.

✓ **G U I D A N C E**

Goal setting

One means of visualising the achievement of therapeutic goals is the **Goal Attainment Scale** (GAS) developed by Kiresuk and Sherman (1968), which was developed to evaluate non-standardised objectives in clinical psychology. The design of the tool is open to the extent that it can be applied irrespective of the substantive context. By setting goals

Goal-Attainment-Scale (GAS)

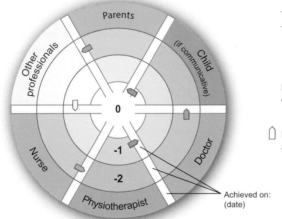

-2 = Baseline
-1 = Partial success
 0 = Achievement of jointly defined
     therapeutic goal

Disc made out of plastic so that the date can be wiped away.

⌂ Movable arrow (magnetic or sliding through a groove)

Linear patient chart

	Goal in line with ICF	Criterion	-2	Achieved on: date	-1	Achieved on: date	0	Achieved on: date
Physiotherapist								
Doctor								
Child								
Parents								
Other professionals, e.g. occupational therapist								
Nurse								

Figure 2.35   Goal Attainment Scale and linear patient chart (© C. Plath, 2013) [M548/L157]

together, the patients become much more involved in the therapeutic process. The newly developed structure of the Goal Attainment Scale provided in ➤ Figure 2.35 aims to actively involve all professional teams and the affected family (parents/child) in the formulation of the objectives. The illustrated circular diagram can be supplemented with movable arrows.
• 0: Those involved agree on a joint therapeutic goal.
• −2: The current baseline situation is set out in writing with a view to the goal (0).
• −1: Potential partial success is set out in writing with a view to the long-term goal (0).
All three circles (−2, −1, 0) are established prior to commencing therapy. Using a slider in a circular motion, each person involved gains an immediate impression of the efficacy of treatment. It is useful in this case to enter the partial goals and long-term goals into a linear patient chart (➤ Figure 2.35).

Treatment plan/interventions:
• Increase frequency to two physiotherapy sessions a week.
• Provide the mother with guidance on the prevention of pressure sores and contractures.
• Position on a wedge and blanket on the floor when supine (improving rotation of the head by reducing the force of gravity).
• Bolster the shoulders (centering in the middle, hand-to-hand contact possible) (Holtz 2004).
• Practise repositioning to the left and right.
• Support the forearms and shift the body's centre of gravity to trigger autonomous locomotion. A wedge-shaped support may be used to protect the tracheostomy.
• Sit upright on the floor with legs extended, supported by the therapist; shift the body's centre of gravity to the left and right, achieving the quadruped position across the therapist's thighs.
• Partial loading of the feet and tactile input on a coarse rug.
• Optimise the position in the therapeutic chair with partial loading of the feet in shoes to improve posture and control of the head, thereby preventing scoliosis. Upper extremities: rolled towels under the upper arms, position the therapy table at different heights (high to support fine motor function; low to promote forearm support).
• Ball games with sister in any position. Aaron responds well to balloons, which he is able to grip and throw/push away with help.
• Activities requiring vigilance are devised in order to enable him to play independently and to develop as well as maintain a physical sense of well-being through improved body image.

As the therapeutic chair cannot be taken with them the father and therapist develop a means of support, using two bars screwed together to create a right angle in which Aaron can sit securely on the floor.

Structure of therapy   Each session of therapy begins and ends with the ritual of singing a greeting and farewell. Aaron's sister is present during his therapy, providing the necessary vigilance and motivation for locomotion. His clothing is not removed, as it gives him security. Aaron responds well to aromas, so a lemon fragrance that his mother has found for him is used during physiotherapy. During the session, a cloth on which the oil has been applied is placed near his head. While this promotes well-being, it may help foster positive memories for the future.

Therapeutic measures for acute deterioration   Aaron returned with his family to their homeland at the age of two and a half years. Since acute deterioration fortunately did not occur over the course of therapy, but could occur at any time, the family needed to be encouraged in their independence. Various activities were devised and practised with the mother for such an eventuality:
• lemon fragrance (olfactory and reminiscent of a ritual);
• tasting (gustatory) various flavours (liquids on a compress);
• decorating the room with black/white, zebra as a cuddly toy, etc (visual);
• hand on the sternum (tactile);
• rocking/singing to favourite music with Aaron in her arms (acoustic);
• positioning under a weighted blanket if restless;
• when bathing, covering or weighing the body down with a warm, wet towel (tactile/proprioceptive);
• positioning with the family (emotion);
• positioning in a hammock (kinaesthetic);

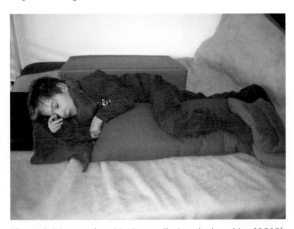

Figure 2.36 Lateral positioning to alleviate the breathing [O595]

- positioning on his side with head slightly elevated to alleviate the breathing (> Figure 2.36), supporting with a rigid foam block behind his back, towel or blanket under the soles of the feet (ideally with the lower shoulders lying freely); supporting the arm and leg lying freely;
- gentle extensions;
- gentle foot massage by his mother;
- mother/father carries Aaron in a sling tied close to the body (socio-emotional level) or sits behind Aaron on the bed, holding him in both arms and performing contact breathing;
- sitting and listening, pure body contact without speaking, are also part of the process.

√ GUIDANCE

Rituals and routine are especially important to young children with limited communication skills, such as a song in greeting and farewell. Older children and adolescents also gain a sense of security and trust from repetitive rituals such as music, touch, speech, aroma.

2.9.5 Conclusion

Physiotherapy in critically and terminally ill children and adolescents has a positive effect not only on the quality of life of the patients, but also their parents and siblings. Bearing in mind the special features of paediatric palliative care, the range of symptoms, setting and therapeutic approach involved, one of the primary goals to the very end of life is to provide the child with encouragement. As members of an interdisciplinary team, therefore, physiotherapists have promising and resourceful options with which to care for children and adolescents, and their families, during the most difficult phase of their lives. Just as Vaclav Havel said: *'Hope is not the conviction that something will turn out well, but the certainty that something makes sense, regardless of how it turns out.'*

2.9.6 Reflective questions

- What does a 'child's autonomy' mean to me? What potential for conflict does this entail for the therapist?
- How can I positively influence the contrast between developing goals and the likelihood of imminent death?
- How can I adapt my therapy to the way in which death and dying are experienced by children at different ages?
- Which options as regards working in a multiprofessional team can I use or expand in my job?

REFERENCES

Breau LM, Camfield C, McGrath PJ, Rosmus C, Finley GA. Measuring pain accurately in children with cognitive impairments. J Pediatrics 2001;138(5):721–727.

Brocke M. Aktuelle Atemtherapie in der Physiotherapiepraxis. München–Bad Kissingen–Berlin–Düsseldorf–Heidelberg: Richard Pflaum, 2003.

Büttner W. Die Erfassung des postoperativen Schmerzes beim Kleinkind, München: Arcis, 1998.

Eddy L, Cruz M. The relationship between fatigue and quality of life in children with chronic health problems – a systematic review. J Spec Pediatr Nurs 2007;12(2):105–114.

Ehrenberg H. Atemtherapie in der Physiotherapie/Krankengymnastik. München–Bad Kissingen–Berlin–Düsseldorf–Heidelberg: Pflaum, 2001.

Hicks CL, von Baeyer CL, Spafford PA, van Korlaar I, Goodenough B. The Faces Pain Scale – Revised: toward a common metric in pediatric pain measurement. Pain 2001;93:173–183

Holtz R. Therapie- und Alltagshilfen für zerebralparetische Kinder. München–Bad Kissingen–Berlin–Düsseldorf–Heidelberg: Pflaum, 2004.

Hunt A, Goldman A, Seers K, Crichton N, Moffat V, Oulton K. Clinical validation of the Paediatric Pain Profile. Dev Med Child Neurol 2004;46: 9–18.

Keller H (Hrsg.). Lehrbuch Entwicklungspsychologie. Bern–Göttingen–Toronto–Seattle: Hans Huber, 1998.

Kiresuk TJ, Sherman RE. Goal Attainment Scale: a general method for evaluating comprehensive community mental health programs. Community Ment Health J 1968;4:443–453.

Largo R. Kinderjahre. München: Piper, 2001.

Largo R. Babyjahre. München: Piper, 2007.

Longaker C. Dem Tod begegnen und Hoffnung finden. Die emotionale und spirituelle Begleitung Sterbender. München: Piper, 1997.

Niethammer D. Das sprachlose Kind. Stuttgart–New York: Schattauer, 2008.

Söller A. Zeig mir, was Du kannst. Ein Buch für Therapeuten, Eltern und Erzieher. München–Bad Kissingen–Berlin–Düsseldorf–Heidelberg: Richard Pflaum, 2007.

Wiesemann C, Dörries A, Wolflast G, Simon A (Hrsg.). Das Kind als Patient. Frankfurt: Campus, 2003.

Zernikow B. Palliativversorgung von Kindern, Jugendlichen und jungen Erwachsenen. Heidelberg: Springer Medizin, 2008.

BIBLIOGRAPHY

Bluebond-Langner M. The private world of dying children. Princeton: Princeton University Press, 1980.

Bluebond-Langner M. Worlds of dying children and their well siblings. Death Stud 1989;13:1–16.

Ebelt-Paprotny G, Preis R. Leitfaden Physiotherapie. München: Elsevier: Urban&Fischer, 2008.

Hüter-Becker A, Dölken M. Physiotherapie in der Pädiatrie. Stuttgart: Georg Thieme, 2005.

Husebö S, Granaas-Elminger V. Liebe und Trauer: Was wir von Kindern lernen können. Freiburg: Lambertus-Verlag, 2005.

Stemme S, von Eickstedt D. Die frühkindliche Bewegungsentwicklung; Vielfalt und Besonderheiten. Düsseldorf: Verlag selbstbestimmtes Leben, 1998.

Viebrock H, Forst B. Therapiekonzepte in der Physiotherapie. Bobath. Stuttgart: Georg Thieme, 2008.

2.10 Physiotherapy in the terminal phase

Brigitte Fiechter Lienert

This chapter addresses the basic features of physiotherapy during the terminal phase of life. A prerequisite of such therapy is the willingness of the physiotherapist to watch and listen attentively in order to comply with the needs and desires of the patient, but also those of the patient's family, during his final days or hours. Knowledge of the most common symptoms at the terminal stage, and optimal clinical reasoning, will help in deciding on the interventions to be undertaken. Questions asked by the physiotherapist such as *"Why am I here?"* and *"What can I do?"* are a pivotal element in the complex, interdisciplinary setting of the palliative care team. By observing the wishes of the patient and/or his primary carers, as well as considering the goals of palliative care as agreed with the patient and his family, the relevance, intensity and nature of the physiotherapeutic interventions to be undertaken in the patient can be determined.

2.10.1 Physiotherapy at end of life – yes or no?

Is there anything more important at the end of life than physiotherapy? Yes, of course. Yet with movement and touch – which are very specific, tangible and therefore 'vivid' experiences – physiotherapy can elicit a feeling of well-being. Whilst certain parts of the body may be disfigured and become weaker and weaker, the patient gains an unbiased, positive physical sensation from physiotherapy. The physiotherapist can reassure the patient and help to palpably reduce muscular tension, an effect which is achieved with various symptoms such as pain, anxiety, agitation or dyspnoea. But readily accepted stimuli and instructions can also be offered, which may be beneficial for instance in the event of fatigue or if there is a feeling of losing control.

An additional task for the physiotherapist is to support the patient's family, such as by explaining the physiotherapeutic interventions that are being carried out. The therapist can also suggest simple 'therapeutic' activities that will leave them feeling less helpless in such a demanding situation. Care must be taken, however, to identify whether the family wishes to get involved in such a way and also whether it is what the patient wants.

In order to ascertain the appropriate moment for respectful and empathic withdrawal, the therapist must give a thought to the prognosis, the potential survival time, the symptoms of imminent death, the needs and desires of the patient and the process of bereavement. As a rule, the patient's desire for withdrawal will be noticeable (National Consensus Project for Quality Palliative Care 2009; Marcant/Rapin 1993). If the therapist notices certain changes in the physical symptoms of the patient (e.g. restlessness, increased breathing rate or greater muscle tone as a possible expression of muscular guarding), this may be a reason for retiring from the therapeutic relationship. This should be communicated openly, and in an appropriate manner. In order not to remove all hope – despite the reality of the situation – it may be helpful for the therapist to make it clear to the patient and family at this stage that he or she remains available. Though there will be no further physiotherapy as such, regular visits to the patient will convey a great deal of respect and attention to all involved.

When does the dying phase begin?

Progression from the terminal to the dying phase is fluid and is not differentiated in all cultures and languages. The **terminal phase** can last **hours, days, weeks or even months.** For example, Twycross and Lichter (2004) use the term 'terminal phase' if death ensues within days; Saunders (1984) understands 'terminal disease' to cover a period of a few hours to weeks or even months, and Nauck (2001) defines the last 72 hours as the 'final phase' compared to the 'terminal phase' that can last weeks to months.

The affected patients become increasingly restricted in their activities despite their symptoms being managed well. Many patients with a terminal illness wish to have as much autonomy and self-rule over their lives as possible. The patient's desire for autonomy, his dignity, and acceptance of his illness and death are basic values that must be wholly respected within the context of palliative care in the terminal phase. The **dying phase/final phase** refers as a rule to the **final hours or days of life,** wherein the following signs often become apparent:

- intense need for sleep;
- reduced awareness of the outside world;
- disorientation;
- reduced intake of fluids and food;
- dwindling excretion;
- cold hands and feet;
- modified breathing pattern (rapid or with pauses);
- pale, waxy skin;
- weak pulse.

Optimal care during the dying phase is reliant on its *recognition* (Coackley/Ellershaw 2007). In diseases that progress slowly and also those in which changes can happen very rapidly, there are challenges and obstacles that complicate recognition of the dying phase.

⚠ C A U T I O N

Factors that hinder an open, realistic vision of the dying phase:
- the hope that the patient could again get better;
- continuation of interventions that have become futile;
- ambivalence between the hope of the family and reality of the palliative care team members in respect of the patient's condition;
- refusal to recognise important symptoms and signs;
- lack of communication between the family and patient;
- fear of curtailing life;
- possible cultural or spiritual barriers.

Is there any sense to physiotherapy in the terminal phase?

If care is initiated by a palliative care team early on, there may be a significant improvement in the quality of life and frame of mind of the patient, with the medical care and treatment undertaken up to the end of the patient's life being less aggressive (Temel et al 2010). The physiotherapist can offer a lot of help by basing his choice of support on the observation of objective and subjective clinical signs. On the basis of such parameters physiotherapeutic intervention may well be indicated in the terminal phase, whereby the setting should be structured deliberately, and the family included in the process as desired by the patient. The resources available to the patient should be acknowledged and put to positive use.

Due to the desire for autonomy, any individual decision on how to use the final days and hours of life must be regarded as paramount. Physiotherapy is not indicated if the patient wishes to use his remaining time in an alternative way.

⚠ C A U T I O N

Physiotherapy may under no circumstances be perceived as a burden, and the patient should be asked every time whether he would like the physiotherapy. If the non-verbal, physical expression of the patient conveys a feeling of stress, indisposition or discomfort, withdrawal from therapy is essential and should be conducted in a respectful and dignified way.

Deciding for or against physiotherapy

How does a physiotherapist decide whether caring for a patient during his final days is wise and expedient?

Actively listening at the first assessment, reflective approaches during treatment, consideration of the patient's opinion as to what best suits him at that time or how the patient's family would view the situation – all these factors are important. Clinical elements are also important to the physiotherapist. Further criteria to be considered in the decision-making process are the point at which the first diagnosis is made, the nature and course of the disease, current stage of the disease, prognosis and personal characteristics of the patient. Patient-centred goals are devised on the basis of such considerations. The decision concerning treatment and care should, whenever possible, be agreed within the care team. What the patient wants comes first and foremost, however. The therapist's own professional constraints and physical symptoms, such as anxiety, muscle tension (➤ Chapter 5) or other signs when dealing with the dying patient, must be identified and pondered.

The following considerations are given as examples, and are important to the decision-making process in physiotherapy:

- **Consider the wishes, opinions and needs of the patient:** What does he need? What would he like best? How does he wish to spend his time? What is most difficult at this time? What does the patient think of physiotherapy? Does he have any experience of physiotherapy?
- **Be aware of resilience or well-being:** Will the patient benefit from physiotherapeutic interventions? Will they alleviate the symptoms? Which interventions does the patient believe are supportive during the terminal phase?
- **Assessments/documentation of clinical signs:** Are the symptoms being relieved, or can the patient cope with them? Are the assessments appropriate and what do they reveal?
- **Apply models in the decision-making process (e. g. clinical reasoning):** What can the physiotherapist do? What should he not do?
- **Interdisciplinary discussion of prognosis and considerations in line with the Liverpool Care Pathway (LCP):** What has the team decided? What should be modified?
- **Consider an inpatient or home-care scenario:** Where and how can the physiotherapist support the care system? Whom in the relevant system can he support? Must it always be the patient?
- **Respect the intuition and experience of the physiotherapist:** To what extent can intuition be trusted? To what degree can the physiotherapist apply the empirical values from his palliative care work when making the decision?

- **Consider specific expertise:** Is the physiotherapist consciously aware of his role? Is he strong enough? How dependable is he? Are the needs of the patient, or those of the physiotherapist of major concern? (Hoskins Michel 2001)

In the complex palliative care situation these 'inter-relationships' between information, observation and clinical evaluation, as well as continuous reflection and feedback from the interventions carried out, are just as much an art as a specific scientific concept (Briggs 2011; Flannery Wainwright et al. 2010).

2.10.2 Physiotherapeutic interventions in the terminal phase

Nobody knows the exact point at which life will end. Fate and time are still unknown factors. Doctors and nurses often use the **Liverpool Care Pathway (LCP)** as a medical guideline for adapting a patient's care and treatment. The discussions held within the palliative care team are an important aspect of this. Their assessments and medical or nursing input have an influence on decision-making processes and interventions.

Moreover, the process of dying as well as the needs of the individual during the final phase of life are very varied. Some patients may die after a long period of intense nursing and a continued loss of autonomy, whereas others may retain a high level of mobility and independence right to the end. For this reason, a palliative care physiotherapist also needs to draw on a **wide range** of specific physiotherapeutic assessments and interventions for managing patients in the terminal phase.

Objectives of physiotherapy

The goal of the initial meeting between the patient and physiotherapist (depending on the setting and agreement of the patient, a relative may also be present) is, amongst others, to **learn about the patient's fears, capabilities and hopes.** This provides a good basis for therapy and also takes into account the physical and emotional needs of the patient. Potential functionality must be evaluated correctly so that the patient can live independently from day to day and remain as autonomous as possible. The primary goals of physiotherapy in the final phase of life are to improve or **optimise the quality of life.** This includes the ideal management of:

- mobility and autonomy;
- pain;
- dyspnoea and respiratory problems;

- joint mobility and muscle strength;
- anxieties and physical unrest;
- fatigue;
- lymphoedema and skin problems.

To some extent the goals are minor. First and foremost are the goals at the participatory level, since *"human dignity also means being able to hold a cup up to one's mouth"* (P. Nieland, unpublished)

Tests and assessments

Examinations can include specific questions on activities, range of symptoms and mobility, plus consideration of tumour locality and potential metastatic processes, where applicable. Standardised or functional assessments can be undertaken, if appropriate, for the purposes of identifying objective inputs concerning mobility, symptoms and quality of life as far as the terminal phase. This routine documentation of functional clinical signs and assessments is essential for evaluating the interventions. They can then be used to adapt goals and estimate any burden. It has been demonstrated that symptoms are variable and unpredictable, depending on the underlying disease and its course as well as the medication administered.

Managing specific symptoms and functional disorders

The evidence in favour of physiotherapeutic interventions has been collected from a number of studies that have demonstrated the effectiveness of individual, supervised exercise programmes for patients in the terminal phase. Improved physical constitution and even an increased life expectancy have been noted. In addition, physical and emotional performance can enhance the quality of life and have a positive effect on pain perception. Such subjective and objective effects provide encouragement in the practice of terminal phase physiotherapy (Oldervoll et al. 2006; Buss et al. 2010; Radbruch et al. 2008).

Mobility and independence

In patients with a short life expectancy, physiotherapy aims to maintain **mobility** and **independence** and facilitate a patient's **participation in life.** The implementation of goals by means of active or actively assisted interventions, focusing on strength and endurance, balance and coordination, as well as ease of movement, can be individually conceived and adapted. Depending on the patient's condition, the treadmill, bicycle ergometer, balls and other therapeutic apparatus can be used until end of life. In accordance with current exercise guidelines (➤ Chapter 2.6), a variety of such activities should be pursued over a prolonged period in order to sustain mobility and independence.

Even if there is not enough time to be able to address a clear training principle, such activities are still useful. Simpler forms of activity (strengthening the muscles in the patient's usual surroundings, walking exercises, etc.) are important and help in maintaining independence for as long as possible. Individual adjustments to aids and appliances may be necessary, and family members may need instruction.

No study could be found, however, in which **'passive mobilisation'** was found to have a positive influence or efficacy in the terminal phase. Nevertheless, such a measure is undertaken with the aim of preventing contractures if the patient is no longer able to assume an active role in therapy. It can be used in addition to positioning and facilitates personal hygiene. Often, the patient perceives the movement and associated physical awareness as very positive. Facial expressions, muscle tension or breathing rate are indicators for determining the intensity and dosage of therapy.

CASE STUDY 1

A 72-year-old male patient with metastatic prostate carcinoma is admitted to hospital for palliative, terminal phase care. He can hardly stand or speak and his breathing is laboured, yet he informs his daughter that he wishes to visit his wife again. She has been living in a care home for several years due to hemiplegia and Alzheimer's disease. He refuses the suggestion that his wife could visit him in the hospital. His desire is to appear smartly dressed at the care home and surprise his wife with a bunch of flowers.

To fulfil this desire, the entire palliative care team has quite a challenge. The nursing team consults with colleagues at the care home. The doctor adjusts the medication for the purposes of the journey, in order to reduce the pain for longer. The family organises the clothes and flowers and are instructed by the physiotherapist how best to support the patient so that he can get up from the wheelchair. The physiotherapist devises a training plan to strengthen the patient's legs and trunk, which includes methods for calming the breathing and dealing with balance and perception, enabling the patient to cope with the journey and rise from the wheelchair into a standing position. The wife is brought into a sitting position in her bed so that the family can push the wheelchair as close to the bed as possible and he needs as few steps as possible to reach the bed with the minimum of effort. He needs help from his family to stand for a few minutes. With tremendous effort, the patient succeeds in handing his wife her bouquet. He beams with delight. He passes away the next day in hospital.

Pain management

In the palliative setting, and during the terminal phase in particular, pain must be viewed within the context of **'total pain'** (total pain, ➤ Chapter 1.3). Physiotherapy can directly or indirectly alter the pain or the experience of pain. Interventions to **support mobility** lead to pain-free movements, improve active or passive motion, and thus prevent secondary problems that can arise from immobility. Depending on the stage of the disease, **cold and heat treatments, electrotherapeutic treatments** (e.g. TENS), **massages, relaxation therapy** and **lymphatic physiotherapy** can be used to alleviate pain (Jolliffe/Bury 2002; Oldervoll et al. 2006; Watson et al. 2009).

Alternative treatments are also used and recommended for reducing pain, such as acupuncture, aroma or music therapy (Pan et al. 2000; Wilkinson et al. 2007; Fellowes/Barnes/Wilkinson 2008; Takahashi 2009). During the dying phase, in the same way as the earlier phases, the use of **pain medication** is crucial to improving quality of life, thus ensuring peace and dignity at end of life.

CASE STUDY 2

Mrs S. is 35 years old and unmarried; her mother, grandmother, stepfather and his daughter are her persons of reference. Mrs S. suffers from acute leukaemia and has developed drug-induced terminal renal failure with extensive complications following a prolonged period of intensive chemotherapy. After an uncertain phase on intensive care she reflects on the time as being unstable, painful, and overlaid with a tremendous fear of dying. She was also fearful during this time of any movement, since the slightest pull on the many lines and tube would induce pain. The tube and the severe physical weakness have left her unable to express herself either verbally or non-verbally. She is helpless and distraught.

After an acute, rehabilitative period of palliative care for 12 months, the patient can initially go home to sheltered accommodation. After a further 14 months, however, her medical condition deteriorates, with exacerbated pain in the lumbar and sternal regions. As a result, Mrs S. can no longer stay at home on her own. She knows the palliative care unit from her previous stays and is highly confident of the palliative care team, including the physiotherapist. On examination, pain is evident due to the advancing renal problems plus muscular components. The general objectives of the palliative care team are to improve the pain scenario by optimising the patient's medication and maintaining her mobility, since Mrs S. wants to return home.

Assessment of the symptoms was restricted to the VAS (9/10). The physiotherapeutic goal of regulating tone was approached by means of alleviating and detonising the tense musculature, improving mobility and gently invigorating the open muscle chains in an active way. The patient's desire was to undertake therapy away from her hospital room. She most preferred to transfer to the therapy room in a wheelchair and pursue enjoyable activities with a person of reference. For example, she would throw a light ball from sitting in the wheelchair, thereby activating an upright posture, responsiveness, and mobility in the thoracic spine and shoulder joints. During such activities, she felt cheerful, distracted, and experienced a different physical sensation. She saw this as a positive side of life, laughing a lot. Such interventions could be continued, with increasing support, until the final day of her life. Mrs S. passed away suddenly in the hospital from renal failure.

Dyspnoea

During the dying phase, the breathing often develops a 'rattling' sound on inspiration and expiration, referred to as **'death rattle'.** These noisy breathing sounds are caused by the fact that patients in their final days or hours are no longer able to swallow or expectorate the secretion and saliva that has collected. The clearance reflex is reduced, primarily in the upper airways, trachea and glottis. Rattling results from the increased production of secretion and mucus due to pulmonary conditions such as infections, tumours, fluid congestion or aspiration and growing loss of the swallowing and cough reflex, but also an increase in exhaustion and impaired consciousness. To relatives, such sounds are frightening and become a lasting memory. The dying patient is probably unaware of the rattling (Albrecht 2004).

Though rattling is a common symptom in the terminal phase, there are no standardised forms of treatment. Early initiation of **pharmacological treatment** in risk patients can have a prophylactic effect (Kass/Ellershaw 2003). Careful **aspiration** from the mouth and upper airways should be undertaken only if absolutely essential. Aspiration of bronchial, deep-lying secretion must certainly not be undertaken as this will stimulate the production of mucus and can cause haemorrhagic lesions (➤ Chapter 2.3). Furthermore, aspiration is highly unpleasant and a further strain to the patient.

Short-term reduction in dyspnoea can be achieved by **physiotherapeutic interventions** such as influencing the breathing pattern or supporting the expectoration of mucus, as well as by optimal positioning (Williams 2011). Physiotherapeutic interventions that have a soothing and detonising effect are advisable (➤ Chapter 2.4).

The airways can also be cleaned and refreshed by repeated **oral hygiene** measures performed by the nursing staff, promoting well-being. Different **complementary therapies** such as aromatherapy, polarity or reflexology can likewise be used to achieve such goals (Pan et al. 2000; Wildiers/Menten 2002).

A change in **position,** if acceptable to the patient and not unreasonable, will improve respiratory function, lymphatic and venous drainage, and alleviate pain. The frequency of positional changes depends on the response of the patient and the resources available.

Fatigue

Physiotherapy can be recommended (➤ Chapter 2.6) since it can significantly relieve the intensity of fatigue during the terminal phase (Buss et al. 2010; Radbruch et al. 2008). **Active physiotherapy** is understood as activities of daily living, activities in bed, as well as mobilisation or individual, supervised exercises for enhancing levels of activity. The objective, namely to influence physical performance and quality of life, remains in place until the very final day provided the patient accepts the physical activities in such a format.

Anxiety and tension

An important goal for the entire palliative care team is to maintain quality of life in the terminal phase, right up to end of life. Experience with patients has revealed that massage (e. g. of the hands, feet, shoulders or back) during the last phase of life and dying phase is associated with positive feelings, inner strength and contentment. Awareness of a loss of autonomy and control over one's own body and its functions is perceived as dependency, anxiety and loneliness. Physical well-being and mental relaxation, achievable with massage, allay the feelings of anxiety which, for their part, can influence pain and relaxation (Corbin 2005) (➤ Chapter 2.7). Physiotherapeutic interventions can also detract from anxiety. If a member of the family is prepared to give a patient a simple massage, then the relaxation and satisfaction that result are a reciprocal benefit to both the family and patient (Osaka et al. 2009; Downey et al. 2009). In such a fragile situation, massage can effect a peaceful atmosphere and provide for periods of inner calm, as well as an atmosphere of attentiveness and respect (Seiger Cronfalk et al. 2009).

Complementary interventions

Interventions from the realms of complementary or alternative medicine, which in part are also employed by physiotherapists, are also valuable options in the terminal phase. Statements can only be made here about acupuncture and aromatherapy.

The impact of **acupuncture** on symptoms such as dyspnoea, fatigue, pain and nausea is mostly described as moderate to significant (Pan et al. 2000; Takahashi

2

2009). The benefits of acupuncture can influence various symptoms without having any side effects. Though patient response can be very varied, there is usually an improvement in activity and mobility as well as increase in energy, which all have a positive effect on quality of life.

Aromatherapy has a positive, short-term effect on mental well-being and therefore can also be used in the terminal or dying phase. The potential beneficial incorporation of other palliative therapies should be contemplated in order to arrive at optimal care and therapy which is tailored to the patient (Tilden/Drach/Tolle 2004; Fellowes/Barnes/Wilkinson 2008; Wilkinson et al. 2007).

Caring for the patient in the last hours or days of life
John Ellershaw, Tamsin McGlinchey

The way we care for dying patients is a reflection of the society we live in (Ellershaw/Wilkinson 2011). A good death has the potential to create positive lasting memory with the people who are left behind. **We only have one (!) opportunity to get care right at this time,** and the Liverpool Care Pathway (LCP) for the dying patient offers one way of improving the way we care for all patients in the last hours or days of life, regardless of diagnosis or place of care. The LCP supports clinical teams in the provision of best quality care at the bedside.

Potential role of the physiotherapist in care in the last hours or days of life

The diagnosis of an expected death and subsequent care delivery may be significantly enhanced by the continued engagement of the physiotherapist with particular emphasis on non-pharmacological aspects of symptom control and advice, which may indeed become more important aspects of care at this time (Booth et al. 2011; Marcant/Rapin 1993; Santiago-Palma/Payne 2001). Additionally, there may be a role for the physiotherapist in empowering the relatives and carers, at the bedside, to be able to deliver care to the patient; for example, how to touch and assist patient movement themselves. Throughout this stage, physiotherapists are frequently involved in offering direct care, advice and support to patients, relatives and carers. As such, physiotherapists constitute a significant part of the MDT – along with doctors, nurses and other allied healthcare professionals – and their views and/or concerns are invaluable.

The Liverpool Care Pathway for the dying patient

The LCP is an example of a best practice model of care, designed to support all healthcare professionals to look after a patient when the MDT has diagnosed dying and believe the patient is now in the last hours or days of life. The LCP is an integrated care pathway (ICP; Vanhaecht et al. 2007) that promotes good record keeping, and provides measurable outcomes of care (Department of Health 2008, 2009; Ellershaw/Ward 2003; Ellershaw et al. 2001). It is a multiprofessional document that provides an evidence-based, best practice model of care, designed to transfer the hospice model of care into generic healthcare settings. The LCP is designed to improve the care provided to dying patients, and it supports the MDT (including physiotherapists) in delivering that care, through joint working and decision making. **Diagnosing dying is a complex process irrespective of previous diagnosis or history, and no one healthcare professional should make this decision in isolation.** There is an algorithm within the LCP, which is designed to support the MDT in formalizing its decision making process regarding diagnosing dying. The algorithm prompts the review and assessment of the patient, and calls for consensus from all healthcare professionals that the patient is imminently dying. **Potential reversible causes for the current condition should be discussed and considered at this time, along with the need for specialist palliative care advice and/or second opinion.** Any decision should be deemed appropriate, discussed with the patient where possible, and always with the relatives or carers. Changes in care at this complex, uncertain time are made in the best interest of the patient and relatives or carers; however, this requires regular review by the MDT.

The LCP, with its goals and supportive prompts designed to promote the close working of all members of the MDT responsible for the care of the patient, incorporates 3 key sections:

• Section 1: The initial assessment: This section emphasizes a holistic approach to patient care, focusing on comfort measures in terms of symptom control, psychosocial and spiritual/religious issues, and good communication with the patients wherever possible, as well as with relatives or carers and other healthcare professionals.

- Section 2: The ongoing assessment: This section documents the patient's ongoing condition and level of physical and emotional comfort, along with the wellbeing of the relatives and carers, as assessed by healthcare professionals. These assessments are promoted at a minimum of 4 hourly intervals in an in-patient unit (each visit in community settings), and prompts the re assessment of the patient and review of the plan of care by the MDT at least every 3 days.
- Section 3: The care after death: This section documents the care and procedures to be followed immediately after the death of a patient, including following appropriate procedures for the care of the patient's body to be treated with dignity and respect, giving information and support to bereaved relatives or carers, and sharing information with appropriate healthcare professionals.

It is imperative that the **use of the LCP is supported by a robust education and training programme,** which includes all members of the MDT, and reflection and learning to drive up the care quality of the dying into the future. The perspective of the physiotherapist is intrinsic to this process.

Although the goals of physiotherapy and palliative care appear to complement each other – in that they aim to optimize quality of life through an holistic approach – it has been suggested that there is a lack of 'interface' between physiotherapy and palliative care (Eva/Wee 2010). This was felt to be possibly attributed to perceptions of physiotherapy as primarily involved actively in promoting function and independence, and palliative care as primarily focusing on managing deterioration and the dying process. **In the care of patients in the last hours or days of life, the LCP may provide one way to improve this interface.** The LCP algorithm serves to bring together all health professionals involved in the patient's care, including physiotherapists where appropriate, to ascertain what is now in the patient's best interest. Physiotherapy expertise can provide valuable input into discussions that take place at this time, which may serve to facilitate improved collaborative working between palliative care and physiotherapy in the longer term.

2.10.3 Conclusion

Brigitte Fiechter Lienert

Physiotherapeutic interventions in the terminal phase of life can have subjective and objective effects on the symptoms and functional limitations that develop during the given period. These effects should embolden the physiotherapist to tackle the different stages of a disease in a variety of ways. The physiotherapist's own fears, helplessness and powerlessness mean that his therapeutic work is highly demanding. Hence it is important for the physiotherapist to be adequately prepared and to confront the subject of death and the palliative care situation, as well as discuss such matters with experienced members of the palliative care team. For personal wellbeing, it is necessary to look at the subject of mortality, trust and the ability to identify one's own limitations. **Respect for life is essential and enables, or prompts, the necessary withdrawal at the appropriate time.** Heroic behaviour is not expected – either by patients, their family, or by therapists and professional colleagues. The ability to respect and reveal one's own feelings at a suitable moment is also important, therefore. It is crucial to reflect on one's own actions and respect one's own role and its constraints.

Aside from acting professionally, the physiotherapist should also trust his own intuition and keep it consciously in check, especially in the case of a long-standing relationship between patient and therapist. Hence, intuition combined with wide-ranging expertise can achieve what is physiotherapeutically and personally appropriate.

2.10.4 Reflective questions

- Have you ever sensed that you were not sure whether to stop or continue with physiotherapy?
- How would you deal with such a situation today?
- How would you describe your role as physiotherapist to patients in the terminal phase of life?
- What experience do you have of assessments in the terminal phase? Did they influence the interdisciplinary teamwork?

REFERENCES

Albrecht E. Symptome in der Sterbephase. In: Bausewein C, Roller S, Voltz R (eds). Leitfaden Palliativmedizin. 2nd ed. München–Jena: Elsevier Urban&Fischer, 2004.

Booth S, Moffat C, Burkin J, Galbraith S, Bausewein C. Non-pharmacological interventions for breathlessness. Curr Opin Support Palliat Care 2011;5:77–86.

Briggs RW. Clinical decision making for physical therapists in patient-centered end-of-life care. Topics Geriatr Rehab 2011;27(1):10–17.

Buss T, de Walden-Galuszko K, Modlinska A, Osowicka M, Lichodziejewska M, Janiszewska J. Kinesitherapy alleviates fatigues in terminal hospice cancer patients – an experimental, controlled study. Support Care Cancer 2010;18:743–749.

Coackley A, Ellershaw J. The terminal phase. Medicine 2007;36(2):105–108.

Corbin L. Safety and efficacy of massage therapy for patients with cancer. Cancer Control 2005;12(3):158–164.

Department of Health. End of Life Care Strategy: Promoting high quality care for all adults at the end of life. London: Department of Health, 2008.

Department of Health. End of Life Care Strategy: Quality markers and measures for end of life care. London: Department of Health, 2009.

Downey L, Diehr P, Standish LJ, et al. Might massage or guided meditation provide „means to a better end"? Primary outcomes from an efficacy trial with patients at the end of life. J Palliat Care 2009;25(2):100–108.

Ellershaw JE, Smith C, Overill S, Walker SE, Aldridge J. Care of the dying: setting standards for symptom control in the last 48 hours of life. J Pain Symptom Manage 2001;21:12–17.

Ellershaw JE, Ward C. Care of the dying patient: the last hours or days of life. Br Med J 2003; 326:30–34.

Ellershaw J, Wilkinson S. Care of the Dying: A Pathway to Excellence. 2nd ed. Oxford: Oxford University Press, 2011.

Eva G, Wee B. Rehabilitation in end of life management. Curr Opin Support Palliat Care 2010; 4:158–162.

Fellowes D, Barnes K, Wilkinson S. Aromatherapy and massage for symptom relief in patients with cancer (review). The Cochrane Collaboration 2008;3.

Flannery Wainwright S, Shepard KF, Harman LB, Stephens J. Novice and experienced physical therapist clinicians: a comparison of how reflection is used to inform the clinical decision-making process. Phys Ther 2010;90:75–88.

Hoskins Michel T. Editorial – Do physiotherapists have a role in palliative care? Physiotherapy Res Int 2001;6(1):iii–iv.

Jolliffe J, Bury T. The effectiveness of physiotherapy in the palliative care of older people: evidence briefing. London: The Chartered Society of Physiotherapy; 2002. www.csp.org.uk.

Kass RM, Ellershaw J. Respiratory tract secretions in the dying patient: a retrospective study. 2003;26(4):897–902.

Marcant D, Rapin CH. Role of the physiotherapist in palliative care. J Pain Symptom Manage 1993;8(2): 68–71.

Nauck F. Symptomkontrolle in der Finalphase. Schmerz 2001;5(15):392–399.

National Consensus Project for Quality Palliative Care. Clinical practice guidelines for quality palliative care. 2nd ed. Pittsburgh: National Consensus Project for Quality Palliative Care

2009. Available at www.nationalconsensusproject.org/Guideline.pdf (last accessed: August 2012).

Oldervoll LM, Loge JH, Paltiel H, et al. The effect of a physical exercise program in palliative care: a phase II study. J Pain Symptom Manage 2006; 31:421–430.

Osaka I, Kurihara Y, Tanaka K, Nishizaki H, Aoki S, Adachi I. Endocrinological evaluations of brief hand massages in palliative care. J Alternat Complement Med 2009;15(9):981–985.

Pan CX, Morrison RS, Ness J, Fugh-Berman A, Leipzig RM. Complementary and alternative medicine in the management of pain, dyspnea and nausea and vomiting near the end of life: a systematic review. J Pain Symptom Manage 2000; 20(5):374–387.

Radbruch L, Strasser F, Elsner F, et al. Fatigue in palliative care patients – an EAPC approach. Palliat Med 2008; 22(1):13–32.

Santiago-Palma J, Payne R. Palliative care and rehabilitation. Cancer 2001;92:1,049–1,052.

Saunders C (ed.). The Management of Terminal Malignant Disease. London: Edward Arnold Publishers, 1984

Seiger Cronfalk B, Strang P, Ternestedt BM, Friedrichsen M. The existential experiences of receiving soft tissue massage in palliative home care – an intervention. Support Care Cancer 2009; 17:1,203–1,211.

Takahashi H. Effects of acupuncture on terminal cancer patients in the home care setting. Medical Acupuncture 2009;21(2):123–129.

Temel JS, Greer JA, Muzikansky A, et al. Early palliative care for patients with metastatic non-small-cell lung cancer. N Engl J Med 2010; 363(8):733–742.

Tilden VP, Drach LL, Tolle SW. Complementary and alternative therapy use at end-of-life in community settings. J Alternat Complement Med 2004;10(5):811–817.

Twycross R, Lichter I. In: Oxford Textbook of Palliative Medicine. 3rd ed. New York: Oxford University Press, 2004: pp. 520–551.

Vanhaecht K, De Witte K, Sermeus W. The impact of clinical pathways on the organisation of care processes. Leuven: ACCO, 2007.

Watson M, Lucas C, Hoy A, Wells J. Oxford Handbook of Palliative Care. 2nd ed. Oxford University Press, 2009: pp. 771–773.

Wildiers H, Menten J. Death rattle: prevalence, prevention and treatment. J Pain Symptom Manage 2002; 23(4):310–317.

Wilkinson SM, Love SB, Westcombe AM, et al. Effectiveness of aromatherapy massage in the management of anxiety and depression in patients with cancer: a multicenter randomized controlled trial. J Clin Oncol 2007; 25(5):532–539.

Williams M. Applicability and generalizability of palliative interventions for dyspnoea: one size fits all, some or none? Curr Opin Support Palliat Care 2011;5:92–100.

Psycho-social aspects

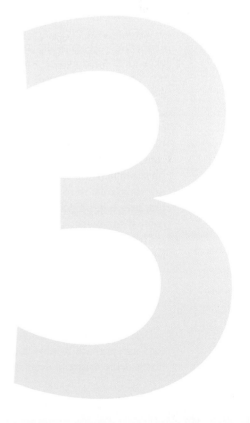

3.1 Communication in palliative care: an introduction

Michael-M. Lippka

The verbalisation of death

The human relationship with death and departure is greatly divided. Human beings are deeply ambivalent around matters of death and dying. This fact is reflected in particular in the language we use. Hence someone has "left us" instead of died and has been "relieved" – usually of "prolonged, but courageously endured suffering" – or even, less formally, has "kicked the bucket". Industrial society views death with a mixture of fascination and horror. Such ambivalence is hardly new: our ancestors would assign words and images to the limitations of physical existence in order to make them more easily digestible. Whether in the context of the Greek God Hades or the Celtic Otherworld – since ancient times, efforts have been made to convey ideas of the afterlife such that they could be meaningfully integrated into both society and religion. Historically we have tales of death gods, and today use characters such as the Grim Reaper as the personification of death.

Personifications and allegories have not only been used to banish man's fear of his own demise, but also as political mechanisms and propaganda. For example, in a number of warrior cultures concepts of a heroic death are commonplace, entailing amongst others the exuberant, otherworldly indemnification for efforts expended. Such a trick was doubly ingenious: firstly the linguistic creation of an otherwordly reality and secondly its vivid representation through religion, mysticism and culture. This has enabled societies to escape – mentally at least – their fear of the ravages of time. Evidently, the idea of the Grim Reaper is easier to cope with than the natural ageing process. Aside from such euphemistic intentions, economic, social or ethical standards were also strengthened and put into practice, e. g. by demonstrating particular bravery in combat situations.

The idea behind this, that is to develop **a truly or allegedly practical concept of the world and to invite the opposite to 'enter into it',** today still remains part of the repertoire of the systemic counsellor. What is actually deemed practical here, however, naturally lies in the eyes of the beholder.

Despite the easily identifiable, seductive nature of such an approach it must in fairness be acknowledged that it is the nature of death itself that encourages such beliefs. Death is beyond reach when we are living. There is no certainty as to what it is like to die on account of the lack of living experts. Man remains reduced to the role of spectator until he himself dies. Such a lack of knowledge comes into play when talking about death, yet one of the purposes of communication is to convey information about that which, in this case, we have no personal experience. Of course this also applies to other subjects such as religion or politics. An important distinction in the case of death, however, is its all-encompassing nature. It affects every living being. An individual may choose to ignore religion or politics, but we all have to die. For centuries man has attempted to compensate for the ambivalence of death by grappling with the subject of mortality in art, culture and customs. Memento mori and images of heaven and hell were popular for a very long time.

That this is no longer the case today is due to the taboo with which the new meritocracy views death. Dead cows don't provide milk; the dying can't go to work, leaving behind a family that is not provided for, with care and disposal causing expense and inconvenience. The superficial inefficiency of dying could also play a part in this system of suppression. Professionalisation in medical care must have a much greater impact. In modern industrial nations, people mainly die in hospitals or homes, and stringent hygiene laws provide for the professional management of dead bodies. Death is thus removed from the focus of society, becoming virtually invisible, odourless and in the figurative sense imperceptible. Death concerns only those who are immediately affected by it, either professionally or privately. Society and religion no longer have generic, ready-made answers; each individual must decide for himself what death fundamentally means.

✓ GUIDANCE

Goal of communication in the palliative care setting

Individuals working professionally with those who are dying and their families are faced with a challenge when confronted by death, having to cope without any guidelines or answers to questions that patients justifiably have concerning their own death. The solution is not to provide the person concerned with answers to their questions regarding the meaning of life and death, but rather to support them in their own search and help them when they need help, and to accept the fact that not everybody finds the answers they are looking for.

Palliative care, as a concept, places the individual quality of life of patients and their families at the centre of every professional action. In such an approach, communication is key: helpful, professional and responsive communication can help to ascertain how the individual concerned defines quality of life and which symptoms are causing the most discomfort in the present situation. In turn this implies that the professional carer must delve into the world of the patient in order to get to know their individual system of values, beliefs, fears and hopes. In doing so, good communication skills are also required: in addition to a professional rapport, the carer/companion can, linguistically speaking, create a space in which the exchange can take place while respecting each other's limits, and thereby establish a protected environment in which the caring relationship can develop.

This communication architecture is based on the considerations briefly addressed below. The concept, namely **systemic communication,** is one of many ways for turning the journey to the limits of human existence into a practical and professional venture.

Systemic communication for beginners

The complex nature of the subject and the taboo surrounding it renders any talk of death very difficult. Hence it is appropriate to gain a broad understanding of the term 'communication'. Communication generally implies anything that can involve an exchange between living beings (Satir 2000). This broad definition allows the purely verbal dimensions (which when working with dying patients are limited) to be expanded in order to draw from the entire repertoire of non-verbal and verbal techniques. Consequently, **body language, facial expressions, gestures** and **touch** can be used as messages, particularly if words are lacking or inadequate.

A systemic understanding of communication is needed in order to increase one's flexibility. Accordingly, dialogue entails the interplay of different elements in a communicative situation. As different machines in a factory work together to produce a particular end product, so the individual elements of a communicative situation work reciprocally and thus permit dialogue to develop. Humans are not machines, of course, and therefore they can neither be programmed nor their behaviour predicted with certainty (Foerster 1998). This situation is of particular importance to professional communication skills: humans respond differently to their surroundings, therefore **any communicative intervention can only be undertaken along the lines of 'trial-and-error', i. e. trying and evaluating.** Hence no philosopher's stone can be found at the heart of professional communication theory and practice – no one model fits all. It is much more a matter of trying, reflecting, evaluating and trying again.

What appears to be painstaking to start with can prove to be a creative, even lively approach. Instead of learning one particular technique or model and then applying it again and again in different situations, new techniques must always be introduced, and individual as well as flexible solutions found. This lack of a right or wrong approach is also reflected in the systemic concept of reality.

Language and imagery – both of which can be learned and forgotten – create reality, a concept that is always individual. In plain language this means that man is constantly confronted with sensory impressions and information. Education, socialisation, experience and similar factors assist him in learning to attribute different levels of importance to such encounters. Over time, therefore, he develops his own concept of the world and how things are related. Such a concept can be described as a '**reality construction**'. It is important in enabling humans to move securely within their own environment and cope in an appropriate way (Neimeyer 2001).

CASE STUDY

Any reality construction depends of course on individual experience and knowledge. A brief example:

- **Mr A.** has been overweight since childhood. More than 30 years ago he took over his parents' snack bar and has managed it successfully ever since. Both his mother and father died at a relatively young age from cardiovascular diseases. Though Mr A. does not yet have any major health problems, he has a fear of heart disease and associated disorders because he believes he is genetically predisposed. Mr A. does not relate the eating habits of his family to the death of his parents. In his world, hearty meals stand for prosperity and happiness.

- **Mr B.,** meanwhile, was born into a vegetarian family. He finds meat eating abhorrent and always looks for organic quality labels when shopping. He is physically very active and never drinks alcohol, smokes or takes drugs. When a routine examination finds Mr B. has a malignant tumour in his lung, he feels deceived by fate.

If in such a situation a supposed truth that guaranteed security and orientation in one's own life is suddenly dissolved, this naturally engenders insecurity and emotional distress. The latter is at times communicated in statements such as *'I've lost all sense of the world'* or *'I don't know anything anymore'* and in evolutionary terms is more than justified: when it came to survival it was important to be well informed, to know that the lion, rather than the gazelle, poses the threat.

Aside from very survival, the **individual self-image** of man is also based on his concept of reality. This encompasses his entire biography and primarily determines the significance he attributes to various life events. Even in his own history, man attempts to create meaningful contexts. He therefore writes his entire life, so to speak, into his biography since only in such a way can he explain to himself and to others who he is, where he comes from and where he is going.

Whether tragedy or adventure – only a **subjective assessment** will lend importance to life-changing events. And such an assessment is expressed in **individual vocabulary.** In other words, whether a witch in the fairytale of one's own life is a justifiably punished child eater or a strange, persecuted old lady in a gingerbread house – this is decided by each individual alone. The terms 'witch' and 'strange old lady' say less about the person being described than about the narrator himself. His choice of words says more about his own opinions, values and attitudes. Only by listening can his counterpart gain an idea of what reality construction lies behind his actions. Above all, the language used by the narrator can create an entire new world in the mind of the listener. 'Witch', 'old lady', 'romance' or 'tragedy' – each of these words can trigger a number of individual images in the head of the listener. So language influences not only one's own concept of reality, but can also alter the ideas of those around us.

> ⚠ **CAUTION**
>
> **Four basic principles of communication and perception**
>
> 1. Communication arises from the interplay of all elements of an underlying communicative situation.
> 2. Living systems are not machines and therefore can only be influenced by the trial-and-error approach.
> 3. Each individual has his own reality construction that determines how he perceives himself and his environment.
> 4. This reality construction is created as well as modified by imagery and language.

These principles form the theoretical basis for practical implementation of systemic communication, as described in the next section.

Communication architecture: how to develop efficient dialogue?

Every professional action undertaken with a view to palliative physiotherapy, as in all related disciplines, is primarily devoted – as already mentioned – to optimising the quality of life of a patient. In very simplified terms this means that the patient should feel he is receiving proper care and support. Aside from any actual physiotherapeutic intervention, skilled and efficient dialogue can be a tremendous help in improving a patient's well-being. The outcome or impact of such communication can never be predicted with certainty, of course, but careful planning can make a difference. The concept is similar to building a house: an architect is not able to guarantee that his clients will experience endless hours of joy in the house he has designed for them, but he can ensure that they will be living in a space where they feel comfortable and which also meets the contracted requirements. In conversations with a patient, the role of the 'architect' is assumed by the professional carer – in this case the physiotherapist. Armed with good communication skills and the task of optimising the patient's well-being, he can structure the conversation in the same way as an architect designs a building.

Communication architecture

The structure of communication generally has no boundaries. Through language, small and claustrophobic conversational cells as well as wide, open corridors full of windows can be created. Such architectural concepts are used by humans on an everyday basis – without giving them much thought. The choice of words, tone of voice, selection of topic and body language can usually be very helpful in creating a conversational setting that is deemed appropriate or beneficial. All of this takes place automatically in most social scenarios. Hardly anyone really considers how they have to behave in a supermarket.

In contrast, deliberate planning and reflection must, can and should be considered in relation to professional communication. By imagining a communicative scenario to be a room, the following elements can be incorporated:

Doors　All professional dialogue requires a good entrance and a clear exit. A good start to the conversation is an ice breaker: relaxed words which, when combined with a greeting, help to melt the ice between the protagonists. Ideally, a smile can be drawn from the face of the person being addressed with statements such as, *'Before we start, let me just look at your flowers …'* or *'Ooh, you have an aroma lamp. I wondered where that lovely smell was coming from …'* – or simply, *'It's so nice to meet you.'* It is also helpful to take the time at the first meeting to provide an explanation of the roles and the assignment, as well as a careful description of physiotherapy in general. This helps to banish any insecurities or anxiety on the part of the patient. Over the further course of therapy, welcoming rituals, standardised greetings or initial physical contact, where appropriate, also prove helpful. They enhance the recognition effect, engender familiarity and signal in a tangible way that physiotherapy is about to begin. A ritual or standard procedure at the end of a therapy session will also provide for structure and clarity. In all events, reference to the next therapy session is wise in order to impart the sense of continuity and counteract feelings of being left alone again.

Floor   All professional dialogue should be built on solid ground. A patient receiving palliative care has every right to expect sound expertise and good communication skills from his professional caregiver. Despite the conventional technique of trial and error in systemic communication, the impression should not be given that the patient is being used as a communication guinea pig. When dealing with the patient directly, all actions should be undertaken with confidence and purpose. This set of skills, as the foundation for any form of professional dialogue, also includes the therapeutic approach. Particularly when working with the terminally ill, whose physical and cognitive abilities often dwindle at a rapid pace, a **resource-based approach** is advantageous. By focusing on what the patient can still do and not what he can no longer do, his motivation to continue with therapy will be strengthened and therapy itself will more likely succeed. Moreover, the systematic use of resources compensates for the natural orientation of the entire health system towards deficits and will have a positive effect on the psychological rapport between patient and physiotherapist. Resource orientation, with respect to one's own attitude, means nothing other than **switching from a mine-sweeping to a treasure-seeking mentality.** The mine-sweeping therapist runs the immediate risk of reducing the patient to a victim and thereby causing frustration. The treasure seeker, on the other hand, can find a hero in the patient who is ready to fight against adverse destiny. He may be impressed by bravery or dexterity, or simply by the relaxed nature with which his hero confronts imminent danger. If the physiotherapist succeeds in becoming a treasure seeker, respect and a belief in the patient come entirely of their own volition.

Walls   Professional dialogue requires form and structure. Walls can provide protection from outside influences, but also form a barrier to the outside world. They create a solid architectural framework in terms of communication, one that stipulates where the conversation takes place, the role each person plays within it, and the timing involved. The more clearly such aspects are defined, the more confident the protagonists will feel in their exchange. The appropriate division of tasks is crucial when erecting these walls. It is usually beneficial for the patient to introduce the topics whilst the physiotherapist is responsible for determining the location and time.

Walls are also symbolic of the limits of responsibility. If the physiotherapist realises that a subject raised by the patient would be better discussed with another member of the multiprofessional team (e.g. a psychologist or spiritual counsellor), he should also be able to broach this matter with the patient. In doing so, the therapist is not only protecting himself but also the patient by offering him truly professional support. If there is no team in the background, it is still important for limits to be set and alternative, professional advisors to be nominated.

Windows   Windows symbolise external factors that play a part in the dialogue and can have an influence on its direction. Being aware of such factors is beneficial to communication architecture. What disruptions can be expected during therapy? Has the telephone been muted? Are family members present or absent during therapy (and is this disruptive, or possibly valuable to further progress)? What is the spatial setting in terms of external influences? These and other similar aspects should be carefully considered and modified, if necessary. **Windows also offer a perspective.** Such perspectives, for example a happy event or the inner energy of the patient (such as his family or a hobby), can be used to provide motivation, suggest a break from conversation or simply introduce a new topic. In certain situations it can even be useful to close the windows, deliberately blocking certain outside influences or omitting certain subjects. The more information the physiotherapist has on a patient, the easier it is for him to identify those perspectives that have a positive effect on well-being and therapeutic progress, and those that are possibly a hindrance.

Ceiling   The ceiling represents the models, techniques and methods along which the physiotherapist navigates his dialogue. The systemic model presented in this article is not the only means of course with which to successfully structure professional dialogue. It does provide a good basis, however, for working in the palliative care setting.

Active listening

The most important method in the approach to professional dialogue is active listening. Theoretically, many professional carers know precisely what active listening is, but seldom actually put it into practice. This could be because active listening is actually very strenuous and requires utmost concentration. It was originally used in psychotherapy and psychosocial counselling but due to its enormous potential has become very well established in a wide variety of fields.

The objective of active listening is to learn more about one's counterpart at the same time as demonstrating respect and understanding. Active listening is therefore the foundation upon which a rapport can be established between the therapist and patient. With active listening, the patient is consciously given a certain amount of time in which to talk about a topic of his own choosing, whilst the role of the physiotherapist is restricted to listening. Such listening is active, for while the patient is talking the physiotherapist has a number of tasks to fulfil. To start with, he should **support the fluency of the patient's narrative** while making note of the content. He can do this on a non-verbal level by creating a comfortable environment (such as appropriate physical closeness or distance between the narrator and listener), using positive body language and nodding the head in support. During breaks in the dialogue, he can respond verbally by **paraphrasing,** i.e. repeating the content of what he has heard in his own words, and **questioning** in order to be sure that what has been said has also been understood. In such a way, the therapist can obtain valuable information on reality construction as well as the patient's biography, goals and desires that can be considered in the care and therapy to follow. He can also display **genuine interest, respect and appreciation,** all of which can positively influence the relationship and the well-being of the patient. He can do this by allowing the narrator to finish talking and then **summarising** everything once the process of active listening is over, thereby signalling that he has really been listening and has also understood. Should the conversation falter, say because the patient's voice begins to fail, the active listener can **verbalise the situation** with a statement such as, '*I can hear you struggling with your voice …*', and continue with the narration. This should not be done too often, however. **Active silence** can also be expedient. Finally, the physiotherapist should avoid the temptation to lead the conversation in a certain direction. One's own interpretations and stories have no place in the concept of active listening. The patient is the focus, and only he may judge and analyse. Active listening is an indispensable element if wanting to be true to the palliative care ideal.

Circular questioning

In the supreme discipline of professional communication, there is one particular **type of questioning above all that can be used to optimise the well-being** of a patient. This is referred to as 'circular' questioning, since the questions are not aimed at a specific answer but rather at the thought process in the consciousness of the person questioned. Circular questions are particularly beneficial when working with severely debilitated patients who due to a high level of distress often experience thinking blocks, i.e. intransigent, negative patterns of thought, that can be unlocked by such a strategy. The idea behind this concept is that the more complex the thought process triggered by a question, the greater the likelihood of eliciting **fresh perspectives or solutions to problems.** For example, the question '*And how would I notice – let's say if I bump into you tomorrow in the corridor – that the pain in your lower abdomen has improved?*', prompts myriad changes in perspective. The formulation 'How would I recognise …' requires the person to look at himself from the outside, whilst 'if I were to bump into you tomorrow' invites him to consider a new perspective in terms of time. By adding '… that the pain in your lower abdomen has improved', the concentration is shifted slightly from the problem towards a solution. The possibilities for asking circular questions are unlimited: '*If I were not now speaking with you but with your children, how would they describe your situation to me and what would they say if I were to ask them how best to deal with you?*' or: '*What would your wife say if you asked her whether the physiotherapy is doing you any good?*'. Circular questions are a matter of practice. The worst that can happen is that you perhaps bewilder the patient. Such questions should be asked sparingly, therefore, so as not to burden the patient and to leave sufficient room for the thought processes to be provoked.

The miracle question

Another very versatile questioning technique is the miracle question. Such questioning is also suitable for giving highly stressed patients a break from intransigent, negative thought patterns. The miracle question invites patients to **mentally escape the prevailing, onerous situation:** '*Imagine that I'm not a physiotherapist but a good fairy, and I could magically enable you to walk again for one hour – where would you go to in that hour?*', or, much simpler: '*If you won the lottery, what would you do with the money?*' The miracle question can be changed in a multitude of ways. The crucial part of this technique is to focus on the desires, hopes and dreams of the patient. Through this type of questioning, the patient can mentally immerse himself in such desires and dreams without building up any false promises or unrealistic hopes: the fairytale nature of the wording (e.g. 'Imagine a fairy …') signals to all involved that we are now in the realms of fantasy. And like any other person, a dying patient is also entitled to dream a little.

Externalisation

In this last technique, **the especially cumbersome elements of life are separated linguistically from the person affected.** In practice it may look like this: instead of asking *'And since when have you not had the confidence to stand up on your own?'*, the physiotherapist asks, *'And since when has this fear been stopping you from standing up on your own?'*, thereby externalising the patient's fear. The difference only appears minimal at first glance. In the first question, we find an anxious patient without the confidence to get up without help. In the second question we have a patient who wants to stand up, but is being hindered – by fear. Shifting the problem outwards or detaching it from the affected individual makes it clear that beyond the deficit there is a normal person: there is life. By doing this, we are not only counteracting the potential loss of self-esteem in the patient, but also putting the problem into perspective. No human consists solely of pain and suffering, or only 'cancer', and no human relationship consists merely of conflict: *'So let's both take a look and see if we can sort this pain out …'*, or, *'And how long has this domestic quarrel been bothering you and your wife?'* – again, the possibilities are almost endless.

The four techniques described are perfectly suitable for entering into systemic dialogue, as they are easy to learn and harmless in their implementation. The practical incorporation of such elements into the communicative space necessitates careful conversational planning prior to therapy, and permanent reflection, including the necessary adjustments after each therapy session. If practised regularly, a certain routine will be established that will transform the dialogue with the patient and family from a mine field into a gold mine.

The last word: silence is golden, speech is silver

Physiotherapists should remain physiotherapists – also when working with palliative care patients. The dividing lines with other caring professions such as psychotherapy or spiritual care must be respected, both by the patient and physiotherapist alike. Nevertheless, professional communication skills and a solid knowledge of communication theory are the tools of the trade of every individual working with the terminally ill and their families. As already mentioned, it is not a case of saying or doing the right thing in every situation. It is more important to listen closely and attentively and only then respond, professionally, in the most helpful way possible. All the given models and techniques can be easily attempted

without a lot of practical training. An exception to this rule is active listening. Nobody becomes a good listener overnight – it requires far too much practice, with 100 % concentration every time. But it does pay off: by listening to a dying patient properly, the physiotherapist not only establishes what the patient needs but also learns a great deal about himself.

Communication illustrated: managing resistance, aggression and violence

The terminally ill and their families generally find themselves in an exceptional situation. The future is uncertain; the suffering and anxiety are often overwhelming. Aggressive behaviour and the search for a putative scapegoat, as a coping strategy, can provide short-term relief. Pent-up frustration is unloaded, by people either harming themselves or taking it out on others. Hence professional carers may be faced with resistance and aggressive behaviour which they have neither provoked nor knowingly caused. In such cases it helps to imagine that the displayed aggression is the basic approach to solving a problem by an overwhelmed, highly stressed individual. Such an approach relieves the professional carer of the inner compulsion of having to justify himself. Thus a decision can be made on a professional, reflective level as to whether to enter into the conflict or work with the resistance. If a situation involving conflict is viewed like a pair of scales that have become imbalanced, then behaviour, statements and changes can be positioned in this scenario like small weights that either maintain the imbalance (and in the figurative sense the conflict) or restore the equilibrium. In practice, it could look something like the case study reported below.

CASE STUDY

The son of a patient in the terminal phase of his life makes forceful complaints about the progress of his father's physiotherapy to date and threatens to lodge a complaint to the hospital management. The therapist, surprised at the accusations, attempts to defend himself – and so the argument takes its inevitable course.

Alternatively, the physiotherapist could react as follows:

Son: *'Again we've been waiting for ten minutes – for absolutely nothing! All these exercises are doing no good at all, my father's getting worse and worse. And anyway, this is the second time you've left us waiting here … it's all so totally unprofessional here! I'm going to complain to the consultant.'*

Therapist (to patient): *'Hello Mr K., how are you? And your son has come to visit …'*

The physiotherapist also offers the son his hand, which is ignored.

Therapist: *'You appear to be very angry …'*

3

Son: *'You can certainly say that. It's hardly surprising with the treatment here. It's an absolute disgrace!'*
Therapist: *'May I ask what's now making you so angry? If you haven't been satisfied with your father's therapy until now, then …'*
Son (getting louder): *'No you may not … I'm going to make a complaint about you!'*
Therapist: *'Of course you can do that, it's perfectly within your rights. We place a lot of importance here on dealing with complaints professionally. If you would like, you can make the call from my phone right now. I can also give you one of our patient satisfaction surveys, then you can hand in your complaint in writing straight away.'*
Son (somewhat undecided): *'Well – I don't know …'*
Therapist: *'Well I'll print the form out for you once the therapy is over, then you can think about it in your own time. But maybe we can talk some of the things through between us. Now, I'd like to spend some time with your father. As you said at the start, he's feeling much worse …'*
Son: *'You can see that: he can hardly talk any more, is no longer eating and is sleeping almost all the time – and he's having a harder time catching his breath …'*
Therapist: *'And you're very worried about it … well let's see …'*
Therapist (to patient, turning to him and touching him gently): *'Mr K., it's me, Mr P. I've come to give you your physiotherapy. Your son just told me he's very worried about you … how is your breathing then?'*
The patient just shakes his head weakly.
Therapist: *'OK, so we'll try to relieve your breathing a little today – and as you have your son here for support, nothing can really go wrong …'*
The patient and his son share a brief smile.
Without denying the son his fury, this mini dialogue means that the physiotherapist has reacted with tact and respect, and has avoided being drawn into an argument. Such a technique does not always work, yet often it does and so is a useful strategy for handling aggression and accusations. However, when using this strategy it is good to remember that it can only work if remaining sincere. If the patient or relative gains the impression that he is not being taken seriously or he is the object of sarcasm, then his anger will only grow.

The following generally applies when managing aggression and violence: aggression is a natural, emotional valve and should be dealt with rather than be suppressed. Violence, whether verbal, physical or sexual, should never be tolerated. If a situation becomes critical, then protecting oneself comes before protecting others. If a patient or his family pose a danger, the therapist must retreat from the situation without delay and only then instigate further measures (such as enlisting the help of a colleague or security staff).

Reflective questions

- What do you admire most about your patients?
- In which professional situations do you believe you are more a treasure seeker, and in which are you more a mine sweeper?
- What benefits do you believe systemic communication skills offer when working with seriously ill or terminally ill patients and their families?
- Think about the situations in your daily professional life in which you can usefully deploy the strategy of active listening.
- Think about your current patients: Which circular questions could you ask the individual patients? Which miracle questions spring to mind with these patients?
- Think back to a successful conversation with a patient. What contributed to the positive air of the dialogue? Can these elements be incorporated into future conversations?
- Try to reflect on your own reality construction. What does death mean to you? And how is this concept of death translated in your work? What does life mean to you?

REFERENCES
Neimeyer RA. Meaning Reconstruction and Loss. In: Neimeyer RA (ed). Meaning Reconstruction and the Experience of Loss. Washington: American Psychological Association, 2001.
Satir V. Selbstwert und Kommunikation. Familientherapie für Berater und zur Selbsthilfe. 14th ed. Vienna, 2000.
von Foerster H. Entdecken oder Erfinden. Wie lässt sich Verstehen verstehen? In: von Foerster, Glasersfeld, Hejl, Schmidt, Watzlawick (eds). Einführung in den Konstruktivismus, Munich, 1998.

BIBLIOGRAPHY
Kindl-Beilfuß C. Fragen können wie Küsse schmecken: Systemische Fragetechniken für Anfänger und Fortgeschrittene. Heidelberg, 2011.

3.2 'Of sad lions that roar' and handling strong emotions
Michael-M. Lippka

Why emotions overflow and the waves they can cause

When it comes to death, most people desire a peaceful end: passing away in old age, right-minded, and free of pain, smiling sweetly surrounded by loved ones – harmony and reverent peace. In a lot of cases the reality is quite different: severe, even fatal illnesses are a burden to those affected and their surroundings, both physically and mentally. Every death is unique. Things happen for which we are not prepared. Anything could suddenly be 'the last time'. Often, those affected find themselves in a world that is completely different to before; processes take place in which quite literally **words fail us** – in a society where the reality of death is still taboo.

In such a demanding life situation, the tolerance of an individual to frustration generally declines. In particular, the often forceful loss of physical functionality and subsequent gradual loss of independence leads to ever-increasing problems. It is no longer possible to get out of bed without help, the legs no longer obey, eating and drinking becomes a real challenge – all this despite intensive medical treatment. Important bodily functions such as digestion or breathing are impaired, triggering justifiable anxiety and anger, embarrassment or even shame.

Increasing physical weakness is often seen as **reduced impulse control.** Suddenly it is no longer possible to hide negative feelings behind a smile or control one's own anger. The diligently acquired, socially preferable concealment of one's own sensitivities disappears and man reacts like most other mammals – from guinea pig to lion – with clearly noticeable expressions of discontent. Screaming, whining, howling or crying are clear signals to the world: something dangerous is happening here, here there is risk – maybe somebody has been injured, someone has been attacked, or someone is suffering. An appeal is made to the world at the same time: someone may need help, but it could also mean that a suffering creature wants to be alone; it may be the final rebellion against something unavoidable. And the world responds: so-called mirror neurons in the brain that cause a yawn to become contagious and the eyes to water when another person cries, trigger a hormonal reaction in the body causing an emotional outbreak in one person to be physically witnessed by another. These mirror neurons are the neurobiological basis, as it were, behind our compassion for others, enabling us to empathise with him. Despite the high evolutionary value – you need only think of the imitation skills of primates or the escapist behaviour of gregarious animals – this ability brings certain challenges with it when viewed in social terms. It permits conflicts to spread, feelings to be transferred and grief to be planted upon someone who may have just now been laughing.

Not only negative sensations are radiated relatively unimpeded during times of crisis. A shrill laugh can be equally unsettling as a loud scream. The distinction made between negative and positive feelings, which quite rightly has been criticised, is in this case useful: feelings such as fear, rage and anger trigger emotional distress in the affected person that in the event of excessive joy, for instance, fails to materialise.

Fundamentally, all such **emotional outbreaks are healthy,** producing short as well as even long-term relief by dispelling the distress. On the other hand, emotional distress directed against oneself can lead to psychological problems, including autoaggressive behaviour and depression. The expression of feelings is a good coping strategy, since it displays the person's suffering and thus elicits help from the outside.

But how should the world deal with such strong emotions when suddenly unleashed? How should the shock be dealt with? What should a physiotherapist do if suddenly confronted during treatment, through no fault of his own, with a fit of crying or outbreak of rage? How far should he wade into this quagmire? What about professional boundaries? At what point should the physiotherapist intervene? And should he, or must he, intervene at all?

Basic tools: acceptance, empathy and credibility

The first step for safely dealing with strong emotions is to accept that they are natural, human, and also logical reactions to the challenges of life. Anyone who has grasped this is relieved of the urge to have to immediately 'extinguish the fire' and does not run the risk of consoling either the patient, his family or himself too hastily. The feelings should not be stopped, but rather be given room and expression. True consolation will come as the emotions progress. **Acceptance** implies the **realisation that strong emotions do have their place when managing palliative care patients.** They are a part of life and also part of the process the patient is going through.

An empathic attitude is closely related to this. **Empathy,** in this context, means **to develop an understanding for the exceptional emotional situation in which patients find themselves.** Such compassion is not the same as sympathy, which tends to be more of a hindrance in crisis situations, since it 'belittles' the patient and reduces him to the level of his suffering. A pitied patient is merely shown regret, i. e. remains passive; if he is to be understood in an empathic way, then working together is key. In other words, to work with a patient you have to engage with him and try to understand what is happening instead of simply feeling sorry for him. Empathy is important to the relationship between the physiotherapist and patient, since it engenders trust. When dealing with strong feelings in particular, which as a rule

3

tend to be rather intimate, trust is the basis for any form of contact with the individual concerned. Being empathic does not mean that everything the patient does or thinks should be proclaimed as good. The point is to be **credible,** i.e. genuine and truthful when dealing with the patient. The physiotherapist cares for a patient with the tools that are available to him. He does not pretend to be a friend. He resists the temptation to replace the spiritual counsellor, and also tries not to mislead the patient as regards his poor health merely to ease his own working environment. **He is what he is, and offers the patient his expertise and experience.** This, in turn, does not mean that he should continually bombard the patient with his own opinions and own take on reality, or even try to convince the patient of such beliefs. A credible therapist acts according to the best of his knowledge. He stands for his professional actions and can identify with everything that he does. As a credible physiotherapist, he is aware of his skills and limitations and is capable of conveying this to the patient accordingly. Credibility promotes trust and security in the professional relationship with a patient.

Carl Rogers assumes that every man naturally has the potential for positive development and for managing a crisis provided he is always shown regard, sincerity and empathy (Rogers 2002). This humanistic image of man is the ideal basis for working with patients in emotionally demanding situations. Regard, empathy and credibility are the foundation for any professional intervention and do justice to the needs of the affected patient and one's one role.

Interventions and other reactions

It should not be forgotten that strong feelings are mostly associated with substantial physical effort on the part of the affected individuals, e.g. hyperventilation, rigidity, tremor, screaming or crying heavily. These physical symptoms offer the attending physiotherapist the opportunity to provide the patient **on a physical level with an exit strategy for such a traumatic state.** Respiratory therapy, manual techniques or activity inducing measures can therefore achieve not only physical, but also psychological relief – all thanks to the relationship between the physical and mental aspects of the patient's condition described above.

A patient with a tremendous fear of imminent death who is suffering from breathlessness will intensify this fear by hyperventilating, which in turn has a negative impact on his breathing. So begins a vicious circle of anxiety from which the patient can hardly escape without help.

Here the attending physiotherapist can offer the patient an exit strategy in response to this desperate situation on a physical level. If it is possible to regulate the breathing using appropriate physiotherapeutic measures, the sensation of asphyxiation subsides and in turn the anxiety is reduced. In such a way, physiotherapeutic interventions can also achieve psychological relief (➤ Chapter 2.3, ➤ Chapter 2.4, ➤ Chapter 2.7).

The speed with which such an offer of help is made should be restricted, however, so as never to give the impression that such outbreaks of emotion are inappropriate or have no place in therapy. Caution is not only the mother of all wisdom, but must always apply in the professional setting to oneself and to others. Hence the physiotherapist should always approach an emotional outbreak – whether in a patient, family member or himself – with caution. In doing so, remember: observation – reflection – contact – reflection – intervention – and again, reflection. Such a 'delaying tactic' is beneficial to the atmosphere, radiating calm and assurance, and thus protecting all involved: it creates a useful distance and permits the therapist to work clearly and methodically, i.e. in a professional way.

First aid or lifeboat? A matter of safety …

Aside from planning ability and transparency, safety is always another aspect of dealing professionally with strong emotions. First and foremost is always the **protection of all involved,** whereby **protecting oneself comes before others.** This implies that if a patient – though due to the often poor state of health this tends to be unlikely, it cannot be ruled out entirely – turns violent during an emotional outbreak or a relative becomes threatening, for example, it is always wise for the attending therapist to first retreat to safety and then immediately enlist the help of a colleague. A helpless carer is of no use to anyone and a black eye can hardly be beneficial to future care. The **safety of the patient and his family** comes second. Should self-harming behaviour develop, such as hitting oneself on the head, etc., then it is likewise appropriate to intervene. Often it is enough to address the patient clearly but calmly in order to halt such self-destructive behaviour.

⚠ **CAUTION**

'Schoolmasterly' reprimands should be avoided in such situations in order not to invoke in the patient the idea of belittlement or abasement. This is extremely important: why should a patient take notice of a therapist who he feels does not understand him and does not take his emotional state seriously?

Strong emotions very much dominate a patient's thoughts. He feels inhibited; 'beside himself'. The emotions demand so much energy that other cognitive functions such as grasping social situations cannot be exercised to the full extent. Confusion and disorientation can result, which leave more room for the emotion itself. Consequently, one objective of addressing or establishing contact with the patient should be to offer **re-orientation.** Simply by saying the patient's name, *'Mrs XY'*, or using a descriptive statement such as *'You're hitting your head quite hard'*, lends a little reality to the situation beyond the realms of the emotional outbreak. Mrs XY is gently reminded that she is Mrs XY and is not merely a ball of pain. Meanwhile, the patient hitting herself on the head might only become aware of her actions through this outward perspective. If the patient is able to do this, then joint reflection is possible, by way of: *'I noticed you were just hitting yourself on the head with your hands. Do you want to tell me what's wrong?'* It is important here not only to put what you have seen into words. The statement, *'I see you're very angry'* may be an obvious interpretation, but can be wrong.

However the patient decides to respond, the therapist should reflect whether or not it is appropriate to intervene. He needs to decide whether to use a **physiotherapeutic intervention** aimed directly at the physical symptoms of the emotional outbreak (such as a massage and exercises for the cervical spine which can become excessively tense during and after highly emotional episodes).

Alternatively, he could also deliberately use a **physical counterpoint,** such as by exercising parts of the body far removed from the area of the body involved in the emotional episode (e.g. exercising the legs of a patient who had beforehand been hitting himself on the head). This would create 'distance' in the true sense of the word.

In some cases it can also be useful to conduct the therapy as planned if the patient has calmed down again and/or indicates that he does not wish to go into what has happened.

There may also be situations in which continued therapy at the given time may not be deemed appropriate because the patient may need rest, for example. In this case it is important to provide an exact explanation so that it is clear that the therapy is not being terminated as 'punishment' for the emotions displayed.

The therapist is a crucial component in the choice of intervention. If he decides on an intervention which makes him feel most safe, ideally this feeling will also be transferred to the patient. The same mirror neurons in the brain that have caused the therapist to react emotionally and physically to the emotional outbreak in the

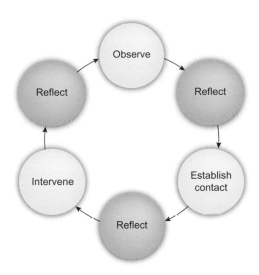

Figure 3.1 Standardised responses to crisis and/or emotional outbursts

patient will now ensure that the assurance radiated by the therapist is also perceived by the patient.

If further outbreaks of emotion ensue during the course of therapy, the standardised mechanism (➤ Figure 3.1) is triggered once more: observe – reflect – make contact – reflect – intervene, etc. The more assured and experienced the therapist appears, the greater the patient's appreciation for the fact that he is in good hands and that his emotions during therapy will be valued. It hardly needs to be mentioned that this will have a positive influence on the therapeutic relationship and in turn the outcome of therapy.

Most important of all

'Speed kills', or in other words: if you go too fast you may lose control – whether of a car or your own actions. If therapists lose control of their own actions, then professionalism is also lost. Of course it is neither hazardous nor disastrous to briefly abandon the professional role – indeed it can sometimes even be beneficial for one's own motivation or the therapeutic process. However, by remaining professional both therapist and patient will be protected in equal measure. This should never be forgotten. Professionalism ensures a healthy relationship between distance and proximity, and prevents overload. It defines the responsibilities of the therapist and those of the patient. Hence it can remind the therapist that the strong emotions being experienced by the patient are not his own. It also reminds him that it is his job as a physiotherapist to care for this person – irrespective of the patient's current disposition.

In terms of timing, i. e. the 'who does what and when', it is important to note how and whether the behaviour displayed by the patient has changed. Certain emotional outbreaks pass fairly quickly, whilst others escalate without intervention.

The timing and intensity of an emotional outbreak is also dictated by the patient. When and whether to intervene at all remains the therapist's decision, regardless of the nature of the outbreak, his current strength and personal experience in dealing with crisis situations. Mostly it is only possible to determine afterwards whether the timing was appropriate or could have been better. The idea that the appropriate speed will be found in a crisis is a good means of self-suggestion which in turn will lead to confidence in managing such demanding situations. The concept that **the patient's behaviour dictates when something should be done** points in a similar direction. This appears to be justified – for it is his own personal dying process.

We end with a quote from the Bible that reflects precisely this feeling of composure:

'Everything has its own time, and there is a specific time (…) for every activity:
a time to be born, and a time to die (…),
a time to weep, and a time to laugh,
a time to mourn, and a time to dance,
a time to cast away stones, and a time to gather stones together,
a time to embrace, and a time to refrain from embracing …'

Book of Ecclesiastes 3:1–5

⚠ **CAUTION**

Even if the emotions unleashed are intense, they become less daunting if instead of fighting them they are given time and attention.

Reflective questions

- What makes you feel confident when dealing with your patients and their families?
- What is healthy about an outbreak of emotion?
- What fierce sensation have you most often encountered so far in your professional capacity?
- Which emotions tend to make you feel helpless and insecure?
- Think about the physical symptoms that can often develop with strong emotions. Which physiotherapeutic measures come to mind?
- How do you react yourself if you are affected by strong feelings or outbreaks of emotion?
- What effect does it have on you when you see a patient crying? What effect does it have on you when you see your own friend or a member of your family crying?
- What do acceptance, empathy and credibility mean to you in your professional work? Where are the boundaries in this respect?
- How do your patients recognise that, as a physiotherapist, you have an empathic, accepting and credible attitude? How is empathy expressed in human relationships? Are there ways of practising attributes such as empathy, credibility and acceptance?

REFERENCES
Rogers C. Entwicklung der Persönlichkeit. Psychotherapie aus der Sicht eines Therapeuten. Stuttgart: Klett, 2002.

BIBLIOGRAPHY
Bärsch T, Rohde M. Deeskalation in der Pflege. Gewaltprävention – Deeskalierende Kommunikation – Schutztechniken. Norderstedt, 2010.

4.1 Ethics and ethical reasoning in palliative physiotherapy
Birgit Jaspers

Ethics and ethical reasoning play a very large part in the palliative care concept. A number of factors are seen as triggers for the intensive preoccupation with ethics and the ethos of the caregiver: the increasing secularisation of the western world, an overall shift in society's values, problems with the ethical justification for rules concerning human action and inaction in pluralistic societies, and the individualisation of lifestyles and values in western industrialised nations. Consequently, not only has the paternalistic nature of the doctor-patient relationship matured into one that respects the self-determination and will of the patient (Eibach/Schäfer 2001), but the self-image of other caregivers has also changed accordingly. Furthermore, the increasing inclusion of palliative care patients into disciplines which tend to have their origins solely in rehabilitation – such as intensive care medicine and also physiotherapy – poses a great challenge to caregivers. The inclusion of physiotherapists is no longer merely a recommendation (Council of Europe 2003, Radbruch/Payne 2011), but in some studies has even been identified as one of the organisational quality indicators for the provision of palliative care (Engels et al. 2010).

Ethics and morality

Ethics (from the Greek *ta ethika* = moral teaching) is a philosophical discipline (Schmidt 1982, p. 170). It is understood to be a reflection of conditions, principles and goals in human social activity. The term should not be confused with **ethos,** which has several connotations: the usual place of life, the epitome of customs and habits (also from *mores,* the Latin for customs) and ultimately attitudes and behaviour, one's personal character (Höffe 2002, p. 30–31). The terms 'morality' and 'ethics' are often used synonymously, thereby causing confusion. In the stricter sense, **morality** describes the phenomenon of habits and customs, and ethics the scientific reflection of this. Man has what is referred to as **moral intuition,** on the basis of which he often makes decisions for or against an action. Moral intuition is founded upon socialisation and on internalised values and moral attitudes which are shared by many, but not all cultures. This includes for example the prohibition of killing, torture, injury, lying, the offer of help in emergency situations, fairness and the virtues (and thus the positive attributes)

of wisdom, strength, prudence, justice, placidity, helpfulness, and many more (von der Pfordten 2010, p. 11).

A basic knowledge of the theories of **normative ethics** is required in order to reflectively consider decisions on what to do. Its role is to lay down criteria for the (moral) rightness and wrongness of actions, the assessment of motives behind our actions and their consequences. Ethical theories and approaches are very diverse, however. In open, pluralistic societies the communication of different ethical approaches is anchored in educational policies. Privately as well as professionally, every individual will find that the decisions and actions encountered in their social and human interactions will always differ depending on moral justification.

In systems such as healthcare, however, there are certain limitations not only to the practical, but also the moral compass of individual decisions. Deviations can be made, of course, but are generally subject to negative sanctions. For example, at a Christian hospital a warning would be issued if a member of the palliative care team organised a prostitute for a severely ill patient because the single man desired some affection prior to his death.

Moral codes may afford patients and carers a degree of safety, but they also pose a challenge when at the same time a patient must be assigned treatments and support that are appropriate and according to their individual preferences. Moreover, a number of principles must be considered in the decision-making process, such as autonomy, justice, beneficence and non-maleficence (Beauchamp/Childress 2001), or different values in relation to a particular procedure. How this should be done and how values can be prioritised are seldom taught in the healthcare professions. An introduction to applied ethics for physiotherapists is offered, amongst others, by a US-American paper (Delany et al. 2010).

Ethical principles for physiotherapists

The *World Confederation for Physical Therapy* (WCPT) with headquarters in London expects its member organisations to have a code of ethics or code of conduct, or supports them in developing such a code. Codes should be published and made available to the general public, to physiotherapist employers, policy makers and health authorities. Members should also develop procedures for dealing with violations against such a code.

In 1995, the World Confederation itself adopted a Declaration of Principle which is binding for all member organisations. Any principles laid down by an organisation should be compatible with this declaration. The Principle was last revised in June 2011, and the next

review is due in 2015. According to the current edition, physiotherapists (WCPT 2011) are expected to:
1. respect the rights and dignity of all individuals;
2. comply with the laws and regulations governing the practice of physical therapy in the country in which they practise;
3. accept responsibility for the exercise of sound judgement;
4. provide honest, competent and accountable professional services;
5. provide quality services;
6. receive a just and fair level of remuneration for their services;
7. provide accurate information to patients/clients, to other agencies and the community about physical therapy and the services physical therapists provide;
8. contribute to the planning and development of services which address the health needs of the community.

Additional explanations are provided on each of these principles. Certain areas – such as palliative care – are never explicitly mentioned, however, though the World Confederation regards its principles as globally applicable to the practice of physiotherapy and as being independent of the political or healthcare systems in which such therapy is undertaken.

A moment's reflection and not least a discussion with others of the first principle will give rise to questions in certain treatment scenarios. What does respecting the rights and dignity of all individuals mean in practice? Knowing the rights that individuals have certainly implies the need to always be aware of the latest requirements. Respecting the dignity of all individuals may at first sound simple, since most people have an idea of what they themselves believe is human dignity. Such notions are by no means identical in each individual, however. What is problematic is the understanding of the concept of dignity in a team or group if the principle of **basic dignity** is not distinguished from that of **personal dignity** (Härle 2006). The commitment to observe the principle of basic dignity is also laid down in article 1, paragraph 1 of the German Constitution: "Human dignity shall be inviolable". All humans have unswerving dignity – regardless of who they are, how they are, what they can do, what they do or possess, whether they believe in such dignity themselves or not. Dignity in this sense is not an objective fact, but the demand of respect for humanity. However, a person may feel totally deprived of their dignity even if it has been respected by others (Härle 2006, Wainwright/Gallagher 2008, Andorno 2011). This is described by victims of rape and torture, but also by people who are critically ill (Chochinov et al. 2002). It may prove difficult to a therapist when

caring for patients if he is unaware that they can be deprived of only personal, but not basic dignity.

CASE STUDY
Part 1

Mrs S. suffers from breast cancer. After excision of her right breast and removal of lymph nodes from the axilla, her husband left her because he was unable to cope with her condition. She finds herself unattractive and it has taken her a long time to find the courage to attend physiotherapy. Though her right arm is very swollen, until now she has never wanted to let anyone except her doctors see her. As she can hardly bear to look at herself, she limits washing to the minimum while keeping her underwear on.
Reflective questions   What do you do if Mrs S. has a different understanding of dignity to her therapists? How can a suitable treatment setting be established? How can therapists respect their patient's privacy? How should they deal with the fact that Mrs S. appears so unhappy and also displays this fact to an obvious degree?

The topics addressed are not only problematic in terms of organisation and verbal as well as non-verbal communication, but primarily entail **ethical questions** that extend far beyond the debate of professional ethics and require fundamental consideration of ethical practice (Partridge 2010).

The same applies to points 2 and 4 of the WCPT principles: to comply with the laws and regulations governing the practice of physical therapy in the country of practice and to provide honest, competent and accountable professional services. These principles imply that values and standards must be acknowledged, such as truthfulness/sincerity, not lying, not taking advantage and honest accounting. Most of these standards and values are not only relevant to professional life.

CASE STUDY
Part 2

Physiotherapist Mr M. has now been treating Mrs S. for five years. She has meanwhile suffered a relapse and her disease has reached a more advanced stage. She is very frail and is cared for by an outpatient palliative care service. The service has called Mr M. to say that Mrs S. would like to continue receiving – now at home – manual lymph drainage treatments from him. She was always very happy with his treatments and a referral has been written.
Mr M. is happy to do this and arrives at the house to find Mrs S. feeling very sleepy. She feels too weak for treatment and would prefer an appointment the following day. However, Mr M. notices that her daughter, who has been providing her mother with a lot of support, is quite exhausted so he offers her a massage within the alloted therapy time. The daughter is very grateful and is visibly more relaxed after the massage. When Mr M. leaves she says she should try to take a little more care of herself.

Reflective questions   What are the ethical implications in Mr M. giving massage therapy to Mrs S.'s daughter? Is there any legal and/or moral justification to enable Mr M.'s employer to bill his work against Mrs S.'s prescription? Should Mr M. even inform his employer?

A competent and accountable service, as suggested by the WCPT principles, certainly also includes continuing professional development and awareness of the latest state of art in terms of therapeutic questions. For example, there is no evidence to confirm the suspected correlation of manual lymph drainage and metastasis, only conflicting statements on the subject in the literature; the sparse evidence that is available generally argues to the contrary (Földi 1994, Godette/Mondry/Johnstone 2006). Consider the following case study:

CASE STUDY
Part 3

Over the course of the long period of treatment, Mrs S.'s breast cancer was found to have metastasised. Mr M. hears from colleagues that this can also be associated with manual lymph drainage. He becomes uncertain as to how he should continue treating Mrs S.
Reflective questions   What do debates concerning the potential outcomes of a treatment, with little or even no evidence, mean to a therapist in terms of accepting responsibility and making mistakes? What does this basically mean with respect to his legal position?

As other therapists and caregivers, also physiotherapists who work in palliative care settings will inevitably be confronted by the subject of death and dying as well as complex ethical issues. In addition, there is a certain intimacy between therapist and patient in physiotherapeutic interventions such as lymph drainage. For those who have reached the end of their lives, who may be lonely or isolated, or who due to visible signs of illness for example have for a long time not felt the touch of others, their treatment can mean a lot more than simply worrying about their symptoms. Furthermore, such treatment scenarios are often characterised by communication between the patient and therapist that can span the most diverse of life's topics. This demands a reflective approach that ultimately is founded upon clear ethical principles and without which communication can sometimes prove very difficult.

CASE STUDY
Part 4

Mrs S. spends the final three weeks of her life in a hospice, where Mr M. visits to administer therapy. Her daughter whispers to him: *'It would be better if Mum would die soon ... but we haven't told her that it could be quite quick.'*
During treatment, while the daughter is in the kitchen, Mrs S. says to Mr M. that she would like to go home again next week, adding, *'that you, as my physiotherapist who I've trusted for a long time, are also treating me while I'm here must be a good sign.'*
Reflective questions   How should Mr M. handle such a situation?

Physiotherapy and ethical research issues

Within the framework of the "*Budapest Commitments*" – a collaboration between the member organisations of the *European Association for Palliative Care* (EAPC) at a congress in Budapest – a number of nations initiated projects and campaigns designed to improve the care of the critically ill and terminally ill (European Association of Palliative Care 2007). Following a two-year period of development, the *Charter for the Care of the Critically Ill and the Dying* was adopted in Germany in 2010 as a contribution to these Commitments (Deutsche Gesellschaft für Palliativmedizin et al. 2010). Over 50 institutions were involved in this process, and more than 150 experts worked on the foundations of this document. Also involved was the *German Physiotherapy Association – Central Association of German Physiotherapists* (ZVK).

The association made the following statement on the collaboration (Deutscher Verband für Physiotherapie 2010): '*This matter is extremely important to us, since we are aware of the tremendous input physiotherapists have in improving the quality of life of such individuals.*'

Point 4 of the charter calls upon physiotherapists, among others, to enter into research. Its argument is that networking the various professional teams in palliative care is not only important to physiotherapy in practice, but also increases the chances of obtaining evidence-based data for practical use. It also states here explicitly that every critically ill or dying individual has the right to be treated in line with generally accepted standards.

The charter likewise states that, for example, the ethical framework for research in critically ill patients must be taken into account. Whether a research project is ethically appropriate is ultimately determined by an ethics panel vote that has to be obtained when research is being planned in humans. To date there have only been relatively few studies in physiotherapy, however, and studies on physiotherapeutic issues related to palliative care and palliative treatment are sparse.

CASE STUDY
Part 5

Mr M. would like to see a study initiated on treatment-related topics – such as on the many female palliative care patients being treated long-term with lymph drainage by him or his colleagues. When talking with his peers, however, doubts were raised as to whether, on ethical grounds, research can be carried out at all into critically ill patients. Most of those with whom he spoke found his idea morally reprehensibe, irrespective of any possible approval to do so.

Reflective questions What could Mr M. have done? At what point during his care for Mrs S. might he have asked whether she would have been prepared to take part in a research project, e.g. into the alleviation of pain by manual lymph drainage? Only at the start, at any point or at the end – or would it have been ethically more acceptable to extract data from the files for a retrospective study?

CASE STUDY
Part 6

Mrs S. died at the hospice. Before she died, she asked a number of times after Mr M. of whom she had become very fond. The hospice director therefore called the practice where Mr M. was working. On the telephone, his employer could find no legitimate clinical reason why Mr M. should change his schedule for that day. He was also reluctant to agree to his employees making private visits during their working hours or taking final leave of a dying patient – viewing it as unrelated to their work and being 'bad for business'.

Reflective questions A number of palliative care patients receive care from a physiotherapist right to the very end of their lives. What reasons are there for prioritising economic factors, and what arguments speak in favour of respecting humanity?

Ethical conflicts and ethical judgements

Ethical conflict is generally understood as the friction between two incompatible norms, both of which are nevertheless acknowledged by an individual (Jaspers 2011). A comprehensive definition of ethical conflicts in healthcare was suggested by the philosopher Hartmut Kliemt at the University of Duisburg-Essen in Germany. Accordingly, '*an ethical conflict (in the stricter sense) can only exist if the following conditions are fulfilled:*

- *An ethically desirable option or one viewed as commendable is opposed by (at least) one ethically likewise desirable or likewise ethically commendable and thus irreconcilable alternative option.*
- *One of the irreconcilable options must be put into practice.*
- *There is a decision-maker who cannot avoid or who at least is authorised to select – 'at the expense of the other' – one of the options.* (Kliemt 2005).

If a team or individual is frequently exposed to such conflicts, the result may be **moral stress** or moral distress ("moral stress" according to Jameton 1984, Rushton 2006). Moral stress occurs, according to the authors, if clinicians believe they cannot carry out what they believe are ethically appropriate measures due to internal or external obstacles. An unresolvable conflict or incongruence thus exists between ethical convictions and the requisite actions. Healthcare professionals often find themselves in such situations. If an individual has to act against his own personal or professional ideals, integrity and authenticity are undermined and can contribute to burnout. Situations involving moral stresses in physiotherapy have been described by Carpenter (2010).

One of the principles of the WCPT states that physiotherapists should assume responsibility for making a sound decision. This is reliant on actually knowing how to make reliable clinical *and* moral judgements and then assuming responsibility for making a decision to the best of one's knowledge. Studies have indicated that decisions involving **moral reasoning** are an important skill required of physiotherapists, whose standing has undergone a huge transition in the last four decades (Swisher 2002). Since the 1980 s efforts have been made to increase the autonomous role of physiotherapists in clinical decision-making and in the healthcare system as a whole (Rose 1989a, 1989b). In doing so, the role of physiotherapists has not only become more complex but has also brought with it more intricate ethical dilemmas and responsibilities (Magistro 1989, Trietzenberg 1996, Praestegaard/Gard 2011).

An American study demonstrated that physiotherapists fare less favourably than other professional groups in the healthcare system when it comes to the complex issues of ethical judgement (Swisher 2010). Even if the reasons for this are unclear, it is presumed that this topic is afforded less relevance in the continuing professional development of physiotherapists than is the case with doctors, carers or medical students and student nurses (Swisher 2010). Studies have shown that the discussion of ethical case examples in small groups enhances moral reasoning skills (Baldwin/Daugherty/Self 1991, Self/Olivarez/Baldwin 1998a, 1998b). A disregard for ethics and for the development of moral reasoning skills may also be related to the fact that physiotherapists were for a long time not regarded as being equal partners in the care of the critically ill, but rather were expected to work to instruction in a role where they were clearly undervalued. To counteract this stance, physiotherapists themselves should urge for increased involvement in decision-making processes and where necessary make it clear to other therapists that they should be regarded as key practitioners in the treatment team.

Decision-making tools for clinical practice

A variety of methods can be employed when making medically and ethically acceptable decisions about particularly difficult treatment scenarios. Important factors to consider when selecting a suitable method, for example, are the setting in which the physiotherapist is working and whether he is part of a team or acting alone.

In the clinical setting, methods involving ethical case discussions and peer consultation have proven successful. Various explanations and instructions can be downloaded in relation to such methods (MTG 2005, Tietze 2010). If an ethical question arises during the treatment of a patient, the physiotherapist could ask the treating doctor to arrange for an ethical case meeting or peer discussion. Physiotherapists who are not part of a formal team (perhaps those who are self-employed and therefore work alone) are generally required to motivate the other protagonists involved in the case to undertake such actions.

In palliative care, the teams caring for a particular patient are not always clearly delineated or do not form one unit that always sees itself as a team. Hence at the beginning Mr M. was part of an informal team when he first got to know Mrs S., through having the initial contact with her general practitioner or oncologist. Later the team was expanded to include the palliative nursing care staff and the daughter as family and carer at home; perhaps a consultation service or outpatient palliative care team was also enlisted. At the hospice the team underwent further changes. **If the team's intentions from the start do not reach as far as including the physiotherapist then his only job is to make himself visible.** This is also one of the ethical challenges a physiotherapist has in the palliative care environment.

Conclusion

All the groups implicated in palliative care, along with the professional associations, have established ethical principles and voluntary commitments. There is no policy, however, that can envisage the subtle complexity even of the most ordinary relationship between two individuals (Pellegrino 1979). Yet ethical principles do

lead practitioners generally to consider the need for their therapeutic work to also be viewed from a moral standpoint. The fact alone that a code of ethics exists is a sign that it should always be borne in mind that working in the healthcare system is not only a technical but also a moral venture. The importance of ethics in the process of professionalisation of physiotherapy differs between countries, however. In Germany, for example, a closer look at the subject is advisable (Jurgons 2009).

REFERENCES

Andorno R. The dual role of human dignity in bioethics. Med Health Care Philos. Dec 16 2011 [Epub ahead of print].

Baldwin DC Jr, Daugherty SR, Self DJ. Changes in moral reasoning during medical school. Academic Med 1991;66(Suppl. 6):S1-S3

Beauchamp TL, Childress JF. Principles of Biomedical Ethics. 5th ed. Oxford: Oxford University Press 2001.

Carpenter C. Moral distress in physical therapy practice. Physiother Theory Pract 2010;26:69–78.

Chochinov HM, Hack T, Hassard T, Kristjanson LJ, McClement S, Harlos M. Dignity in the terminally ill: a cross-sectional, cohort study. Lancet 2002;360:2,026–2,030.

Council of Europe: Recommendation Rec(2003)24 of the Committee of Ministers to member states on the organisation of palliative care. Adopted by the Committee of Ministers on 12 November 2003 at the 860th meeting of the Ministers' Deputies, Strasbourg 2003. Available at: http://www.coe.int/t/dg3/health/Source/Rec(2003)24_en.pdf (last accessed August 2012).

Delany CM, Edwards I, Jensen GM, Skinner E. Closing the gap between ethics knowledge and practice through active engagement: an applied model of physical therapy ethics. Phys Ther 2010;90:1,068–1,078.

Deutsche Gesellschaft für Palliativmedizin e. V., Deutscher Hospiz- und PalliativVerband e. V., Bundesärztekammer (Hrsg.). Charta zur Betreuung und Begleitung schwerstkranker und sterbender Menschen, 2010. Available at: http://www.charta-zur-betreuung-sterbender.de/tl_files/dokumente/Charta-08-09-2010.pdf (last accessed July 2012).

Deutscher Verband für Physiotherapie – Zentralverband der Physiotherapeuten/Krankengymnasten (ZVK). Unterversorgung im Bereich der Palliativmedizin. Available at: https://www.zvk.org/bundesverband/fachkreise/news/einzelansicht/artikel/Barmer-GEK-Heil-und-Hilfsmittelreport-2010-in-Berlin-praesentiert.html (last accessed July 2012).

Eibach U, Schäfer K. Patientenautonomie und Patientenwünsche. Ergebnisse und ethische Reflexion von Patientenbefragungen zur selbstbestimmten Behandlung in Krisensituationen. MedR Medizinrecht 2001;19:21–28.

Engels Y, Vanbeek K, Woitha K, et al. Development of an indicator set for the organisation of palliative care in Europe. In: Ahmedzai S, Gómez-Batiste X, Engels Y, et al. (eds). Assessing organisations to improve palliative care in Europe. Nijmegen: Vantilt Publishers 2010, S. 73–90.

European Association of Palliative Care. Budapest Commitments, 2007. Available at: http://www.eapcnet.eu/Themes/Policy/Budapestcommitments.aspx (last accessed July 2012).

Földi M. Treatment of lymphedema (Editorial). Lymphology 1994;27:1–5.

Földi M. Editorial. Hat die manuelle Lymphdrainage Einfluss auf die Rezidivhäufigkeit des Mammakarzinoms? Földi Newsletter Juli 2009, S. 1.

Godette K, Mondry TE, Johnstone PA. Can manual treatment of lymphedema promote metastasis? Review. J Soc Integr Oncol 2006;4: 8–12.

Härle W. Menschenwürde – Zentrales Element des christlichen Menschenbildes. Evangelische Verantwortung G5931Februar 2006:1–11. Available at: http://www.eak-cducsu.de/content-system/upload/ev/10_2_2006–12_58_49-EAK-EV-02–2006.pdf (last accessed July 2012).

Höffe O. Medizin ohne Ethik? Frankfurt: Suhrkamp, 2002.

Jameton A. Nursing Practice. The Ethical Issues. Prentice-Hall: Englewood Cliffs, 1984.

Jaspers B. Ethische Entscheidungen am Lebensende bei Palliativpatienten in Deutschland – Eine prospektive Untersuchung anhand von Daten aus der Kerndokumentation 2005 und 2006. Radbruch L, Elsner F (Hrsg.). Reihe Aachener Dissertationen zur Palliativmedizin, Band 3. Aachen: Shaker Verlag, 2011.

Jurgons S. Die Bedeutung der Ethik im Professionalisierungsprozess der Physiotherapie. Ein Vergleich zwischen den USA und Deutschland. pt_Zeitschrift für Physiotherapeuten 2009;61. Available at: www.physiotherapeuten.de/antje-hueter-becker-preis/jurgons01.pdf (last accessed July 2012).

Kliemt H. Ethische Konflikte im Gesundheitswesen. Oral presentation on 31 August 2005. Available at: http://www.socialpolitik.org/docs/oldtag/2005/Kliemt%20Vortrag.pdf (last accessed July 2012).

Magistro CM. Clinical decision-making in physical therapy: a practitioner's perspective. Phys Ther 1989;69:525–534.

MTG Malteser Trägergesellschaft gGmbH (ed). Ethische Fallbesprechung. Eine interdisziplinäre Form klinischer Ethikberatung. Cologne: MTG, 2005. Available at: http://www.malteser-krankenhaus-stcarolus.de/06.Das_Krankenhaus/06.02.Ethik/ethischeFallbesprechung.pdf (last accessed July 2012).

Partridge CJ. Does ethical practice in physiotherapy matter? Editorial. Physiother Res Int 2010;15:65–68.

Pellegrino ED. Towards a reconstruction of medical morality: the primacy of the profession and the fact of illness. J Med Philos 1979;4:32–56.

Praestegaard J, Gard G. The perceptions of Danish physiotherapists on the ethical issues related to the physiotherapist-patient relationship during the first session: a phenomenological approach. BMC Med Ethics 2011;12:21.

Radbruch L, Payne S. Standards und Richtlinien für Hospiz- und Palliativversorgung in Europa. Part 2: Weißbuch zu Empfehlungen der Europäischen Gesellschaft für Palliative Care (EAPC) Z Palliativmed 2011;12:260–270.

Rose SJ. Editor's note: Gathering storms. Phys Ther 1989a;69:354–355.

Rose SJ. Editor's note: Our body of knowledge revisited. Phys Ther 1989b;69:297–298.

Rushton C. Defining and addressing moral distress – tools for critical care nursing leaders. AACN Advanced Critical Care 2006;17:161–168.

Schmidt H. Philosophisches Wörterbuch. Neu bearbeitet von Georg Schischkoff. 21st ed. Stuttgart: Kröner, 1982.

Self DJ, Olivarez M, Baldwin DC Jr. Clarifying the relationship of medical education and moral development. Academic Med 1998a;73(5):517–520.

Self DJ, Olivarez M, Baldwin DC Jr. The amount of small-group case study discussion needed to improve moral reasoning skills of medical students. Academic Med 1998b;73(5):521–523.

Swisher LL. A retrospective analysis of ethics knowledge in physical therapy (1970–2000). J Phys Ther Educ 2002;82:692–706.

Swisher LL. Moral reasoning among physical therapists. Results of the Defining Issues Test. Physiother Res Int 2010;15:69–79.

Tietze KO. Kollegiale Beratung. Hamburg 2010. Available at: http://www.kollegiale-beratung.de/index.html (last accessed July 2012).

Trietzenberg HL. The identification of ethical issues in physical therapy practice. Phys Ther. 1996;76:1,097–1,107.

von der Pfordten D. Normative Ethik. Berlin: Walter de Gruyter, 2010.

Wainwright P, Gallagher A. On different types of dignity in nursing care: a critique of Nordenfelt. Nurs Philos 2008;9:46–54.

World Confederation for Physical Therapy (WCPT). Ethical responsibilities of physical therapists and WCPT members, 2011. Available at: http://www.wcpt.org/sites/wcpt.org/files/files/PS_Ethical_Principles_Sept2011.pdf (last accessed July 2012).

4.2 The interface between function and meaning
Andrew Goodhead

A physiotherapist colleague at St Christopher's Hospice, London, UK described physiotherapists as 'can-do people', meaning that physiotherapists are trained to enable patients to regain muscle tone or mobility after illness or trauma. In palliative care, physiotherapy has a different aim. A physiotherapist's task is as much to rehabilitate an individual to their optimum ability – even if that means a limited functionality – as to enable a patient to recognize that illness means that function will become increasingly limited and to work within those changing limits. Dahlin and Heiwe (2009, p. 12) suggest this of the physiotherapist's role: '*Physical therapists use physical approaches in order to promote, maintain, and restore physical, psychological, and social well-being. Physical therapy in palliative care is often directed toward controlling symptoms and compensating for lost functions.*'

Another aspect of the physiotherapist's role in palliative care is to work with a patient to improve breathing when disease has limited lung function and, through that, to enable the patient to mobilize more comfortably, albeit within a limited range. One patient, Mary, experienced such a marked change when encouraged to exercise she said: '*This week is the first time in four months I've been out by myself. I went out without oxygen. This circuit class has given me confidence. It energizes me. I see this gym as a place of hope.'*

Mary's life, or her spiritual understanding of her life, encapsulated in the need to be active, meant her personal meaning or narrative changed through the physiotherapist's involvement.

'Making meaning', that is rediscovering purpose, or dealing with issues around 'who am I?' in the illness journey could be limited only to conversation and therefore restricted in scope to certain staff who have a psychospiritual or counselling approach to their practice. To hold this view limits the way men and women make meaning matter and identify themselves to themselves and to others.

As the chaplain at the hospice, part of my role is to sit with patients who are facing the process of dying and to listen to the changes that they have experienced in their life through disease progression. Often those conversations relate to meaning: how a person recounts themselves in the present to their past; how change can be lived with, and how a sense of purpose – even with the knowledge of a limited prognosis – is possible. I have observed physiotherapists at St Christopher's Hospice working one to one with patients, assessing function and planning future interventions, either on a continuing one to one basis, or in a physiotherapy group in the rehabilitation gym. This work requires the skilled physiotherapist to be a listener to what is said by the patient, as much as what is unsaid, and then – as far as possible – to set mutual goals. **Good physiotherapy is achieved by the active listening and responses of the professional to far more than the symptoms of debility.** The chaplain's role involves giving attention, listening and responding appropriately, and not always in speech. This, however, is only one approach to 'making meaning'. In this chapter I set out ways in which physiotherapists have an important role in enabling the body to give meaning through function, however limited. Mary exemplified a positive outcome of the physiotherapist's work.

Our common task is to be both attentive and responsive to those we meet and to experience with them a sense of 'being with' at its deepest level. In any encounter with a man or woman seeking to express or find meaning, it is the need of those whom we are with that needs to be found and expressed. Our task is somehow to be a conduit for that expression. This chapter does not use the word spirituality to describe the creation of meaning, yet it is concerned with the spirituality or philosophical outlook of the patient who is seeking to create new meaning through function. To use the word 'function' is to normalize the experience of the patient's

meaning-making process and to ground this in practical responses and enable open conversation.

4.2.1 What does society tell us about our bodies?

In 2005, five women, patients at St Christopher's Hospice discussed together how they could no longer find clothes that fitted following surgery for breast cancer. Their discussion centred on how they wanted to be remembered. From that conversation, a project with a London fashion college began. They talked with the fashion students, chose materials, designed and made dresses. The project ended with a hospice fashion show with family, friends and hospice staff present. Each of the participants walked the catwalk in their dress. The atmosphere was electric and the event deeply moving. One participant recognized that she would not marry and designed a wedding dress in vibrant orange.

For each of these women, their ability to make meaning was engaged with in the designing and making of dresses. Although society might not make buying clothes on the high street a pleasurable experience for those who have undergone surgery, alienating them from the ideal presented as the norm, this project gave them dignity and a sense of who they were at that particular time. Two participants chose to be buried in the dress that they had designed.

Western society seems obsessed with retaining physical attraction or physical ability. Magazines, advertisements, billboards, shop counter displays and other means of promotion almost shout out that to remain fully human every effort must be made to hold back the ageing process and deny the advance of years its inevitable toll on physical capacity. Beauty has been idealized and has become a totem for all those who wish to remain desirable to others. The increase in cosmetic surgical procedures gives a clear indication that the pursuit of retaining 'youth' and attraction is a major goal for some individuals. In 2005, over 22,000 procedures were carried out in the UK, a rise of more than 34 % on the previous year. Interviewed by the BBC in 2005, Adam Searle, a consultant plastic surgeon, stated: *'These figures [for 2005] appear to represent a growing acceptance of aesthetic surgery, particularly in maintaining appearance with age'* (BBC 2006). In 2010, 38,274 cosmetic procedures took place in the UK (British Association of Aesthetic Plastic Surgeons 2011).

Health and fitness also feature as a popular leisure pastime for many. This industry is now worth £3.77 billion annually. The chief executive of the UK Fitness Industry Association, Andree Deane, said in 2009 that *'fitness and exercise is now perceived by consumers to be a vital part of their lives and well-being and not a luxury expenditure'* (Leisure Database Company 2009). Maintaining fitness is good for overall health and well-being, but the question remains how much meaning do individuals, consciously or otherwise, give to the ongoing pursuit of a 'young' body? Mount (2010, p. 75) suggests that *'no single thing is more striking about men and women in the modern world than their obsessive concern for their physical well-being and flourishing. There is a limitless appetite for miracle medicines, cures for the incurable, sure-fire routes to spectacular weight loss, life-changing therapies, surgical breakthroughs and diagnostic techniques that solve all medical mysteries.'*

Mount does not imply that these pursuits tend towards finding meaning. Rather they suggest an interest in avoiding decline and death.

4.2.2 To what is the healthy body an antidote?

A healthy body that retains physical attractiveness, and ability may be an attempt to seek a retreat from, or denial of, death. In the UK, the number of people over the age of 80 is predicted to more than double between 2010 and 2035, and those over 100 will increase sevenfold to over 80,000 people (Office for National Statistics 2009).

The 2008 *End of Life Care Strategy* for England and Wales recognized that for many people *'death cannot be spoken of: the reality of death and dying is rarely discussed in modern society. Many consider death to be the last great taboo in our society'* (UK Department of Health 2008). Talking about death and personal wishes often remain unspoken within families. An American study of mortality attitudes eloquently reveals a marked change in the discussion of death as an aspect of the human condition. Quoting Ariès the study noted, *'death has now not only disappeared, but become shameful and forbidden'* (Lundgren/Houseman 2010).

The desire for the body presented to society in a variety of media, and the personal quest for health and fitness and growth in gym membership, indicate a death denying society. As an ordained minister, I wonder whether denying death is a result of increasing secularity in Western Europe. At a recent conference (NCPC 2010), Douglas Davies suggested that religion exists to deal with the problem of death. It is true that major world faiths hold an understanding of death and existence after death as central tenets of belief. In the Christian tradition, a belief in Jesus Christ as saviour is a means of continuing to live after death. Other religions also deal with concepts of suffering, illness and ageing. It is not clear that secularity has any way of contextualizing illness and death in a coherent manner: I am not saying that religious belief systems are the answer to understanding and being comfortable with death, but I am not sure that secularity has yet reached a common understanding of dying beyond a religious framework. Steve Bruce, writing about secularity in Britain, tellingly noted that just because people do not have a religious structure in which dead people achieve eternal salvation or damnation does not mean that for the bereaved, dead people simply cease to exist: *'To say, 'Ethel has died and is no more' is to imply other possibilities: Ethel has gone to another world; Ethel's body has died but we can still communicate with Ethel-ness; Ethel has not died but has gone into hiding and will reappear when we deserve her; the essence of Ethel has left her worn-out frame and reappeared in a baby born the same day as she died, and so on'* (Bruce 2002, p. 43).

4.2.3 Function and meaning

Given that men and women seek to retain physical function and independence – and through that make sense of themselves in their world – the interface, or boundary between function and meaning may be blurred. The interface, or point at which being able 'to do' interrelates with being able 'to be', is a liminal point. **The physiotherapist's task in palliative care is to stand at the limen and enable the patient to cross the threshold safely, recognizing that their meaning is embraced by function.** Such a point is almost indefinable, and without a boundary. Function and meaning are of necessity liminal to each other, for one emerges from the other. When illness comes, meaning may be lost to function, as function is limited.

Tony Walter indicated how to cope with the body as a purely mechanistic device: medicine often views the patient *'primarily as a malfunctioning machine, rather than as a whole person'* (Walter 1997, unpublished). Palliative medicine challenged this view following Dame Cicely Saunders' introduction of multi-professional working as a means of meeting the whole person through the interactions of a number of disciplines, each of which brings a unique contribution to the meeting (Saunders 2006). Walter makes the startling point that the human body cannot be disposed of until a doctor has signed a medical certificate. Once signed, a body can be buried or cremated without rites or rituals (Walter 1997).

At death, the corpse has no societal meaning as its usefulness has been spent; yet, in reality, no matter how a body is disposed of, whether in a religious or secular manner, the dead person is endowed with significant meaning and disposed of with appropriate formality: a dead person is more than just a body.

A helpful way to consider more fully the interface between function and meaning is through the approach of phenomenology. This is a philosophical understanding initially presented by Edmund Husserl, but developed by Maurice Merleau-Ponty, amongst others. Merleau-Ponty developed the theories of phenomenology, and saw the body as one of the important aspects of being. Phenomenology is a philosophical approach to understanding consciousness. The interface between function and meaning can be understood using this approach since phenomenologists make clear that the body and human consciousness are integral. Men and women understand their bodies in two ways: that we have bodies (an 'object body') and that we are our bodies (a 'lived body'). Bullington (2009) uses these terms and clearly differentiates the 'object body' (i.e. the body as a material, functioning object) from the 'lived body' (i.e. the mind, body and world as experienced). Merleau-Ponty argued that the facets of the lived body cannot be understood separately, yet different aspects of the 'mind/body/ world' lived body may come to the fore at different times to cope with different situations (Carman 2008) He described this as a harmony of situations, enabling each circumstance to be understood and dealt with. Bullington helpfully explains this concept: *'The harmony of situations is 'sedimented', to use Merleau-Ponty's language, in terms of so-called structures, which allow the world to be apprehended in a rudimentary organization which we already understand … His development of the concept was to describe structure as an 'in-between' phenomenon, that is, neither in things nor in subjects, but created in the meeting between the two'* (Bullington 2009, p. 105).

I have already used the word liminal to describe a similar concept. It is 'sedimentation' that offers the physiotherapist a means of understanding what a patient experiences during rehabilitation or a physiotherapy consultation. Using the concept of 'sedimentation', there is an opportunity for the physiotherapist to engage with the alleviation of a patient's physical distress, which may be brought on by decreasing mobility or increasing fatigue and breathlessness. Working with the idea that an individual makes sense of themselves in 'layers', by enabling some of those layers that feel lost to the patient to be restored (e.g. using various therapeutic exercises, breathing control techniques with pacing of activity, simple yet sustained exercise, etc.), even if only for a short time, assists with the reconstruction of personal meaning. Neimeyer, taking a constructivist view of bereavement and mourning, suggests a useful insight into making meaning, stating that people *'attempt to "emplot" the various episodes of [their] life story within a broader framework of meaning that makes them both intelligible and significant. The result of this evolving effort is a self-narrative'* (Neimeyer 2006). This process is similar to sedimentation, or to the recognition that meaning is made in liminal places. The case study illustrates.

CASE STUDY
Understanding a patient

David was a 42-year-old white male with a diagnosis of motor neurone disease. For David the maintenance of strength and agility had been long-term goals. He had resisted the progression of his disease through exercise. David was keen to use the rehabilitation gym on every visit to the hospice, particularly so when he was an inpatient for several weeks. David was keen to use a motorized upper/lower limb resistance machine and parallel bars to maintain his function and standing. When he became less able to function, David became tearful and frustrated; he became particularly tearful when he considered his future. On one occasion, David was unable to exercise in the gym. He became frustrated and angry with himself, his disease and the therapist, returning from the gym to his room and locking himself in his bathroom. Subsequently David was a day-care patient, and continued to request physiotherapy input and time in the rehabilitation gym.

David experienced a fundamental change in his experience of sedimentation. He was unable to view the world in a way that made sense for him. The 'in-between' or liminal aspects of his meaning making were lost. David experienced an alienation from his pre-illness self, and this continued. David was no longer able to 'emplot' himself into a broader picture of himself and his life. The physiotherapist's task with a patient like David was not to talk about an 'object body' (i.e. that which is viewed externally), but to engage with his 'lived body' (i.e. that which experiences the mind/body/world and seeks to make sense in the relationships between each aspect). For the physiotherapist, the task might be – through reduced exercise and reflection on diminishing mobility – to help David understand that the world of the lived body which he used to know has fundamentally changed, and a transformation of what is possible needs to be taken into the experience of the lived body. David's world changed, but he entered a new understanding of self and meaning which lives with restriction, unsteadiness and consequently pain.

The physiotherapist is a skilled professional who is able to sustain conversation around debility and change from a functional perspective and, with care, to set those issues into the broader sense of loss experienced by a patient. A relationship of mutuality exists between the physiotherapist and the patient. This relationship is built upon trust that the physiotherapist will not abandon the patient's goals, and the trust that there will be honest reassessment from day to day as to the feasibility of those goals.

Bullington, writing about chronic pain, insightfully states that *'the dis-articulation of the world found in chronic pain can also be understood in terms of an alienation from one's pre-pain self, as well as an alienation from others who do not have pain'* (Bullington 2009).

Alienation may take the form of anger or blame directed toward the physiotherapist, who is viewed by the patient as the bearer of functional knowledge (➤ Chapter 3.2). Clark picks this theme up: *'Chronic pain in advanced, terminal disease ... posed particular challenges at the level of meaning'* (Clark 1999). Clark reviewed the model of total pain articulated by Saunders in her early writing. At the outset of Saunders' research and subsequent writing, for the patient pain caused an interruption to the ability to make sense of the world, i.e. the past, the present, guilt, loss and the future: all these are aspects of meaning.

Niemeyer, writing about the manner in which bereaved people re-make meaning following the death of a family member or friend has suggested that meaning reconstruction is a task of mourning. Taking Saunders'model of 'total pain' and particularly spiritual pain as one aspect of that model, might it be that spiritual pain contains some pre-bereavement grieving? If so, then Niemeyer's comment that *'human beings are inveterate meaning makers, weavers of narratives that give thematic significance to the plot structures of their lives'* (Niemeyer 2005) is applicable to those who, used to making meaning with their body, are no longer able to do so. That the human body can be a means of making sense of the self within the world offers physiotherapists an opportunity to engage in discussion and the journey of personal meaning reconstruction.

4.2.4 The use of narrative: A key approach for the physiotherapist

Within end of life care, a key component of the role of the physiotherapist is to solve a problem by listening to the patient. Such an approach opens another model for the physiotherapist: the use of narrative. Listening to patients for their whole story and being with them as they reinterpret or renegotiate that story for the present is important. Rasmussen and co-workers, in a discussion following a literature review of the personal experiences of deteriorating bodies of cancer patients, adopt as their leading approach the Asklepian tradition of healthcare (Rasmussen/Tishelman/Lindqvist 2010). This tradition, based upon the myth of Asklepios, the Greek god of medicine, seeks to listen to the patient and to act upon what is heard for the promotion of well-being. The Asklepian tra-

dition complements the Hippocratic tradition, derived from Hippocrates, an ancient Greek physician. 'Hippocratic medicine' works with a logical, scientific approach. Of particular interest in this model of healthcare is the value of the relationship between the body and distress: *'Suffering occurs when a state of distress threatens the "intactness" of a person. Narrative research supports this understanding by showing how bodily deterioration and symptoms undermine identity and dignity'.* Rasmussen et al. highlight one phenomenological study, which supports Bullington's arguments above. Individuals in late palliative phases of cancer lose their taken for granted" body [lived bodies] or, to use Rasmussen et al.'s term, the body they *'felt at home with'* (Rasmussen/Tishelman/Lindqvist 2010). Michael Kearney draws on the Asklepian tradition, suggesting an approach to holistic care for patients. He notes that the use of Asklepian principles is *'primarily subjective and refers to what is happening within, rather than outside, the patient'* (Kearney 2000). Asklepian philosophy asks the clinician working with the patient to enter into the patient's suffering; to do so is not to experience the patient's distress or pain, but to offer empathy and to recognize one's own experience of pain: *'It is impossible to help patients in suffering without entering their experience with them, and because this inevitably brings carers into their own experience of suffering, Asklepian healing involves 'clinical subjectivity!' The dictum, 'physician, know thyself' applies here'* (Kearney 2000).

It is by listening to the patient's own narrative and seeking to understand this, that an Asklepian approach helps the physiotherapist working with patients to hear what the nature of patients' losses are, and through rehabilitation to recover lost function (or rediscover lost function), and through that to discover 'meaning'.

4.2.5 Conclusion

The process of making 'meaning' or finding spiritual peace in palliative illness is undoubtedly complex. This chapter is presented in the hope that practitioners will explore further how, as physiotherapists in palliative units or hospices, their task is understood and transmitted to colleagues as more than a 'can do' concept. Physiotherapy as any intervention in palliative care has an integral role in meeting the spiritual need of patients when taking a total or holistic model of care seriously.

In this chapter, I have suggested that against a societal milieu that values only perfection, or at least the ideal of perfection, the rehabilitative role of physiotherapy can play an important role in giving back – through the patient's own work and the physiotherapist's support – the patient's sense of themselves as human beings with dignity and value. **Phenomenological and narrative approaches enable the patient to re-inhabit the 'lived body' with all its frailty and even its pain, so that sense can once again be made of the world.**

Like Mary, who re-found meaning in her ability to go for a walk, or David struggling with physical change, **the physiotherapist is a central professional in enabling a sense of meaning to be established in the 'here and now',** which can sustain and improve individual quality of life. Every patient works to establish meaning at the liminal places of life where mind/body/world interact. The physiotherapist may see the physical improvement a patient experiences through rehabilitation and not see that their work has played an important part in the patient's re-engaging with others and understanding themselves again. Yet, it is through function that meaning can be found or re-found just as much as through any other disciplinary approach. Bullington concludes: *'Rehabilitation must ultimately have as its goal the opening up of new horizons. If this is accomplished through physiotherapy, psychotherapy, dance therapy, music therapy or supportive therapy is unimportant. Even if it is not possible to eliminate pain, it is nevertheless possible to live a stimulating life'* (Bullington 2009).

4.2.6 Reflective questions

In this chapter imagine, if you can, when reading the two case studies that you are the patient, not the physiotherapist. Try to place yourself in the shoes of both patients and then read the case study:

- What do you think you would want to gain from a physiotherapy intervention?
- What loss of function have you already experienced and how has this impacted on making sense of your world?
- How would a loss of function inhibit your ability to make meaning of your own self?

Having done that read the case studies again and put yourself in the role you are familiar with. Then ask yourself:

- How you would address the issues beyond those functional matters that are initially presented to you by the patient?
- Would you undertake an intervention differently having imagined yourself in the place of the patient?

REFERENCES

BBC. Big Rise in Cosmetic Surgery Ops. London: BBC News Website, January 2006. Available at: http://news.bbc.co.uk/1/hi/health/4609166.stm (last accessed August 2012).

British Association of Aesthetic Plastic Surgeons. Moobs and boobs: Double DD'igit rise. Press release. London: British Association of Aesthetic Plastic Surgeons, January 2011. Available at: http://www.baaps.org.uk/about-us/press-releases/855-moobs-and-boobs-double-digit-rise (last accessed August 2012).

Bruce S. God is Dead: Secularization in the West. Oxford: Blackwell Publishing, 2002.

Bullington J. Embodiment and chronic pain: implications for rehabilitation practice. Health Care Anal 2009;17:100–109.

Carman T. Merleau-Ponty. London: Routledge, 2008.

Clark D. 'Total pain': disciplinary power and the body in the world of Cicely Saunders, 1958–1967. Soc Sci Med 1999;49:727–736.

Dahlin Y, Heiwe S. Patients' experiences of physical therapy within palliative cancer care. J Palliat Care 2009;25:12–20.

Davies D. Oral presentation at the Conference 'Spirituality – The missing piece'. National Council for Palliative Care, 2010.

Department of Health. End of life care strategy: Promoting high quality care for all adults at the end of life. London: UK Department of Health, 2008. Available at: http://www.cpa.org.uk/cpa/End_of_Life_Care_Strategy.pdf (last accessed August 2012).

Kearney M. A Place of Healing: Working with Suffering in Living and Dying. Oxford: Oxford University Press, 2000.

Leisure Database Company. Resilience in the fitness sector. Pressemitteilung. London: The Leisure Database Company, 2009. Aus: http://www.theleisuredatabase.com/news/news-archive/resilience-in-the-fitness-sector (letzter Zugriff: August 2012).

Lundgren BS, Houseman CA. Banishing death: the disappearance of the appreciation of mortality. Omega 2010;61:223–249.

Mount F. Full Circle: How the Classical World Came Back to Us. London: Simon & Schuster, 2010 (especially Chp. 2 'The gym', pp. 49–79).

Neimeyer R. Grief, loss, and the quest for meaning: Narrative contributions to bereavement care. Bereavement Care 2005;24:27–30.

Neimeyer R. Making meaning in the midst of loss. Grief Matters 2006;9:62–65.

Office for National Statistics. National population projections, 2008-based projections. London: UK Office for National Statistics; 2009. Available at: http://www.ons.gov.uk/ons/rel/npp/national-population-projections/2008-based-projections/index.html (last accessed August 2012).

Rasmussen BH, Tishelman C, Lindqvist O. Experiences of living with a deteriorating body in late palliative phases of cancer. Curr Opin Support Palliat Care 2010;4:153–157.

Walter T. Popular afterlife beliefs in the modern west. Unpublished manuscript, 1997.

4.3 With respect and openness: intercultural competence in palliative physiotherapy
In-Sun Kim

The study of migration is very much complicated by a number of issues. Even determining the exact number of migrants in a country is not as easy as it would seem.

This is due in part to the fact that the European Union does not have a specific definition for the term 'migrant'. In some member states immigrants are termed as such only after having resided in a country for one year and only then are added to the relevant statistics. Other nations calculate on the basis of the actual period of residence, whilst others take into consideration the length of time and the reason why an individual intends to stay in the country. Also, in EU member states with a colonial past, immigrants from former colonies can be naturalised very easily and therefore are not included in any official 'alien' statistics. Some member states, such as France, make no records of immigration. Countries like Greece or Portugal, meanwhile, take quite some time to establish their own statistics. As if such technical and defining features were not enough, the methods for compiling the statistics also differ (Bundeszentrale für politische Bildung 2008).

When the first foreign workers arrived in Europe it was presumed that they would only remain in the relevant country for a limited period of time. The **first generation of migrants** in particular, who arrived many years ago, came with the intention of earning enough money to establish their own livelihoods and so return to their homelands. This desire to return home, which was upheld for decades, was not compatible with a future in the country of residence. Acquiring the language of that country and behavioural strategies for solving problems, as well as integrating into a foreign and unusual world, often did not seem relevant in view of the awaited repatriation. Indeed, my own life story – shaped by a migratory background – and my own present status has often been disjointed or felt negated, frequently resulting in inner psychological turmoil. A life of migration became "permanently temporary" and consequently integration was often lacking.

Now, as the first-generation migrants grow older, they are becoming a growing part of the palliative care world in all its various guises. Like all other patients, they come complete with their memories, life histories and different ways of life. Yet unlike many patients without a migratory background, such memories are not only of individual, emotional significance. The memories of the first migrants arriving to embark on a new life in a different country should serve to help preserve the way of life reminiscent of their native land. Since they have not been wholly integrated into the system of standards and values of their country of residence, they can only determine what is right and wrong, how to live and how challenges are to be dealt with. Memories create a form of homeland for people who themselves still feel like strangers in their present surroundings.

Whilst the first generation has preserved a specific cultural identity with established behavioural patterns, the **subsequent generations,** having grown up in the country of residence, often have the sense of a broken relationship – both with their culture of origin and the culture in the country in which they are living. They are constantly faced with the dilemma of choosing between the standards and values of their parents and those of the society in which they live. They also will one day be patients with their own standards and values who, unlike their parents, will no longer necessarily have much in common with the true culture of their homeland. **Their cultural identity does not originate from their own memories,** but rather from a mixture of the memories and ways of life of their parents and grandparents (who are decades older) along with their own experiences in their country of residence which are often dominated by a sense of being different. To also account for such cultural complexity in the palliative care of patients with a migratory background, the physiotherapist must possess a whole range of skills that can be consolidated under the term **intercultural competence.**

This set of skills encompasses all the expert knowledge and every social skill necessary for facilitating the appropriate, respectful and empathic management of individuals from different cultures to one's own. Of vital importance of course are a sound knowledge of the function and impact of cultures and traditions as well as linguistic expertise and the ability to reflect (Bolten 2007). Furthermore, in the case of physiotherapy specific awareness of the **role of the body in different cultures** is paramount.

The meaning of culture

Culture (from the Latin cultura, meaning cultivation or improvement) in the broadest sense is **anything an individual creates in his own way,** as opposed to the natural surroundings that he has neither created nor modified (Duden 1963). The term culture refers not only to all creative skills and activities in general, but also to the individual way in which they are used in a particular society at a particular time, and in a particular place. In spite of globalisation it can hardly be denied that the majority of inhabitants in New Delhi, India, differ in the way they live, dress, earn a living, eat, etc., from the majority of inhabitants in Washington, USA. It is not only location, however, but also time that makes a cultural difference. Today, nobody in Egypt is buried in a pyramid, orphanages such as in Oliver Twist's time luckily no longer exist in the UK, and the Forbidden City in Beijing is now open to tourists. Cultural change takes place wherever culture exists, therefore. It is seldom viewed as a true change, however, because cultures possess much longer life spans than human life itself.

Tradition as a cultural memory

Human societies are reliant on cultural skills in order to survive and satisfy their needs. In order for such skills to become available to future generations, one generation must pass on its standards, values, religion, language and institutions – often referred to under the generic term of tradition – to the next by means of education.

Tradition is often claimed as a pure truth, meaning that other traditions are frequently perceived as strange and incomprehensible. Whilst one's own tradition needs no justification, another is seen as inexplicable. Such an encounter can either lead to isolation of the alien concept or acceptance of individual parts thereof, or even to a critique of tradition that questions one's own rites, habits, customs and standards.

Appreciation of a different culture necessitates an understanding of one's own biography and orientation in terms of time and habitat, i. e. an awareness of one's own traditions.

The experience of the author, as a nurse and hospice manager, has revealed that the ideals and cultures of individuals are versatile and, in the long term, adaptable. In modern societies, culture is understood as the product of the collective actions of society and the reasoning of individuals.

Viewed in such a context, culture can be learned, defined by social norms and values, and continually adapted by one's own perceptions, thoughts and judgements.

An individual arriving and staying in a new country – whether straight from their homeland or after many years of flight – is inevitably confronted with other ideals and traditions. Whether and to what extent such a confrontation may lead to one's own original culture being questioned and perhaps broken, and the degree to which new cultural aspects are taken on board, can only be examined and experienced through openness on the part of the physiotherapist.

The human body in different cultures

The way in which cultural and biographical histories can influence physical contact with other people – in this case staff at a hospice – is illustrated by two case studies.

CASE STUDIES

Mrs K.

Mrs K., 65 years old and of Japanese descent, had breast cancer. She had undergone surgery for removal of the left breast and chemotherapy, plus 33 sessions of radiotherapy. Her doctor had prescribed regular lymph drainage, which Mrs K. refused because she was unwilling to expose her body during physiotherapy.

Mrs K. was married to a German for 20 years and lived in Berlin for 40 years. Since her divorce she had lived alone and seldom received visitors. She also talked very little about herself.

Mrs K. was pleased when visited by a team member of the hospice who respected her sense of shame; she was always polite but maintained a distance. Mrs K. wanted to organise a lot of things for herself, such as her burial at sea and a living will. But there was always a boundary created by embarrassment and distance: despite intensive efforts, Mrs K. died before ever allowing lymph drainage to take place.

Mr S.

This is not the case with Mr S., a 59-year-old patient from Korea who had leukaemia and was ultimately undergoing palliative care. He definitely wanted to die at home. He and his wife, a former nurse, were Christians who came to Germany 35 years ago and married in Berlin.

The author, who was caring for these patients, had known him for a long time and there was a great deal of trust between her and the family. During the final phase of his life, the flow of energy was activated in his body – in agreement with his wife – by massaging his hands and feet, and acupressure. It was quite apparent that Mr S. became more and more relaxed from these gentle massages, allowing his breathing to deepen. After initially **'enduring' the tranquil approach, rather than lapsing into activity, being passive resulted over time in enjoyable encounters** that not only touched the therapist very much on a spiritual level, but were also welcomed by Mr S. and his wife as soothing and beneficial. By maintaining a certain distance and respecting the etiquette of the culture of origin (by obtaining the wife's agreement), the treatment achieved the desired outcome.

Based on these two cases it is evident that patients, and in particular individuals with a migratory background, can be reached by respecting their culture. Body-contact therapists, especially, must **consider the relevance of physicality in different cultures when drawing up a therapeutic strategy:** it is therefore important to consider the biographical side of a patient when it comes to physical contact. The desire for touch and physical contact is a profoundly human element unrelated to age and disease. Dying patients can be very sensitive to touch – unpleasant or even traumatic sensations could be triggered. Whether individuals come from a culture in which physical contact is minimal, or they have come to regard physical contact as threatening due to experiences of warfare and fleeing, the possibility that even the 'best-intentioned' approach could prove counterproductive must always be taken into account.

It is useful to remain open to any encounter and ask what the patient wants. In doing so it will be clear whether touch is perceived as pleasant and where it is welcomed. If (as is often the case in the dying phase) this is not possible verbally, it is important to look for non-verbal signs.

Though the subject of 'touch' is very prevalent in physiotherapy, what has been discussed above naturally also applies to other therapies – whether in training, 'sport' or the use of certain aids. Whether the interventions are indicated and accepted does not solely depend on personal, but also cultural coping strategies.

Cultural family characteristics

Experience to date has revealed that there is by no means a generally accepted code for a therapist to follow when dealing with individuals from different cultures and their bodies. Below, aspects of Asian cultures are used to illustrate the approaches that can help to promote reciprocity between the individuals involved. These thoughts are designed to help the therapist make individual decisions when caring for others, regardless of cultural background.

Cultural heritage in Korea, Japan, China and Vietnam

Confucius was a Chinese philosopher believed to have lived from 551 BC to 479 BC. He was the founder of Confucianism, a system based on the belief of social order; and according to Confucius, this is achieved by respecting others and worshipping our ancestors. The primary virtues of Confucianism are mutual love, righteousness, honesty and support. In addition, there are social obligations: filial piety (meaning ancestor worship), modesty and customs. The sum of all virtues is understood to be true humanity. Anyone observing all these rules is not only acting ethically to the highest degree, according to Confucianism, but is also influencing the entire universe through his actions.

People originating from countries shaped by Confucianism see themselves more as components of a family system or society rather than as individuals. As a result, they often have difficulty orienting themselves in an individualistic society.

Individuals brought up on the teachings of Confucius therefore tend to think collectively. Issues are preferably resolved within the family and are not shared with the outside world. This often leads to the refusal or inability to accept professional help or advice.

Integration of the family into one's professional work is therefore essential. If a patient is critically ill, the head of the family (usually the father or brother) or a religious authority in the community must first be consulted. If someone is seriously ill or dying in a foreign country and the head of the family is not immediately available, the local parish priest can usually fulfil this role. In the case of Buddhists, this should usually be a monk.

Such Asian traditions, as an example, can be found in other parts of the world in modified form. Yet even with a sound knowledge of the different aspects of dying in the patient's own culture, the physiotherapist should still remain alert. Not all customs are necessarily still observed; this applies not only to industrial nations but also to the rest of the world. Who today still covers their mirrors on the death of a relative? How many Christians and Jews still bury their urns despite the fact that such a practice was totally rejected by monotheistic religions way into the 19th century?

The cultural practices a patient pursues and those he does not must also be questioned individually.

Personal cultural background and how it influences your work

To understand different cultures in terms of religious rituals, consciousness of the body and touch, physiotherapists must acquire and practise special intercultural skills. This also entails, as already described above, reflecting on one's own culture and personal background. Important questions and reflective topics include:

- writing your own biography: Where do you come from, where do you stand, where do you want to go?
- finding out about your own cultural background;
- being clear about how your cultural background influences your own actions;
- being aware of the relativity of values;
- developing an ability to express yourself appropriately in both cultures, verbally and non-verbally;
- talking with people from different cultures about shared realities and possible solutions;
- being open to other cultures;
- being clear about your own needs and preconceptions;
- taking your own needs and feelings seriously;
- loving others;
- having a positive attitude and being tolerant;
- confronting the subject of 'dying'.

Cultural similarities in the process of dying

Surveys have shown that 80 % to 90 % of all persons questioned in western industrial nations would prefer to die at home. Desire and reality are two very different things, however: only 10 % to 20 % of all people (in Germany's cities) actually do die at home, whilst the rest end their lives in hospitals and care institutions. This is a clear indication of how difficult the situation has now become in terms of the dying (Deutsche Hospiz-Stiftung 2001).

60 % of the population would like a fast and sudden death. However, a lot of people evidently would also like to be able to bid their family and friends farewell while spending the final stage of their life in familiar surroundings.

Collaborative solutions at end of life

Terminal care

Terminal care as the term used to describe the care and treatment of terminally ill and dying patients includes physical care, quenching hunger and thirst, reducing symptoms of nausea, anxiety, pain and breathlessness. But it also offers personal attention and spiritual support to the dying patient and his family. A key objective therefore must be to preserve the ability of the patient to express his own will even during the dying phase – for as long as is medically (whether in the conventional, alternative or traditional Chinese medicine sense, for example) feasible, and for as long as tolerable and desirable for the affected individual.

Therapy at end of life

Treatments at end of life include all medical interventions, including palliative care, that help to reduce suffering during the final phase. Irrespective of cultural background, the wishes of the patient take priority over medical options during all stages of end-of-life therapy, thereby concentrating on the patient's quality of life and respecting his personal history.

Conclusion

In addition to specialised skills, personal reflection on subjects such as communication, spirituality, dying, death and bereavement is a prerequisite for working well as a physiotherapist in palliative care.

In future, the treatment and care of those with a migratory background who are critically ill and dying will become an everyday feature of both outpatient and inpatient physiotherapy. To meet such requirements, it is important that physiotherapists have intercultural skills that they have acquired either through learning or drawn from their own migratory background. The subject should therefore be covered by continuing professional development courses.

Physiotherapists must also be open and able to offer alternative treatment methods based on orthodox medicine (such as energy treatments). Also, more room should be given in the application of physiotherapy to the elements of self-reflection and biography, as well as supervision and confrontation with one's own psychohygiene.

One of the most important resources when caring for critically ill and dying patients from different cultures is teamwork: being part of an interprofessional – and perhaps even intercultural – palliative care team.

REFERENCES

Bolten J. Interkulturelle Kompetenz. Erfurt: Landeszentrale für politische Bildung Thüringen, 2007.

Deutsche Hospiz Stiftung (German Hospice Foundation). Meinungen zum Sterben. Emnid Survey, 2001. Available at: http://www.hospize.de/docs/stellungnahmen/08.pdf (last accessed May 2012).

Der Große Duden. Etymologie. Mannheim: Dudenverlag, 1963.

Bundeszentrale für politische Bildung (German Federal Central Office for Political Education). Migration im europäischen Vergleich – Zahlen, Daten, Fakten? 2008. Available at http://www.bpb.de/themen/KAGJSA,0,0,Migration_im_europäischen_Vergleich_Zahlen_Daten_Fakten.html (last accessed May 2012).

5 "Self care" for Physiotherapists

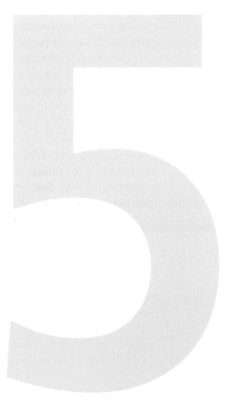

5.1 "How am I really feeling?" – questions and suggestions for (self-)supervision
Wolf Schönleiter

Prelude to supervision or: when the body leads the way

'How am I really feeling?' – this self-reflective question was the response of a physiotherapist (Mr A.) who wanted to work out for himself the extent to which one-on-one supervision could be a useful and beneficial way of helping him to understand and modify the increasing dissatisfaction he was experiencing in his professional work. He had been working for about two years in palliative care, making home visits or attending geriatric facilities for an outpatient care service, without being incorporated into a fixed team.

Having discussed a few important aspects concerning the underlying conditions during our initial telephone call, we arranged a first appointment. Only then would a commitment be made concerning further one-on-one supervision.

His question was the response to my enquiry after his well-being shortly after starting this first session: 'So now that we're here together, how are you feeling?' Mr A. initially responded non-verbally, with a look of shock and quizzical helplessness. Then came his verbal 'reply' – one which initially left my question unanswered by posing a counter-question, namely whether this was actually an element of the supervision.

I confirmed this and then repeated my question about his well-being. This wasn't at all easy for him to answer and in fact he replied that he wasn't quite sure how he was actually feeling. I haven't asked you a very simple question and you don't want to give me a simple answer. You seem to be taking this very seriously, which I appreciate and which is why I also don't want you to feel pressurised by my asking after your well-being. You alone can determine whether and if you have anything to say. One rule of supervision is that there's no obligation to answer, though it's almost impossible not to …'

Mr A. interrupted to assure me that he wanted to say something, but it wasn't easy and at the moment it appeared that he couldn't quite find the right words, which seemed to be causing a 'simmering' within him. I hooked onto this image of 'simmering', believing that my question and what he seemed to think it entailed had not left him cold. Simmering, for me, conjures up images of cooking and heating so inwardly he could have become heated – which in turn I could interpret as some form of

response to my question: 'That's what I just meant by suggesting that it's not actually possible to not reply. You've given at least two answers; one was a counter-question and the other the suggestion of simmering. To be precise, there were actually three answers, since your body language in response to my question about your well-being could be interpreted as a mixture of disbelief, surprise and mistrust, as if you can't believe that my question can really be serious.'

At this, Mr A. smiled, somewhat embarrassed; in doing so he appeared less tense than at the start of the conversation and then repeated my question in his own words: 'Well, how am I really feeling?' – again, his tenseness appeared to grow, to the extent in fact that he was silent and no words would cross his lips, and he was visibly making an effort to maintain his composure.'

My appraisal was that it would be inexpedient and detrimental to further progress to allow the silence to grow and wait for a verbalised response or indeed insist on one. Instead I drew my subject's attention to the fact that he had now repeated my question and in such a way had asked himself the same question, though I noticed that his version had placed particular emphasis on the 'am', thus turning it in his own particular way into his own question, making it more acceptable. In response to his asking, with curiosity and visible concern, what in my opinion the stress he had placed on the question could have implied, I responded: 'It suggested taking the formulation literally, and so I'd like to suggest you answer by just being, calmly without any words: if you try to be, as you are, then you would basically be inviting your body to find a response. I particularly like this idea because as a physiotherapist you are in fact a specialist in matters of the body. So you could in fact let your body speak for itself. We can still talk about it later in words, if you want.'

Mr A. responded that he liked this idea and was very open to it, since he was a great believer in using the body as a source of information: 'also realise that I often deal with patients in such a way if they find it difficult to speak, reading a lot into their posture and facial expressions as to how they feel and what mood they are in.'

It was then quite impressive to see how Mr A. went on to express his well-being physically – not only by 'being', but also by assuming a variety of positions including lying on the floor. He appeared to be clearly relieved by the chance to perceive and acknowledge with the help of time and space his own sorrow, the simultaneous feelings of aggression and his annoyance at everything he had 'bottled up' since working with palliative care patients. It was then clear to him that by continuing to consult with a supervisor he wanted to discover what working as a physiotherapist in the palliative care setting was doing to him and whether in future it could be an occupational area in which he would feel confident. A practical tip he gained from this first session of supervision was to again observe and listen more intently and consciously. To commit to patient relationships in such a way thus appeared to him to be less onerous than to attempt, through silence, to avoid and fend off a relationship, which in any case would not work. In one of the following sessions he realised that he had increasingly developed behavioural strategies vis-a-vis his patients, to whom he was trying not to get too close. In doing so he felt himself being ruled by fear, overcome by pity when coming too close, incapacitated and thus deeply ashamed.

Mr A. repeatedly referred to the opening scene of the supervisory session, gaining knowledge that he believed would facilitate his work. He once reported, for instance, that the seriousness and insistence of my question had both annoyed and impressed him such that he realised he had increasingly avoided, and out of embarrassment had virtually banned himself from asking explicitly how his patients were feeling. He also added that words failed him when colleagues or other professionals would ask patients 'insincerely' and disrespectfully, *'So how are we today?'* That this could be an unfortunate strategy in one or another case for establishing proximity – embarrassing on the one hand, cringing on the other – was reason enough not only for him to look for other ways to establish contact with his patients, but also to dare to enter into a critical discussion with colleagues in which he would explain his feelings. Later he again appeared to be relieved that such discussions could lead to an intensive dialogue about feelings of embarrassment when working with palliative care patients.

⚠ CAUTION
Closeness and discomfort

The condescending, artificial closeness employed (by those in professions that focus on the body) in order to regulate the balance between distance and proximity is often 'greeted' by patients by means of 'counter-diminishment' (grumbling, complaining, rudeness, non-compliance, etc.) designed to again create distance. The classic lack of detachment common in physiotherapy is what I call the verbal or communicative 'we-us', e.g. *'We'll now put our foot …'* or: *'So how is life treating us today?'*
The failure to manage closeness and distance in physiotherapy is documented in a supervision case study by Schönleiter (2002).

Simply to be reminded of the fact that communication between himself and his patients takes place on a linguistic as well as – much more intensive – physical level was to Mr A. a means of rediscovering a wealth of knowledge. The concept of maintaining as well as expanding such knowledge and applying it with greater intensity and deliberation, appeared to him to be a resource that could facilitate his work in palliative care. He now looked at such palliative care work, which in the last two years had come to be an increasing burden, as motivation for his future as a physiotherapist insofar as he could understand and put it into practice as a special form of learning, namely 'reading the body'. He attributed his perception of relationships with patients as being closer (and in parallel less cumbersome) to the acknowledgement of his increasing ability to see patients not primarily as 'illnesses' but as living bodies, with whom he could refine his art of body reading. After demanding work sessions he would undertake special bodily journeys as rituals for relaxation and relief.

Suggested exercise

- Why, and in what subjects, would you want to enlist help, advice or supervision?
- When did you first or last have help in relation to your work?
- When have you ever used your own body as a helpful tool, e.g. as an emergency source of inspiration during a complex, cumbersome, anxiety-inducing situation?
- Do you have a close or a more distanced relationship with your own body?

✓ GUIDANCE
Resources for supervision

The theory and practice of supervision in physiotherapy are illustrated in the writings of Schönleiter (2002), Schönleiter/ Steinhoff (2006) and Nieland/Schönleiter (2012). Easily accessible information on the various forms and practicalities of supervision can be found on the websites of professional associations for supervision (➤ References).

The unlikelihood of a stress-free environment in palliative care

It would appear unlikely that members of palliative care facilities will *not* be exposed to considerable strain when pursuing their professional activities. Physiotherapists in a wide variety of palliative care institutions are also affected by this potentially stressful normality, attention to which – focusing on the specific stresses experienced by physiotherapists on the palliative care unit – has been drawn by Helfenbein (2012).

There is no lack of evidence concerning the extent to which daily contact with the terminally and incurably ill, and constant encounters with death, can lead to serious psychological, physical and social strain. To focus the necessary attention so that the psychological equilibrium and also the motivation, interest and pleasure in such work is not permanently jeopardised, meanwhile, is a constant challenge to palliative care physiotherapists.

How could such a challenge be dealt with successfully? A simple, straight answer could be: immediately rise to the challenge and establish your personal work-life balance. It could be helpful here to fall back on self-assessment proposals which can be found on the Internet under keywords such as "health", "stress", "strain" or "burnout check", as well as in the wealth of literature that has been written on the subject. Similarly, concepts and methods that promise strategies for coping with strain, stress and self-management at work and on a daily basis, as well as advice on managing the risks of burnout, can be selected and reviewed with an eye on how they could be of personal use.

Suggested exercise: burnout check

The following questions can give clues as to whether the motivation for, and enjoyment of your work has already become fragile and also can reveal the extent to which burnout could have occurred or could be a risk. Self-assessment, by responding to the questions below, should give you an idea whether you feel you are exposed to the given strains:

- Do you approach your work and/or palliative care activities with considerable resistance?
- Are your palliative care activities accompanied by feelings of failure, reluctance, annoyance and/or guilt?
- Do you feel disheartened and indifferent in relation to your occupational demands?
- Is your professional work overlaid with defeatism and negativism?
- Do you feel isolated from others, avoid socialising and withdraw from social contact?
- Do you regularly, or always feel tired and exhausted during your work and/or afterwards?
- Do you sense a loss of perspective, dismay, pity, depression and despondency taking you over in relation to your work?
- Do you get the feeling when you are working that time just simply won't pass?
- Have you lost any positive feelings for your patients?
- Do you try to shirk (certain types of) contact with patients?

- Do you perceive contact/relationships with patients/relatives/colleagues (increasingly) as inconvenient, unpleasant, disturbing?
- Do you harbour prejudices against patients?
- Do you find it difficult to concentrate on patients, listen to them or give them your attention?
- Are there situations during your working hours in which you feel numb and no longer capable?
- To what extent do you feel annoyance, disinterest, anger or senselessness when you think about your work and working environment?
- Are your responses to patients and/or their family cynical, reproachful, harsh, unsympathetic and castigatory?
- Do you see yourself wanting to only do what is absolutely necessary and preferring to 'work to rule'?
- Do you avoid conversations and discussions with colleagues?
- Can you recognise a tendency to mostly be preoccupied with yourself?
- Are you aware that you are experiencing psychosomatic reactions (headache, neck pain, back ache, gastrointestinal disorders, sleep disorders, nausea or other physical abnormalities)?
- Could it be that any consumption of stimulants could be a negative and self-damaging attempt to cope with your occupational stress?
- Do you think a lot at home about patients and/or matters arising in your work?
- Do you believe that your enjoyment of life is being negatively influenced by your professional commitment to palliative care?

It is not the absolute number of yes and no answers that makes a difference here. Even if you have only answered yes to one question, this should prompt you to look at the stress you are under very seriously – such as by leaving a little time and then repeating the questions or/and discussing the matter with somebody. If you notice that you are starting to bargain, qualify, make light of the situation or console yourself along the lines of, "it'll all be alright", "*one* yes is *not* really a yes", "it's not all that bad", "others are worse off than me", this could be a sign that you do not want to believe or accept. You are practically devaluing your individual experience by making light of it using normative constructions. This could indicate that you prefer to keep going and suffer without complaining – perhaps because to you it always seems **easier, more beneficial and rewarding to suffer than to make a change.**

As a supervisor and advisor, I use the responses to the listed self-assessment questions along with further more differentiating questions, particularly when a risk of burnout seems to be imminent, in order to decide on topics to address during supervision and the extent to which additional expert help (medical, therapeutic or otherwise) should be enlisted. The questions were developed from a brief synopsis of the symptoms of burnout written by Burisch in 1989. Another tool for examining one's own burnout potential, using a self-test, is the *Maslach Burnout Inventory* (MBI), which requires yes and no answers to the items 'emotional exhaustion', 'de-personalisation' and 'own performance appraisal' (Fengler 1991).

Stress is normal

Burnout or the 'disease of over-commitment' (Freuden-berger/North 1994) can be understood as the final stage of a development process. By looking at the specific strains in palliative care environments, an attenuating effect can be achieved simply by not allowing oneself to become primarily obsessed with the potential risk of reaching this outcome. However, the temptation here is huge, since burnout now appears to be 'en vogue' in public discourse, where alarmingly we can only find fatigued, burned out and helpless individuals.

In a deliberate attempt not to dramatise, and instead take a more relaxed approach, questions such as those listed below could help to define individual encounters and personal experience as responses to the normal strains arising from the various fields of palliative care:

- May I even admit that there are also things that cause me stress?
- What do I perceive as *more,* and what do I see as *less* stressful?
- Can I detect any *differences,* and what would they be in terms of the nature of the stress?
- How can I identify the sources of stress and strain within the context of my occupational demands? Do they lie within me, in the way I organise myself and my lack of resilience? What importance do the various target groups and people have with whom I come into contact and have to deal with professionally? Are there elements of pressure and stress arising from my inclusion or non-inclusion in a team? Could there be family/private stress factors that are having an impact on my work?
- You could also ask why you deal with matters which are a strain or stressful to you in the way that you do. Do you approach dealing with the matter seriously, play it down, or find it unpleasant? Could you imagine inviting the stresses in as guests?

Perhaps you believe the question about the personally stressful situations to be selfish and inconsistent in light of the high goals associated with your professional commitment in the palliative field, meaning that you see the question as more appropriate and permissible in so far as you, as the physiotherapist, can continue to display the 'right' behaviour vis-a-vis your patients, their families, your colleagues, etc. It could also be that the question about what could cause you stress is quickly answered by the very simple and quite commonplace reaction: stressed, who isn't?

Self-image, shame and potential fears with respect to the repercussions sometimes complicate the perspective of stress such that they are not even registered to begin with or at best are theoretically taken into consideration and conceded.

An important condition for accepting the normality of a stressful existence would be not to see it as an outwardly determined necessity that is prescribed and specified, whether by experts in palliative care or other disciplines. You, the reader of this article, are the expert being addressed here. Only you can decide whether to rise to this challenge. Such self-commitment can release the energy that is required in order not to recoil from questions and insights that perhaps are uncomfortable or make you anxious. Once the thought of stress is no longer viewed as an inconvenient and redundant obligation or as an outwardly dictated necessity, and thus is befriended and not perceived as a declaration of war, then an important and fundamental step has been taken towards finding or developing ways to cope with stress. This will be beneficial to your own well-being.

On the one hand we can talk generally about the high levels of stress to which the palliative care physiotherapist is subjected, but on the other hand it is still true that stress is a subjective and individual experience. The experience of stress and dismay is not the same to everyone, but is very varied. Age, personal and professional background or sex are just some of the factors that create such diversity. Only personal experience and individual awareness guide and dictate our actions when it comes to dealing with stress. Stress is only ever understandable on an individual level and likewise only modifiable on an individual level based on self-perception. In this respect, the sensory awareness of palliative care physiotherapists in the context of a consistent work ethic cannot be regarded highly enough.

'Integrity of perception' (Dörner/Plog 1992) – or the constant endeavour to be as wholly insightful as possible – is an important requirement in identifying and understanding stress, and not suffering from it permanently or even reaching the feeling and state of burnout and exhaustion. Conducive to this method of perception is the **adoption of a searching attitude,** allowing for questions and leading to questions, confronting them and then dealing with them. In doing so, questions at the **knowledge or content level** must be distinguished from those on an **emotional or relational level.**

In practical terms this can mean to also direct your perception and searching attitude towards the personal motives and desires that are associated with your own palliative care work:

- What do I want as a physiotherapist in palliative care, what am I hoping for as a person from this occupation?
- How did I even end up working in this area: was I in control, or were there others who influenced my decision to work here, or did coincidence play a part?
- How do I see professional physiotherapeutic help in the context of palliative care?
- How do I feel before, during and after treating a patient?
- Where do the impulses come from that make me want to help?
- Can I help myself? How easy or perhaps difficult do I find it?
- How do I feel, being dependent on others?
- Is there help that is better or worse for me?
- How do I approach the issues that confront me as a palliative carer?
- In which situations or concerning what subjects do I notice an open attitude in encounters with patients, families, colleagues – and where and when is reticence more likely to guide me?
- Where do my opinions, appraisals and ideas with regard to the requisite handling of patients differ from those of my colleagues, the patients themselves or even their families?
- If I were a palliative care patient myself, what would be my attitude, preferences and demands regarding how I and my family are treated?
- Could it ever be that I would contemplate suicide or that I would beg or urge to be left to die or kill myself?
- What would my approach be with relatives or friends if they were to become palliative care patients?
- What are my beliefs regarding the dignified treatment of palliative care patients?
- Are there scenarios from my professional practice in which my ideas of the respectful and dignified treatment of palliative care patients clearly differ from those of my social environment or of my colleagues and other professionals?
- How do I deal with the differences? How important to me are the similarities in terms of the concepts of dignity, morality and ethics when dealing with dying patients?

Answers to such questions can bring relief to the extent that they help with self-reflection and self-assurance. Unresolved attitudes and opinions can be given shape, facilitating a clearer understanding not only of oneself, but also of what is happening in a relationship, and of communication and interaction processes between all those involved in palliative care.

Suggested exercise

What enables you, and what enables others (who?), in your opinion, to recognise that your basic attitude as a palliative care physiotherapist is to be as highly perceptive as possible? How would you explain to a colleague, for instance, why you strive for total perception and what you understand this to mean? Look again to see whether it could be useful to write a stress diary, or whether another form of documenting and recording your experiences in the palliative care environment would be conceivable.

Using your own body as a supervisor

The way in which physiotherapists could expand their skills in (as far as possible) total perception and total communication has been described for physiotherapists by a female colleague in the context of her deliberations concerning self-management: *'One's own fears and involvement in stressful situations inhibit the ability to assist the patient. It is helpful as a therapist to know and to be able to recognise the congestion one's own body can create in such environments. In my opinion, your own body is the best supervisor you can have and it is freely available at any time. In addition, your own body demonstrates to the patient, at the non-verbal level, the 'true' world view that his therapist has. Mixed messages in such situations can block the patient's access to his own resources and cause anxiety'* (Mehne 2002).

The following questions could be used as an exercise to sharpen one's own **physiognomic self-perception** in order to incorporate it into the **art of body reading** and physiological examination, thereby making one's palliative work easier:

- What posture (position of mouth, line of sight, etc.) do I assume when I am concentrating on my work, and when I am relaxed in my work?
- What posture do I assume if I feel embarrassed, uncertain, anxious or am making an effort to try to prevent errors or conceal them?
- Am I aware of certain body language that tells me I am about to ignore a breaking point?

- How can I use my body language, for example, to compensate for abnormal physical sensations?
- Could I imagine conferring with the various organs in my own body?
- How can I put this into practice in a treatment situation?

Suggested exercise
How can you find out how to potentially use your physical competencies in a better way than before? Could specific forms of physical engagement also be a possibility here? The range of approaches, from A for autogenic training to Z for zen meditation, and various sports such as yoga, archery, dancing and many more, is far too broad to be able to even begin listing them all here.

Could it be both interesting and relaxing for you to approach your body differently from how you have before? How do you relax? How do you achieve a relaxing muscular state, and how do you manage to relax mentally? What would a suitable, as it were perfectly customised tension/relaxation training programme look like in your case?

Linguistic dexterity as a useful resource

Attentiveness and accuracy in terms of physical perception are not the only effective therapeutic resources when it comes to easing the relationship with the patient. The careful and sensitive use of language can also help to loosen or buffer difficult, stressful situations. An example is the so-called **exacerbation or catastrophe question** that can be posed by the therapist: '*Which formulations and words could I use, as a therapist, to sustain or even worsen a situation that is perceived as difficult and stressful?*' Answers to such a question could look like this (Mehne 2002):

- By using words that focus too much and too quickly on change and thus one-sidedly emphasise the lack of change or the recognition of the situation as it is.
- By using words that describe too vaguely what is understood by changing and not changing, and how this can be recognised.
- By using words that do not adequately acknowledge what the patient is undergoing in order to alleviate the awkward situation.
- By using phrases that have triggered conflicts of loyalty between the patient, his family and other members of the multidisciplinary team.
- By making remarks to suggest that everyone else knows better than the patient himself.

- By using ambiguous words that disguise mixed messages in order to hide anxiety, insecurity, mortification or other feelings.

Through questions and answers it becomes clear that the realms of palliative care should be used, as it were, as a permanent **training ground for precise reasoning, coherence and respectful language.** Exoneration and relief are the rewards, creating a respectful environment in which both you and the patient are treated with dignity.

Suggested exercise
- How do you feel after exploring such a course of action?
- What thoughts occur to you in relation to the language you use? How do you talk with patients? What choice of words is characteristic to you? When do words fail you?
- Can you imagine enhancing your linguistic potential in a different way and to more effect than before? Could it in fact be helpful to create a picture of yourself as a tuneful orchestra incorporating all the creative tools you have at your fingertips?

Anxiety and its management

If the greatest possible level of perception is required when dealing with stressful situations, experiences and events, then self-perception plus a focus on one's feelings are of tremendous importance. Whether you are a lone fighter or team player, feelings that develop in a patient can fundamentally be experienced by anyone working in palliative care. Hence, **self-sensitisation leads simultaneously to sensitisation in the patient:** '*Self-perception is not achieved by categorising, through observation, the way in which events are perceived, i. e. hands-off, at a distance, treated as an object. Rather, the question should be asked: do I and my peers also have such feelings, how do they experience them, evaluate them, what do they do with them, and what stops us from having such feelings?*' (Dörner/Plog 1992, S. 41).

The potential spectrum of feelings is too broad to be able to list them all here. Anxiety, however, is one aspect at least that should be addressed since it is an important, primary feeling that itself can emerge in the most varied of hues and guises. The list of potential anxieties arising in palliative care physiotherapists illustrates the strains and stresses to which they feel they are exposed. For instance, the following 'fears' (Schönleiter 2002) can be identified:

- Fear of feeling powerless, helpless and swamped as an individual and as the caregiver (not being able to prevent death)
- Fear of having learned and also understood a lot, but not being able to put this to practical and helpful use
- Fear of not being able to satisfy the patient, even after a professional development course
- Fear that continuing professional development could bring further stress
- Fear of not recognising certain symptoms in a patient, thereby treating them inappropriately and harming them unnecessarily
- Fear of being reminded of one's own experiences or those of people close to you that are associated with illness, being a patient, dying and death
- Fear of being viewed by the patient and his family as incompetent and being rejected
- Fear of failure during therapy and hurting the patient
- Fear that patients could instil feelings of guilt and cause offence
- Fear of not coping with the different degrees of intimacy, severity of the disease or injury and the level of responsibility that results
- Fear of not being able to adequately cope with dying and death, suffering and pain, aggression, or feeling squeamish or embarrassed
- Fear of responding to aggressive patients with counter-aggression
- Fear of not treating the patient fairly (e. g. because of a lack of time and staff)
- Fear related to increased cases of death or protracted and particularly inexorable processes of dying
- Fear associated with the expectations of the family
- Fear regarding the need to cooperate with other professional teams
- Fear of too intense an emotional demand in light of being permanently confronted with the fate of the terminally ill
- Fear related to feelings of guilt ('continuing to live yourself'; 'wishing death on the patient')
- Fear associated with the unpredictability of death (the patient could die during a treatment session or as a result of treatment)
- Fear of being aloof (saying no)
- Fear that one's own feelings related to grief could have a negative effect on one's private life
- Fear of making (being part of) the wrong decision in relation to ethical questions
- Fear of straining one's private life too much due to the lack of opportunities to relax during working hours

- Fear in relation to the preoccuption with one's own life philosophy and one's own death
- Fear of anxiety

Irrespective of the fears involved in any particular situation, it is important in palliative physiotherapy to always remember that when dealing with fear (as with all feelings) it is a matter of **not counteracting them, but working with them and making something out of them.** To suppress and work against the anxiety and feelings only makes them worse, more intense and more stressful. The fundamental step in the *'emotionally healthy management of fear, therefore, is to register fear,'* and thus also to admit *'that you feel powerless and helpless. This must replace the attitude whereby you want to do something about the fear. Fear can be understood just as little as the ability to do something about it. Conversely, fear can help me to understand myself better. In a relationship this means that I can't take your fear away and I also can't combat it, but I can be there so that you can establish what your fear is saying to you; for you have to realise this yourself, take possession of your fear and make it a part of yourself'* (Dörner/Plog 1992, S. 41).

The less room it is afforded, the greater the potential for fear, as a source of stress, to become a permanent burden in palliative care work. To qualify fear as superfluous or senseless proves to be a rather unfortunate approach, whilst interpreting fear and stress as useful and meaningful can be an initial step towards resolution:

- What could be the positive aspect to feelings of fear and stess?
- What could my fears be trying to tell me?
- Assuming my fears have good intentions: what could their message be?
- What does my fear stop me from doing and what does it want to enable me to do?
- What answers could my body, as the supervisor, give me in response to my fears?
- If I were to ask a valued colleague or friend what my fears could mean – what would their response be?
- What impact, in behavioural terms, do certain fears have on me and others?
- Consider for a moment the assumption that your interest in professional development could also help in warding off fears or keep them in check.
- What effect would it have if your fears or one particular fear suddenly no longer existed?
- How would you converse with your fear if it were sitting in the chair opposite?
- What questions would you ask your fear?

Whatever the individual fears, topics or stresses may be, they must be **afforded space and time** in order that they can be acknowledged, reflected upon and processed.

In association with basic existential experiences such as farewells, grief, death, it becomes quite clear that they are not subject matters to be appropriated. This does not preclude the possibility that knowledge of bereavement phenomena and processes, as documented for example – with no particular esoteric or pseudo-religious slant – in the writings of Kübler-Ross (1997), Kast (2011) and Worden (2011), can be a helpful means of achieving relief. Moreover, in the context of being as wholly perceptive as possible, it is a matter of giving these feelings the space and time that is believed to be necessary and appropriate. This does not mean solely talking about it. **Silence, fright, crying, even laughing and many other forms of expression are some of the finite possibilities with which pain, departure, grief and death can be experienced.** Anyone who is perceptive to their experience here is 'right' in his observations and 'authoritative' in the meaningful sense of the word. This may happen in a variety of pre-defined, secure spatial situations, as can be the case with all types of supervision, conversations with peers or even friends, professional development courses, and therapeutic and advisory settings. The use of such space is always tied to the question of where and to whom I can and would like to reveal my trust as well as my vulnerability. If such space can be incorporated into the (working) schedule and institutional framework of professional palliative care itself, then options for first-rate socio-psychological relief would be available to members of staff which often are overlooked merely because they should be used during leisure or private time (which then tends to be regarded as further stress).

Being aware of one's own grief and other existential experiences creates the necessary supportive structure for witnessing, enduring and attending to pain, dying, death and bereavement with dignity, and without suffering any spiritual harm oneself.

Suggested exercise

It is not only the final questions in this article, below, that should encourage you to always ask which important question(s) for you has (have) remained unspoken.

- With what level of attention, interest, curiosity, ambivalence do you deal with your feelings of grief, pain, anger, desperation?
- What questions do you ask yourself in relation to death?
- How does the room appear in which you could imagine being able to talk about departure, death and bereavement?
- What do you understand by a fulfilled life?
- Do you take time to make an inventory of the experience(s) you have made with personal loss?

- What does it mean to you – and expressed in your own words or perhaps using creative media – that death and grief are part of life?
- Does death mean the end of life, salvation, outrage, a terrible event …?
- The deaths of which patients have touched you in which way?
- Have the deaths of any of your patients remained in your mind for a long time?
- Are there rituals that you find/have found helpful when dealing with death, departure or grief (lighting candles, creating a table of mementos, displaying books of memories or mourning, etc.)?
- What would help you personally and do you good when it comes to dealing with departure, grief and death?
- Could you imagine that certain items or symbols would give you strength and assurance, meaning you would incorporate them as useful aids when dealing with grief in your daily (professional) activities?
- Try to establish the difference between managing and overcoming grief, and registering as well as allowing grief and other feelings to surface.
- Would you like to live forever and for instance have your body plastinated or preserved using cryonics?
- What sense would you like to give to your life and your death?

This last question was examined at various stages of the supervision process by the physiotherapist receiving guidance at the beginning of this chapter, knowing that he could review the coherence of his responses and the associated feelings in his own way using his body as a guide. The way in which he tried to embody his sense of life and death was a living expression of the fact that the serious reflection of existential questions and their answers can be a useful means of allowing ease, pleasure and enjoyment to thrive in stressful professional disciplines such as palliative care.

This chapter is littered with questions, however it is by no means designed as a manual but rather as an invitation. I would like to end by describing a case of life *and* death. In both cases there were questions and of course answers that decided between life and death: *'Once upon a time, so the story goes, a young farmgirl from Desha took a nap at lunchtime in the field. Her husband sat beside her and pondered how he could be rid of his wife. Lady Midday suddenly appeared and presented him with various questions. The more questions he answered, the more new questions she had for him. As the bell struck one o'clock, his heart stood still. Lady Midday had questioned him to death.'* (E. Canetti 1980).

5.2 Closeness and distance, to touch and be touched; the physiotherapeutic dynamic

Michael-M. Lippka, Rainer Simader

Contact is a major feature of therapeutic relationships. Only in such a way can the therapist and patient establish an honest, empathic and respectful relationship. Working on the relationship, in turn, is pivotal to the desired efficacy of therapy.

Contact can be achieved non-verbally, verbally and/or by touch. Physiotherapists have a decisive advantage over many other professions in that touch is a major element in their therapeutic interventions. Aside from the purely physiotherapeutic effects, touch and the closeness this engenders are always accompanied by an emotional and social component. This may not be understimated in sometimes very isolated individuals, as can often be the case with palliative care patients. However:

> ⚠ **CAUTION**
> Touch is not a one-way street.

Closeness and touch are always associated with a reduction in distance and space – also as concerns the therapist.

Mirror neurons, which are found in the cranial motor nerves and are also activated in dealings of an emotional nature, are partly responsible for the body responding to empathic carers in very 'intimate' situations. This can range from automatic reflections (e.g. unconsciously adopting a similar posture) to physical and symptomatic reactions (refer to the literature on secondary traumatisation). Those physiotherapists who are confronted *simultaneously* with movement and sometimes emotionally demanding and challenging topics should be aware of the significance of consciously managing closeness and distance.

Since physiotherapeutic interventions always pursue a goal and in doing so are distinct from non-professional intervention, the following observations should be made concerning the **psycho-hygiene of the therapist** as well as considered when making decisions during the therapeutic process or during one's therapy-free time:

Clear pursuit of therapeutic goals versus intermixing roles

At facilities in which the therapist is provided with support by other members of a multiprofessional team, and in which responsibilities are clearly assigned, it is easier to exercise a purely physiotherapeutic role. The challenge is greater in a setting where the physiotherapist is working alone or in the private sphere of the patient. It is important that the therapist remains aware of this situation and clearly defines as well as observes his position, work, and also the boundaries.

Active versus passive treatments

It has been mentioned that the patient should be as actively involved in the therapy as possible in order to counteract the threat of the patient relinquishing control (➤ Chapter 2.7). Such an approach – if therapeutically indicated – also prevents excessive physical closeness and in turn an emotional loss of control on the part of the therapist. It is important to clearly determine whether hands-on or hands-off techniques are indicated, and whether they are the only, primary means of achieving the goal.

Empathy versus sympathy

Compassion on a professional level (empathy) is an important requirement for achieving therapeutic success. Becoming emotionally involved or affected by fate is likewise a natural reaction. If the motivation or outcome of the therapeutic process, however, is to 'suffer with' the patient, such an approach should be reflected upon and modifed for one's own protection. Sympathy reduces the distance from the patient and possibly leads to (excessively) strong emotional and physical closeness.

Conscious perception versus dissociation

During treatment, the *conscious* differentiation between the patient and therapist is decisive. This means being aware of your own body and physical processes during treatment. Dissociative behaviour (e.g. 'ignoring' topics that are emotionally stressful, feelings of 'merging with the patient' or a lack of awareness of one's own body during treatment) can render the therapist vulnerable. The physiotherapist must be aware of both general psycho-hygiene (e.g. rituals following treatment, leisure activities, supervision, etc.) and ways in which he can protect himself in a stressful situation.

Needs of one's own body versus needs of the patient

A physiotherapist must ask himself regularly whether there is a suitable balance between his obligation to the bodies of his patients and the obligation he has to his own body's well-being. Personal training (e.g. endurance training, weights or relaxation) or compensatory activities (e.g. massages) are important psycho-hygienic activities especially for those who are caring for the physical needs of others and whose work is to a considerable extent physically demanding.

REFERENCES

Burisch M. Das Burnout-Syndrom. Theorie der inneren Erschöpfung. Berlin–Heidelberg–New York: Springer, 1989.

Canetti E. Crowds and Power. London: Victor Gollancz, 1962.

Dörner K, Plog U. Irren ist menschlich. Lehrbuch der Psychiatrie, Psychotherapie. Bonn: Psychiatrie Verlag, 1992.

Ehrenberg A. Das erschöpfte Selbst. Depression und Gesellschaft in der Gegenwart. Frankfurt am Main: Campus Verlag, 2004.

Fengler J. Helfen macht müde. Zur Analyse und Bewältigung von Burnout und beruflicher Deformation. München: Verlag J. Pfeiffer, 1991.

Freudenberger H, North G. Burn-out bei Frauen. Frankfurt am Main: Fischer Verlag, 1994.

Helfenbein L. Belastungserleben im physiotherapeutischen Berufsalltag auf der Palliativstation – eine qualitative Studie. Bachelor thesis (unpublished), Hochschule Osnabrück, 2012.

Kast V. Trauern. Phasen und Chancen des psychischen Prozesses. Freiburg: Kreuz Verlag, 2011.

Kübler-Ross E. Interviews mit Sterbenden. Stuttgart: Kreuz Verlag, 1997.

Mehne S. Die Kraft der Gedanken – SYS PT für langzeit-, schwer- und todkranke Patienten. In: Mehne S, Haupter, L (eds). Vom Tun und Lassen: Grundlagen der Systemischen Physiotherapie – SYS PT®. München: Pflaum, 2002: pp. 216–251.

Nieland P, Schönleiter W. Physiotherapie und physikalische Therapie. In: Aulbert E, Nauck F, Radbruch L (eds). Lehrbuch der Palliativmedizin. Stuttgart: Schattauer, 2012.

Schönleiter W. Was macht das Nichtwissen, wenn es versteckt wird? SYS PT in der Supervision von Physiotherapeuten. In: Mehne S, Haupter, L (eds). Vom Tun und Lassen: Grundlagen der Systemischen Physiotherapie – SYS PT®. München: Pflaum, 2002: pp. 319–357.

Schönleiter W, Steinhoff D. Integrierte Supervision in der Physiotherapieausbildung: Das Bonner Supervisionsmodell – SuperPhysioVision (SPV). Beiträge zu Unterricht und Ausbildung. Krankengymnastik – Zeitschrift für Physiotherapeuten 2006;30(2):19–26.

Worden WJ. Beratung und Therapie in Trauerfällen. Ein Handbuch. Bern: Verlag Hans Huber, 2011.

INTERNET LINKS

Association of National Organizations for Supervision in Europe (ANSE): www.anse.eu

Swiss Professional Association for Supervision, Organisational Consultancy and Coaching (Berufsverband für Coaching, Supervision und Organisationsberatung, BSO): www.bso.ch

British Association for Supervision and Research (BASPR): www.baspr.co.uk

German Association for Supervision (Deutsche Gesellschaft für Supervision e. V., DGSv): www.dgsv.de

Austrian Association for Supervision (Österreichische Vereinigung für Supervision, ÖVS): www.oevs.or.at

5

Index